Principles and practice of

Clinical Physics and Dosimetry

Michael L.F. Lim, CMD, ACT

Advanced Medical Publishing, Inc., USA

2006

Published by:
Advanced Medical Publishing, Inc.
P.O. Box 5046
Madison, WI 53705, USA

Phone: 608-833-2599
Fax   : 608-833-2255
Website: http//www.advmedpub.com
e-mail: info@advmedpub.com

Advanced Medical Publishing, Inc., USA

ISBN: 1-883526-11-6 Hardcover-Clothbound

Cover design by Siamak Shahabi, Teri Gehin, & Michael L. F. Lim
Inetrior design by Advanced Medical Publishing , Inc.

Acknowldgement

I would like to thank Dr. Siamak Shahabi, chief technical editor of Advanced Medical Publishing for his tireless effort in formatting the layout of the book and in improving and enhancing the image quality of the diagrams.

Michael L.F. Lim, CMD, ACT
May, 2006

Contents

Preface

Several radiation oncology and radiation physics textbooks have been written over the years, each with their strength. Most of these textbooks are biased heavily on radiation physics or radiation oncology with few detailed practical examples. There is a need for a textbook dealing with practical step-by-step dose calculation methods and manual dose distribution planning. Furthermore, there are considerable interests in a textbook of dose distribution atlas of every site in the human body. This is such a textbook.

In this textbook, basic treatment planning concepts are defined and explained in detail. Following the definition and explanation, the concepts are applied in clinical situations. The detailed step-by-step dose calculation methods and the examples of manual dose distribution planning would especially benefit dosimetrist trainees, radiation therapy students and junior physicists. The comprehensive atlas of dose distribution of every site in the human body would serve as a good reference source for dosimetrists, physicists, radiation oncologists, residents and radiation therapists. In addition, the dosimetric problems would provide additional practice in problem solving.

Finally, I wish to express my gratitude to my dear wife, Sad Eng Lim, for the quiet time to work on this book and for her constant encouragement.

Michael L.F. Lim, CMD, ACT
May, 2006

Dedication

This book is dedicated to all the cancer patients who put their trust in us as health care providers.

—— *CHAPTER 1* ——

Principles of Treatment Planning

I. INTRODUCTION

The aim of radiation therapy in cancer management is to deliver the maximum radiation dose to the target volume *(tumor plus margin)* but minimum radiation dose to the surrounding normal tissues and vital organs in order to minimize normal tissue complications. In order to achieve this aim, the patient's radiation treatment must be carefully planned before delivery of the radiation.

Treatment planning includes localization and delineation of the target volume and surrounding vital organs, computer generated dose distribution plan, and verification of the plan using the simulator and or port films or portal imaging.

II. LOCALIZATION AND DELINEATION

Localization and delineation of target volume starts at the simulator. Diagnostic studies such as diagnostic X-Rays, CT, MRI, post-operative reports, etc are on hand to guide the radiation oncologist in the localization and delineation of the target volume.

The patient is set up on the simulator couch in the treatment position. If the treatment site is in a location where critical organs such as optic chiasm, optic nerve, brain stem, etc are near by, an immobilization shell *(cast)* may be fabricated to help maintain the patient position to minimize patient movement and aid in the reproducibility for daily treatment.

The radiation oncologist visualizes the target area under fluoroscope. Visualization may be enhanced in some cases by contrast agents such as barium in the localization of esophageal tumors. The field size is set to adequately cover the target volume. An anterior and a lateral orthogonal X-Ray films are taken for referencing in CT planning. Field centers are marked on the patient's skin or on the immobilization shell *(cast)* for the anterior and lateral portals.

A. Non-CT Planning

If the patient does not require CT planning, a contour is taken manually on the simulator. The contour is traced onto paper. The target volume and vital organ such as the spinal cord are delineated on the contour using the anterior and lateral simulator X-Ray films.

B. CT Planning

If CT planning is required, the patient is transferred to the simulator CT. The patient lies in the same position as at simulation, on a flat table top insert on the CT couch. Radio-opaque catheters are taped onto the patient's skin sagitally along the simulated field center on the anterior and lateral centers. The catheters show up on CT images for referencing during treatment planning. CT slices are obtained at 0.2 cm slice increment to 1cm slice increment. This variation in slice increment depends on the accuracy required for the site. For example, sites in the head and neck region usually require finer slice increments due to vital structures such as the optic nerve, optic chiasm near by. Sites in the pelvic region may only require 1 cm slice increments. The central slice is slice 0 for referencing.

After CT, the CT slices are exported to the planning computer. The planning computer imports the CT images. The radiation oncologist delineates the target volume and the organs at risk. Commonly, the gross target volumes *(GTV)* are delineated on each CT slice. Margin may be added to the GTV to form a CTV and a further margin may be added to form the PTV for planning.

III. GROSS TUMOR VOLUME (GTV)

The Gross Tumor Volume *(GTV)* is the gross palpable or visible/ demonstrable extent and location of malignant growth. *(ICRU 50)*

IV. CLINICAL TARGET VOLUME (CTV)

The Clinical Target Volume *(CTV)* is a tissue volume that contains a demonstrable GTV and/or subclinical microscopic malignant disease, which has to be eliminated. This volume thus has to be treated adequately in order to achieve the aim of therapy, cure or palliation. *(ICRU50)*

V. PLANNING TARGET VOLUME (PTV)

The Planning Target Volume is a geometrical concept, and it is defined to select appropriate bean sizes and beam arrangements, taking into consideration the net effect of all the possible geometrical variations, in order to ensure that the prescribed dose is actually absorbed in the CTV. *(ICRU50)*

VI. TREATED VOLUME

The Treated Volume is the volume enclosed by an isodose surface, selected and specified by the radiation oncologist as being appropriate to achieve the purpose of treatment *(e.g., tumor eradication, palliation). (ICRU50)*

VII. IRRADIATED VOLUME

The Irradiated Volume is that tissue volume which receives a dose that is considered significant in relation to normal tissue tolerance. *(ICRU50)*

VIII. TREATMENT PLANNING

Treatment planning is done via a treatment planning computer. Beam energy, field size, open or wedged field, gantry angle, weighting, etc are used in combination to cover the target volume with maximum uniform dose encompassing the target volume and minimum dose to surrounding normal tissues and organs at risk. A hard copy of the plan is plotted for the radiation oncologist's approval and dose prescription. The beams' eye views are exported to the treatment machine for conformation with port films and the MultiLeaf are exported to the treatment machine for daily treatment.

Plan data such as field size, wedge angle, weighting, energy, gantry angle, field depth, and etc. are documented in the plan and in the patient's treatment prescription.

IX. VERIFICATION OF PLAN

The patient is re-simulated to verify the plan. The field parameters from the treatment plan are reproduced to verify the plan. X-Ray films are taken for documentation. Reference marks are placed on the patients' skin or shell for treatment set up.

The patient's chart is completed with calculation of the MU for each of the treatment field and the beam data are exported to the treatment unit. The MUs are printed for double checks by the dosimetrist and physicist and forms the documentation for the treatment.

X. REPRODUCTION OF PLAN ON TREATMENT UNIT

The patient's set up is reproduced on the treatment unit. It is prudent to take port films on day one of treatment to verify the treatment fields before treatment.

— *CHAPTER 2* —

Quantitative Dosimetry

I. INVERSE SQUARE LAW

This law relates the intensity of the radiation to the distance from the radiation source. The intensity of the radiation is inversely proportional to the square of the distance between the radiation source and the point of interest.

$$\left(\frac{I}{I_o}\right) = \left(\frac{d_1}{d_2}\right)^2$$

where;

I = Intensity at point of interest; d_1 = Distance at which I_0 is measured

I_0 = Original intensity at distance d_1; and d_2 = Distance at point of interest

Example:

If the original intensity at 80 cm is 120 cGy/min, calculate the intensity at 160 cm.

$$I = I_o \times \left(\frac{d_1}{d_2}\right)^2 = 120 \times \left(\frac{80}{160}\right)^2 = 30 \quad cGy / \min$$

Notice by doubling the distance, the intensity is decreased by four times. This is important in radiation protection.

II. EQUIVALENT SQUARE

Equivalent square is defined as the square field having the same values of % depth dose, TAR, etc as a given rectangular field of the same radiation quality.

When data such as TAR, depth dose, etc. are measured for treatment units, square fields are usually used in the measurements. However, when patients are treated, the fields are usually not square. They are often rectangular.

Data for every possible rectangle would be very time consuming and would not be practical. Equivalent square for rectangular field may be calculated by the formula,

$$Equivalent \quad square = 4 \times \left(\frac{A}{P}\right)$$

where A is area and P is the perimeter.

Example:

Calculate the equivalent square for 10 ×13 cm^2.

$$Eq.Sq = 4 \times \left(\frac{10 \times 13}{10 + 10 + 13 + 13} \right) = 11.3\,cm^2$$

III. D$_{max}$ (Depth of maximum)

This is defined as the depth where maximum dose is deposited in tissue. The D$_{max}$ is also called the build-up depth and also called depth at which electronic equilibrium occurs. It is this build-up region which gives rise to the characteristic shoulders of depth dose curves for high energy beams. This region of build-up also provides the skin sparing effect of the beams.

Table 2.1 Table of D$_{max}$ for various photon energies.

Treatment Unit	D$_{max}$
SXR(100 kV)	Surface
DXR(200 kV)	2-3 mm
Cobalt-60	5 mm
6 MV	1.5 cm
10 MV	2.5 cm*
15 MV	3 cm*

* The depth of D$_{max}$ changes with field size due to scatter from the collimator.

IV. BEAM PROFILE

Beam profile is an intensity profile across the principle axis of the beam. The profiles shown are profiles across A to B at 5 cm depth for Cobalt-60 and 6 MV photon beam. The dose at central axis is normalized to 100%.

Beam profile can be very useful in determining the dose fall off towards the beam edge. This is useful in off-axis calculation and in field matching.

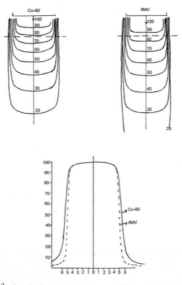

Figure 2.1 Isodose chart (10 × 10 cm^2) for Cobalt-60 at 80 cm SSD and 6 MV photon beam at 100 cm SSD. Beam profiles are at 5 cm depth.

V. PENUMBRA

Penumbra is the region between the 90% and the 10% isodose line across the beam edge. Penumbra is caused by the source or focal spot size and by lateral scatter. The penumbra for the Cobalt-60 is larger than that for 10 MV photon beam because the source size for the Cobalt-60 is 1.5 cm whereas the size of the focal spot for the 10 MV is 2 mm though in practice it is larger than this due to diffusion of the focal spot by the beam flattening filter. Another reason for the larger penumbra on the Cobalt-60 is the larger lateral scatter compared to that from 10 MV photon beam where most scatter are in the forward direction.

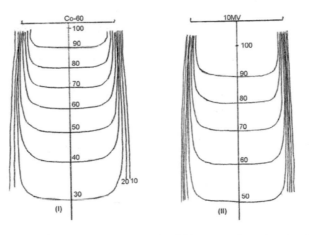

Figure 2.2 10 × 10 cm² isodose chart from (I) Cobalt-60 at 80 cm SSD and (II) (10 MV photon beam) at 100 cm SSD showing the difference in the width of the penumbra.

By simple geometry, it can be shown that: 1) the larger the source, the larger the penumbra; 2) the greater the SSD the larger the penumbra; and 3) the greater the source diaphragm distance (SDD), the smaller the penumbra.

As stated, the smaller the source size the smaller the penumbra but in practice this is not very practical for Cobalt-60 units because reducing the source size also reduces the output. Decreasing the SSD decreases the penumbra but also decreases the % depth dose. Increasing the source diaphragm distance decreases the penumbra but the closer the diaphragm patient distance, the greater the electron contamination from the diaphragm scatter. Hence, a compromise has to be reached between output, source size, SSD, SDD, and an acceptable penumbra.

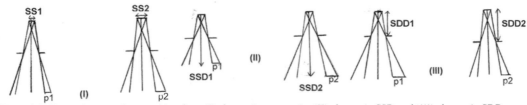

Figure 2.3 Change in penumbra resulting from (I) change in source size (II) change in SSD and (III) change in SDD.

A. Calculate the penumbra for the given parameters

The penumbra can be calculated if the SSD, SDD, and source size are known. Where the, SS, source size is 1.5 cm, SSD, source skin distance is 80 cm, SDD, source diaphragm distance is 45 cm, and DSD, diaphragm skin distance is 35 cm.

Therefor,

$$\left(\frac{p}{SS}\right) = \left(\frac{DSD}{SDD}\right) \rightarrow \left(\frac{p}{1.5}\right) = \left(\frac{35}{45}\right) \rightarrow p = \left(\frac{1.5 \times 35}{45}\right) = 1.17\,cm$$

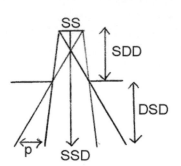

Figure 2.4 Geometry of penumbra.

VI. ADVANTAGES AND DISADVANTAGES OF PENUMBRA

i. Advantages

For matching fields, the larger the penumbra the better because the problem of over or under dosage is not as severe compared to small penumbral width. This may be observed in Figure 2.5 and 2.6. For Cobalt-60 beams with large penumbra, where a small movement of beam 2 towards beam 1 causes a small overdose at point x. For the Linac beams with small penumbral width, the same small movement of beam 2 towards beam 1 causes a larger overdose at point x. The reverse is true if beam 2 is moved away from beam 1.

ii. Disadvantages

When an area that is close to a critical organ (e.g., lens) is treated, a sharper beam (i.e., smaller penumbra) is highly desirable to limit the dose to the critical organ.

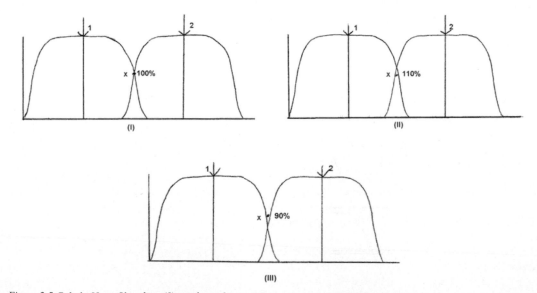

Figure 2.5 Cobalt-60 profiles show (I) good match at x, (II) overdose at x, and (III) underdose at x.

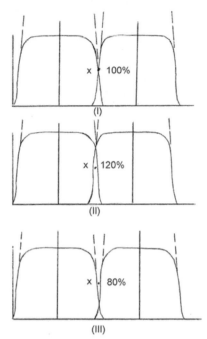

Figure 2.6 (10 MV photons) profiles show (I) good match at x, (II) overdose at x, and (III) underdose at x.

VII. FIELD GAP

Due to the divergence of radiation beams, a gap must be set between adjoining fields if over-dosing is to be avoided. The treatment distance, field length and depth of the match are needed to calculate the gap.

A. Two Fields on the Same Side

Where, a = 24 cm, b = 20 cm, d = 6 cm, and SSD = 100 cm.

$$\left(\frac{x}{(1/2)a}\right) = \left(\frac{d}{100}\right) \rightarrow x = \left(\frac{12 \times 6}{100}\right) = 0.72\,cm$$

and similarly,

$$y = \left(\frac{10 \times 6}{100}\right) = 0.60\quad cm$$

Therefore total gap between the two fields on the surface = 0.72+0.60 = 1.32 cm.

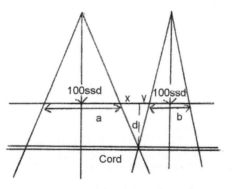

Figure 2.7 Gap between fields.

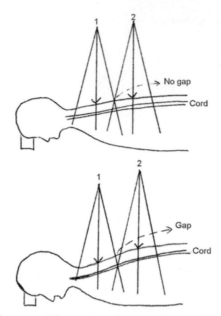

Figure 2.8 Diagrams show overdose to cord if no gap is set between adjoining fields and no overdose to cord if correct gap on skin is set.

B. Two Fields From Anterior and Two Fields From Posterior

Due to the slope of the patient's contour, the separation for the superior field is different to that for the inferior field. Matching for the four fields is calculated at the two different separations (Figure 2.9) or at a common separation (Figure 2.10).

i) Field match at two different separation

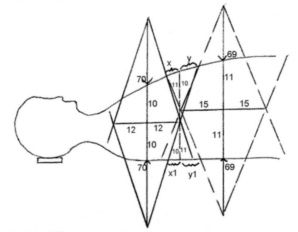

Figure 2.9 Field match at two different separations.

Referring to Figure 2.9,

$$x = \frac{11 \times 12}{80} = 1.65\,cm \qquad and \rightarrow \quad y = \frac{10 \times 15}{80} = 1.88\ \ cm$$

$$x_1 = \frac{10 \times 12}{80} = 1.50\,cm \qquad and \rightarrow \quad y_1 = \frac{11 \times 15}{80} = 2.06\ \ cm$$

Therefore the gaps are: (a) between the anterior fields = 1.65+1.88 = 3.53 cm, and (b) between the posteri-or fields = 1.50+2.06 = 3.56 cm.

ii) Field match at common separation

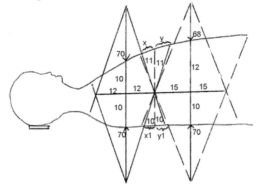

Figure 2.10 Field match at a common separation.

Referring to Figure 2.10,

$$x = \frac{11 \times 12}{80} = 1.65\,cm \qquad and \rightarrow \quad y = \frac{11 \times 15}{80} = 2.06 \quad cm$$

$$x_1 = \frac{10 \times 12}{80} = 1.50\,cm \qquad and \rightarrow \quad y_1 = \frac{10 \times 15}{80} = 1.88 \quad cm$$

Therefore the gaps are: (a) between the anterior fields – 1.65+2.06 = 3.71 cm, and (b) between the posterior fields = 1.50+1.88 = 3.38 cm.

If the treatment distance is increased, the gaps are decreased as shown in Figure 2.11.

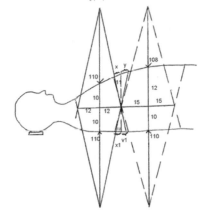

Figure 2.11 Decreased gap with increased SSD.

Referring to Figure 2.11,

$$x = \frac{11 \times 12}{120} = 1.10\,cm \qquad and \rightarrow \quad y = \frac{11 \times 15}{120} = 1.38 \quad cm$$

$$x_1 = \frac{10 \times 12}{120} = 1.00\,cm \qquad and \rightarrow \quad y_1 = \frac{10 \times 15}{120} = 1.25 \quad cm$$

Therefore the gaps are: (a) between the anterior fields = 1.10+1.38 = 2.48 cm, and (b) between the posterior fields = 1.00+1.25 = 2.25 cm.

Due to the gap between fields, there is a small region anterior to the match where the dose is lower. Care must be taken by the radiation oncologist to ensure that there is no disease in this region. By moving the junction, the dose in the region can be improved.

C. One Posterior Field and Two Lateral Fields

Referring to Figure 2.12, it is not necessary to have a gap between the posterior field and the lateral fields because the divergence of the posterior spinal field is matched to the lateral skull fields by angling the collimator for the lateral fields.

The collimator angle is obtained as follows;

$$Tan\theta = \left(\frac{1/2(length)}{SSD}\right) = \frac{27}{110} \rightarrow \theta = 13.8^\circ$$

The collimator angle for the opposite lateral field is the reverse of this.

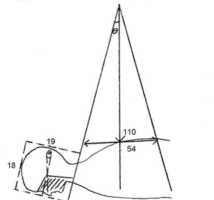

Figure 2.12 Collimator angled by θ degree to match divergence of posterior spinal field.

Referring to Figure 2.13, the divergence of the lateral fields may be matched to the posterior spinal field by angling the floor.

The floor angle is calculated as follows;

$$Tan\theta = \left(\frac{9.5}{100}\right) \rightarrow \theta = 5.4^\circ$$

The opposite lateral field is the reverse of this.

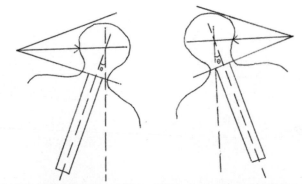

Figure 2.13 Floor angled by θ to match divergence of lateral fields to posterior spinal field.

D. One Anterior, One Posterior and Two Lateral Fields

Referring to Figure 2.14, the collimator for the lateral fields are not angled because of the opposing anterior-posterior fields. Instead, a gap (a) is calculated between the superior edge of the anterior-posterior fields and the inferior edge of the lateral fields.

In this example,
$$Gap = \left(\frac{x}{1/2(length)} \right) = \left(\frac{d}{SAD} \right) \rightarrow x = \left(\frac{7 \times 5}{80} \right) = 0.44 \quad cm$$

where L = 14 cm is the length of anterior-posterior fields, d = 5 cm, the depth, and SAD = 80 cm

This gap of 0.44 cm from the superior edge of the anterior field is marked at mid-line. The divergence of the lateral fields are matched to this mark by angling the floor as described in the previous section (Figure 2.14.)

In this example, the floor angle is caculated as follows;
$$Tan\theta = \left(\frac{7.5}{80} \right) \rightarrow \theta = 5.4^{\circ}$$

Another method to work out the gap is to move the couch longitudinally from the center of the anterior field by half the field length of the anterior filed using the central axis of the field. This point is marked on the shell and the lateral fields are matched to this mark as described above.

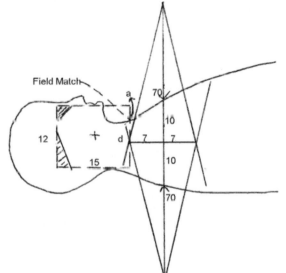

Figure 2.14 Match of anterior-posterior and lateral fields at depth d. Gap is a.

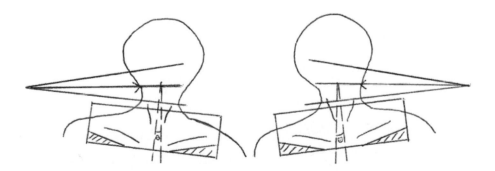

Figure 2.15 Floor angled to match divergence of lateral fields to anterior-posterior fields.

VIII. HALF-VALUE LAYER (HVL) OR HALF-VALUE THICKNESS (HVT)

Half value layer is the layer or thickness of attenuator required to reduce the quantity of radiation to half its original intensity. The HVL is a measure of the quality of a beam for low energy radiation such as the superficial. High energy units like the Cobalt-60 or Linear Accelerators are not quantified by HVL but by the energies that they emit. For example, the average energy for Cobalt-60 is 1.25 MV.

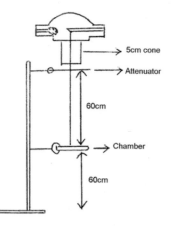

Figure 2.16 Set-up to measure HVL for DXR unit.

To measure the HVL, an exposure is measured without attenuator. Layer by layer of an attenuator is then added between the target and the measuring probe. The measurements are continued until very little radiation is measured. The measurements are normalized to the measurement without attenuator. A semi-log graph is plotted with the exposure on the vertical axis and the thickness of the attenuator on the horizontal axis. The thickness of the attenuator required to reduce the radiation to half its original value can be read off the graph.

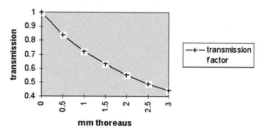

Figure 2.17 Graph of Thoraeus attenuator for DXR 250 kV 15 mA.

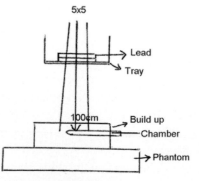

Figure 2.18 Set-up to measure HVL for 6 MV photon unit.

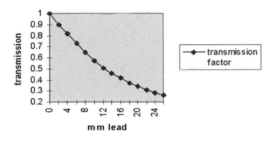

Figure 2.19 Pb attenuator for 6 MV photon unit.

Generally, for superficial units, the HVL is in mm Al. Even though high energy units like the Cobalt-60 and linear accelerators are not quantified by HVL but by the energies, HVL for these high energy units are useful to have in order to determine the thickness for shielding purposes. The HVL for these high energy units are in mm of Pb.

IX. LINEAR ATTENUATION COEFFICIENT (μ)

Linear attenuation coefficient is defined as that fraction of radiation that is attenuated by unit thickness of the attenuator. Linear attenuation coefficient u is related to HVL by $\mu = 0.693/\text{HVL}$. Knowing the HVL, the μ can be calculated.

Example:

HVL for Cobalt-60 = 1.1 cm of lead. $\mu = 0.693/1.1 = 0.63$

Where; I_p = present intensity, I_o = original intensity, e = base of natural log, μ = linear attenuation coefficient, and x = thickness of attenuator, I_o = 100 cGy, x = 5.5 cm, and μ = 0.63.

Therefore, $$I_\rho = I_\theta \, e^{-\mu x} \rightarrow I_\rho = 100 \times e^{-0.63 \times 5.5} = 3.1 \ cGy$$

In other words, for 100 cGy passing through 5.5 cm lead, 96.9 cGy is attenuated by the lead.

X. ISOCENTER

Most modern high energy treatment units are constructed with the capability to rotate about a point that is the intersection of the central axis and the axis of rotation. This point of intersection is the isocenter. The isocenter is usually at 80 cm for Cobalt-60 units and 100 cm for high energy photon beams.

Isocentric unit is very useful in treating multifields because after one field is set-up, other fields may be set-up by just changing the gantry angles.

Referring to Figure 2.20, the isocenter is set-up by setting to a pre-determined depth as planned. Fields #2 and #3 are set-up by just rotating the gantry to 9° and 279° respectively.

Isocenters should be checked regularly by either using a mechanical pointer set at isocenter and rotating the gantry to check coincidence of central axis cross hair with the pointer or by taking "star shot" using a film. A very narrow beam ($0.1 \times 0.1 \ cm^2$) is set on the collimator and a film (in paper covering) is set in a vertical position to the gantry. The film is exposed with the gantry positions at 30°, 60°, 90°, 120°, 150°, 180°, 210°, 240°, 270°, 300°, 330°, and 360°.

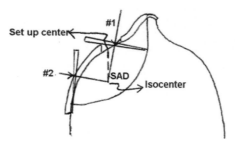

Figure 2.20 Isocentric set-up.

The film is developed and a fine pencil line is drawn through the center of each of the beams. The intersection of the pencil lines determines if the isocenter is within the tolerance.

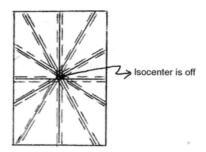

Figure 2.21 "Star shot" to check isocenter of a treatment unit.

XI. TIMER CORRECTION (SHUTTER TIME)

For Cobalt-60, this is the time taken for the Cobalt-60 source to move from its safe position to treatment position to start the timer. For the superficial and deep x-ray units, it is the time taken for the emission of radiation from the x-ray unit to the start of the timer.

XII. MEASUREMENT OF TIMER CORRECTION

A. Formula Method

The timer correction for a treatment unit should be routinely checked to verify optimum performance of the pneumatic system and source drawer for the Cobalt-60 unit or to verify optimum performance of the timer for the SXR and DXR units.

Using an Ion chamber, an exposure in Roentgen(R) is taken for 1 minute. This is repeated for 0.2 min each for 5 readings.

$$Timer\ correction = \left(\frac{M_1 T_2 - M_2 T_1}{M_1 N - M_2} \right)$$

Where; M_1 *is total exposure in R collected in time* T_1, T_1 *is time of single exposure in 1 min,* M_2 *is total exposure in R collected over five exposures,* T_2 *is total time of 5 × 0.2 min exposures, and N is no. of small* T_2.

Example:

If M_1 = 30.75R, T_1 = 1 min, M_2 (sum of 5.57R, 5.57R, 5.58R, 5.57R, 5.56R) = 27.85R, T_2 = 0.2 × 5 = 1 min, N = 5, and T_1 = T_2. The Timer Correction is calculated as follows:

$$Timer\ correction = \left(\frac{30.75(1) - 27.85(1)}{30.75(5) - 27.85} \right) = +\ 0.023 \quad min$$

The timer correction may be positive in which case this is added to the treatment time setting. It may be negative in which case this is subtracted from the treatment time setting.

B. Graph Method

A number of R readings with small times are taken. The results are plotted and extrapolated to zero dose. The slope is propotional to the exposure rate. The intercept on the horizontal axis is the timer correction. This method depends upon the linearity of the measuring instrument.

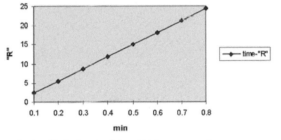

Figure 2.22 Cumulative exposure against multiple time to determine timer correction.

XIII. CONTOUR

Contour is an outline of the patient. Contour may be in the cross sectional *(transverse)* plane or sagittal plane or coronal plane. Contours may be obtained with. 1) lead wire; 2) plaster of Paris bandage strip; 3) optical distance indicator *(ODI)* on the simulator or treatment unit; 4) formulator; 5) multipurpose projector; 6) pantograph; 7) ultrasound, 8) CT; and 9) MRI.

1. Lead wire

The easiest way to take a body contour is to wrap a piece of lead wire around the body and transfer the wire shape onto graph paper. Care must be taken to ensure that the shape of the wire does not change or get tilted during the transfer. Due to the lack of rigidity of the wire, lateral and anterior-posterior separation may be confirmed with a caliper. Table top height to reference points helps improve the accuracy of the contour.

2. Plaster of Paris Bandage Strip

The plaster of Paris bandage strip does the same job as the lead wire. A wet strip plaster of Paris bandage is molded around the body contour. This is left to dry for a few minutes before removal from the patient. The shape is transfer onto graph paper.

3. ODI

The optical distance indicator *(or ODI)* is a more accurate method to obtain contour. This can be done on the simulator with the patient in the treatment position. With the gantry at zero degree, the isocenter is set to approximately mid depth in the patient. The SSD is noted The gantry is rotated every 10° and the SSD is noted and documented in a contour table. The SSD readings are converted to depth by subtracting the SSD readings from 100 cm SAD. The depths are joined together to obtain the contour.

Table 2.2 Table of depths against gantry angles.

Gantry	SSD	depth	Gantry	SSD	depth
0	90	10	350	90	10
10	89.8	10.2	340	90	11
20	89.6	10.4	330	88	12
30	89	11	320	87.2	12.8
40	88.4	11.6	310	86.4	13.6
50	87.6	12.4	300	85.5	14.5
60	86.6	13.4	290	84.8	15.2
70	85.6	14.4	280	84.2	15.8
80	84.4	15.6	270	83.5	16.5
90	83	17	260	84	16
100	82.7	17.3	250	84.3	15.7
110	83.2	16.8	240	84.4	15.6
120	83.8	16.2	230	84.8	15.2
130	84.3	15.7			

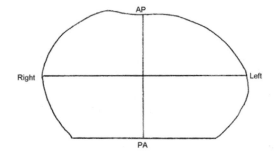

Figure 2.23 Contour generated from the Table 2.2.

4. Formulator

The formulator is made up of vertical rods bound together. These rods are free to move vertically until each rod touches the patient's skin. The rods are then secured by tightening the binding that holds the rods. The contour is taken by tracing along the ends of the rods.

5. Multipurpose projector

The multipurpose projector consists of a mounting device in which the patient's immobilization shell or cast may be mounted on. The mounting allows for collimator rotation by tilting the shell to the simulated collimator angle. The contour is taken from the shell using a horizontal pointer mounted on a vertical stem. The pointer lines up with a hole drilled through the pointer base so that each point taken along the shell outline may be marked onto paper.

6. Pantograph

This is a mechanical or electro-mechanical device in which the contour may be taken by using one end to trace the patient outline and the other end to trace the contour onto paper.

7. Ultrasound

Reasonable contours may be obtained from ultrasound. In addition to obtaining the contour, some internal structures may also be localized; example the lung interface with the chest wall. This is helpful in determining the thickness of the chest wall in tangential planning.

8. CT and MRI

All the methods described above for taking contour are generally acceptable and are used to a greater or lesser extent in most centers, but they are not as accurate as one would like them to be. The inaccuracy increases if multi-plane contours are needed as when there is large contour difference from plane to plane.

In addition, they do not provide localizations of the tumor and important internal organs such as the kidney, liver, cord, lens, etc.

This is where the CT and MRI images have the advantage. Not only do the images provide very accurate body contours in any plane but the images also display the tumor and other internal organs.

XIV. HALF-BLOCK OR BEAM SPLITTER OR ASYMETTRIC JAW

Due to the divergence of radiation beams, a gap must be allowed between adjoining fields if overdosing is to be avoided. If a non-diverging beam is available, the problem of field overlap is absent. Such non diverging beam may be produced from half-block system or from asymmetric collimation system of newer therapy machines.

The half block is machined from a lead block and is mounted on a perspex shielding tray. It is machined with a 3° slant at the border of the unblocked edge. This is to prevent a steep cold spot if the half block is slightly across the central axis or a steep hot spot if the half block is slightly away from the central axis. With this 3° angle at the edge of the block, a slight over or under lap is not as critical and does not produce a dramatic change in the dose at the junction of the fields. The half block is set to match the adjoining field at a pre-determined depth.

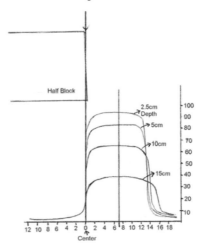

Figure 2.24 Beam profiles for half-block (Cobalt-60).

In the example where the half block is used in the treatment of nasopharyngeal carcinoma, the anterior, posterior fields are treated with the half-block shielding the superior half of the field. For the left and right lateral fields, the half block shields the inferior half of the field. In this way, the set-up center is the same for four fields and the junction is well matched with a sharp edge and there is no divergence problem.

Nowadays, new Linear Accelerators are equipped with asymmetric jaws that may be closed independently. One set of jaws is closed to the center of the field axis to mimic the beam splitter to treat one half of the field. The other half of the field is treated by opening the opposite jaw and closing the previous jaw to central axis.

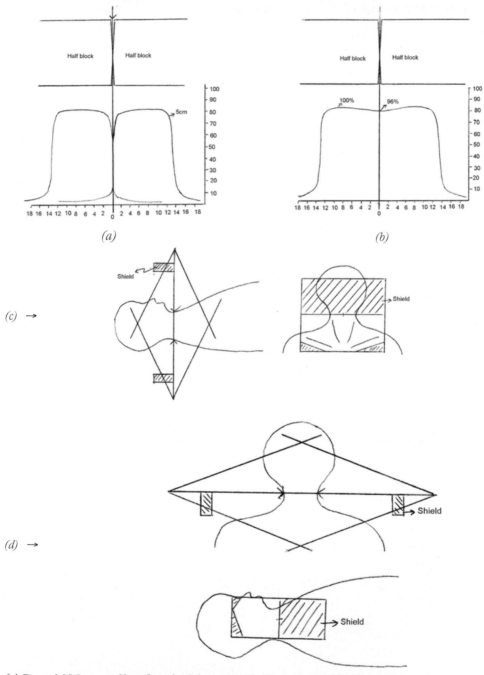

(a) *Figure 2.25 Beam profile at 5 cm depth for each half of the unblocked field (Cobalt-60.)*
(b) *Figure 2.26 Summation of each half of the unblocked field at 5 cm depth (Cobalt-60).*
(c) *Figure 2.27 Lateral and anterior view of treatment using half-block. Inferior half is treated and superior half is shielded.*
(d) *Figure 2.28 Anterior and lateral view of treatment using half-block. Superior half is treated and inferior half is shielded.*

XV. PERCENTAGE DEPTH DOSE (%DD)

A. Definition and Measurement

Percentage depth dose is defined as the ratio of the dose at a point in phantom to the maximum depth dose. This maximum depth dose is also called the D_{max}.

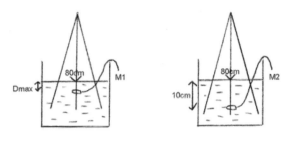

Figure 2.29 Set-up to measure %DD.

$$Percent\ Depth\ Dose(PPD) \rightarrow \%DD\ (10 \times 10\ cm^2,\ 10\ cm\ depth) = \left(\frac{Dose(10cm)}{Dose(D_{max})} \right) \times 100$$

Table 2.3. Table of %DD for Cobalt-60.

FS→	5(cm)	7(cm)	10(cm)	12(cm)	15(cm)
Depth(cm)					
0.5	100	100	100	100	100
1	97.3	97.6	98	98.1	98.2
2	91.6	92.5	93.4	93.8	94.1
3	85.8	87.1	88.4	89	89.6
4	80	81.7	83.3	84.1	84.9
5	74.5	76.3	78.2	79.1	80
6	69.1	71.1	73.2	74.3	75.4
7	64.1	66.2	68.4	69.6	70.8
8	59.4	61.5	63.9	65	66.5
9	54.9	57.1	59.5	60.8	62.3
10	50.8	52.9	55.5	56.8	58.4
11	46.9	49.1	51.6	53	54.6
12	43.4	45.5	48	49.4	51.1
13	40.1	42.2	44.7	46.1	47.9
14	37	39	41.6	43	44.8
15	34.2	36.2	38.7	40.1	41.9
16	31.6	33.5	36	37.4	39.2
17	29.2	31.1	33.5	34.9	36.7
18	27	28.8	31.2	32.6	34.3
19	24.9	26.7	29	30.3	32.2
20	23	24.8	27	28.3	30.1

B. Factors Affecting %DD

i. Depth

Percentage depth dose decreases with depth due to increased distance from the source and increase attenuation through the phantom. For Cobalt-60, the %DD for 10×10 cm^2 at 5 cm depth is 78.2% and at 10 cm depth, it is 55.5%.

ii. Field Size

Percentage depth dose increases with field size due to increase scatter. The effect of scatter on %DD decreases with increase photon energy. Thus for higher energy photon beams, the %DD increase with increase in field size is less pronounced.

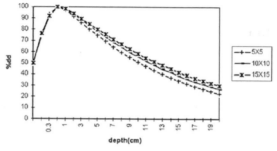

Figure 2.30 %DD for Cobalt-60.

iii. SSD

Percentage depth dose increases with increase source skin distance (SSD). This is because the reduction in dose rate with increase SSD is less severe at depth than at D$_{max}$. A commonly used method to calculate the change in %DD with SSD change is the Mayneord Factor method.

Example:

%DD (for 10×10 cm^2 at 10 cm depth at 90 cm SSD) =Mayneord Factor $\times$ %DD (10×10 cm^2 at 10 cm depth at 80 cm SSD)

Therefore the PDD is calculated as follows;

$$\%DD(10 \times 10cm^2, d = 10cm, SSD = 90cm) = \left(\frac{SSD + D_{max}}{SSD + depth} \right)^2 \times \left(\frac{80 + depth}{80 + D_{max}} \right)^2 \times \%DD(10 \times 10cm^2, d = 10cm, SSD = 80cm)$$

$$= \left(\frac{90 + 0.5}{90 + 10} \right)^2 \times \left(\frac{80 + 10}{80 + 0.5} \right)^2 \times 55.5 = 56.8\%$$

(iv) Energy

Percentage depth dose increases with energy due to increase penetration of the higher energy photon.

C. Calculation Using %DD

Example:

A patient is being treated on the Cobalt-60 unit using parallel-opposed fields of 15×15 cm^2 at 80 cm SSD. If 4000 cGy in 20 treatments is prescribed to mid-depth, what is the total dose to the spinal cord? The separation of the patient is 18cm and the spinal cord is 6 cm from the posterior.

Calculation:

The %DD to mid depth at 9 cm for 15 × 15 cm² field = 62.3%

The %DD to the cord at 12 cm from the AP = 51.1%

Tumor dose from the AP at mid depth = 2000 cGy

$$The\ dose\ to\ the\ cord\ from\ AP\ field = \left(\frac{51.1}{62.3}\right) \times 2000 = 1640\ cGy$$

The %DD to the cord at 6cm from the PA = 75.4%

Tumor dose from the PA at mid depth = 2000 cGy

$$The\ dose\ to\ the\ cord\ from\ AP\ field = \left(\frac{51.1}{62.3}\right) \times 2000 = 1640\ cGy$$

Therefore the total dose to spinal cord = 1640 + 2421 = 4061 cGy

XVI. TISSUE-AIR RATIO (TAR)

A. Definition and Measurement

Most modern treatment units are isocentric units. Patients are planned and treated using isocentric techniques. For an isocentric technique, all treatment fields have the same source axis distance (SAD) but because of the different treatment depths, the source skin distances (SSD) are different. Due to this change in SSD, the %DD changes for each field making it very cumbersome to calculate dose and treatment time. TAR replaces the %DD in the calculation of treatment time.

Tissue-air ratio is defined as the ratio of the dose at a point in phantom to the dose in air at the same point. TAR is measured by taking an ion chamber reading in air at a distance of 80 cm from source to chamber. This is repeated with the chamber at the same distance at D_{max} in a phantom (such as water tank). Readings for different depths are taken by increasing the water level keeping the source to chamber distance at 80 cm. The whole process is repeated for various field sizes.

Where TAR is defined as:
$$TAR = \left(\frac{Dose(depth)}{Dose(air)}\right)$$

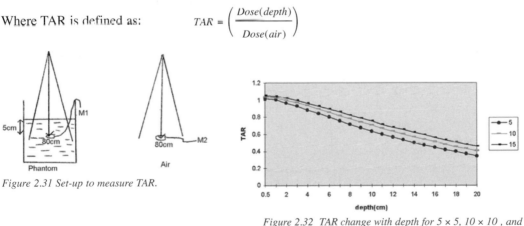

Figure 2.31 Set-up to measure TAR.

Figure 2.32 TAR change with depth for 5 × 5, 10 × 10, and 15 × 15 cm² field size (Cobalt-60).

B. Factors Affecting TAR

(i) Depth

TAR decreases with depth due to attenuation of the beam as it traverses more phantom.

(ii) Distance

TAR is independent of distance because the dose in phantom and in air are at the same point (*i.e.*, same distance from source.)

(iii) Field Size

    TAR increases with field size due to increase scatter.

Table 2.4. TAR table for Cobalt-60.

FS →	5(cm)	7(cm)	10(cm)	12(cm)	15(cm)
Depth(cm)					
0.5	1.018	1.025	1.035	1.041	1.049
1	1.003	1.013	1.026	1.034	1.043
2	0.967	0.983	1.000	1.012	1.023
3	0.927	0.948	0.971	0.983	0.997
4	0.885	0.909	0.936	0.950	0.966
5	0.842	0.868	0.898	0.914	0.932
6	0.799	0.826	0.859	0.876	0.897
7	0.756	0.785	0.819	0.838	0.86
8	0.715	0.745	0.780	0.800	0.824
9	0.675	0.705	0.742	0.762	0.788
10	0.637	0.667	0.705	0.726	0.752
11	0.600	0.631	0.669	0.690	0.717
12	0.566	0.596	0.634	0.656	0.684
13	0.533	0.562	0.600	0.622	0.651
14	0.501	0.53	0.568	0.590	0.620
15	0.472	0.500	0.538	0.560	0.590
16	0.444	0.472	0.509	0.531	0.560
17	0.418	0.445	0.481	0.503	0.533
18	0.396	0.419	0.455	0.477	0.506
19	0.369	0.395	0.43	0.451	0.481
20	0.347	0.372	0.406	0.427	0.456

C. Use of TAR in Calculation

Example:

    A patient is treated with a pair of anterior-posterior fields using a field size of 15×15 cm^2 at 80 cm SAD. The separation of the patient is 20 cm and the daily tumor dose to mid depth is 100 cGy from each field. Calculate the treatment time for each of the fields.

Solution:

Daily tumor dose (DTD) from each field = 100 cGy

TAR for 15×15 cm^2 at 10 cm depth = 0.752

Air dose rate at 80 cm SAD = 145.8 cGy/min

Timer correction (TC) = +0.02 min

$$Treatment\ time = \left(\frac{DTD}{ADR \times TAR} \right) + TC = \left(\frac{100}{145.8 \times 0.752} \right) + 0.02 = 0.93\ \ min$$

D. Relationship Between %DD and TAR

%DD and TAR are are related as shown in the equations below.

$$\% DD = \left(\frac{SSD + D_{max}}{SSD + depth} \right)^2 \times TAR \; \left(\frac{1}{PSF} \right) \times 100$$

$$TAR = \left(\frac{SSD + depth}{SSD + D_{max}} \right)^2 \times \% DD \; \times \left(\frac{PSF}{1} \right) \times \left(\frac{1}{100} \right)$$

E. Calculation of %DD Given TAR (80 cm SSD)

Point P is at 10 cm depth in a 80 cm SSD set-up with $10 \times 10 \; cm^2$ field size. If the TAR at P is known, the %DD at P can be calculated. Since TAR is dependent on field size, the field size at P *(10 cm depth in this example)* must be calculated first.

The field size at 80 cm SSD is $10 \times 10 \; cm^2$. Point p is at 10 cm depth that is 90 cm from the source.

$$\text{Therefore the field size} \; \rightarrow P = \left(\frac{90}{80} \right) \times 10 = \; 11.25 \; cm^2$$

From the table, TAR at 10 cm depth = 0.718.

$$\text{Field size at } D_{max} = \left(\frac{80.5}{80} \right) \times 10 = \; 10.1 \; cm^2$$

$$PSF \text{ for } 10.1 \; cm^2 = 1.035$$

$$\text{Therefore } \% DD \text{ at } P = \left(\frac{80 + 0.5}{80 + 10} \right)^2 \times (0.718) \times \left(\frac{1}{1.035} \right) \times 100 = 55.5\%$$

F. Calculation of TAR Given %DD (80 cm SSD)

From %DD table, (%DD $10 \times 10 \; cm^2$, 10 cm depth) = 55.5%.

$$\text{Therefore} \rightarrow TAR = \left(\frac{80 + 10}{80 + 0.5} \right)^2 \times (55.5) \times \left(\frac{1.035}{1} \right) \times \left(\frac{1}{100} \right) = 0.718$$

G. Calculation of %DD Given TAR (80 cm SAD)

The field size at P is $10 \times 10 \; cm^2$ and the TAR (10 cm depth) = 0.705.

$$\text{Field size at } D_{max} = \left(\frac{70.5}{80} \right) \times 10 = \; 8.8 \; cm^2$$

$$PSF \text{ at } 0.5cm \text{ depth for } 8.8 \; cm^2 = 1.031$$

$$\text{Therefore } \% DD \text{ at } P = \left(\frac{70 + 0.5}{70 + 10} \right)^2 \times (0.705) \times \left(\frac{1}{1.031} \right) \times 100 = 53.1\%$$

H. Calculation of TAR Given %DD (80 cm SAD)

$$\text{Field size at } D_{max} = \left(\frac{70.5}{80} \right) \times 10 = \; 8.8 \; cm^2$$

%DD from the 80 cm SSD depth dose Table at 10 cm depth for $8.8 \times 8.8 \; cm^2$ = 54.5% and applying the Mayneord correction for 70 cm SSD, the corrected percent depth dose (%DD);

$$\%DD = \left(\frac{80+10}{80+0.5}\right)^2 \times \left(\frac{70+0.5}{70+10}\right)^2 \times (54.5) = 52.9\%$$

$$Therefore \quad \rightarrow \quad TAR = \left(\frac{70+10}{70+0.5}\right)^2 \times (52.9) \times (1.031) \times \left(\frac{1}{100}\right) = 0.702$$

Note that the calculated TAR of 0.702 is different from the table TAR of 0.705. This is because the corrected %DD of 52.9% used in the calculation was approximated using the Mayneord correction.

I. Calculation of %DD for Extended SSD Using TAR
<u>i) 110 cm SSD</u>

Point p is at 10 cm depth at 110 cm SSD set-up with a collimator setting of 10 × 10 cm².

$$Field\ size\ at\ P = \left(\frac{120}{110}\right) \times 10 = 10.9\ cm^2$$

$$TAR\ at\ 10cm\ depth\ for\ 10.9\ cm^2 = 0.714$$

$$Field\ size\ at\ D_{max} = \left(\frac{110.5}{110}\right) \times 10 = 10.05\ cm^2$$

$$PSF\ for\ 10.05\ cm^2 = 1.035$$

$$Therefore\ \%DD\ at\ P = \left(\frac{110+0.5}{110+10}\right)^2 \times (0.714) \times \left(\frac{1}{1.035}\right) \times 100 = 58.5\%$$

XVII. PEAK SCATTER FACTOR (PSF) BACK SCATTER FACTOR (BSF)

A. Definition and Measurement

Peak scatter factor is the ratio of the dose at D_{max} to the dose in air at the same point. PSF is really the TAR at D_{max}. PSF increases with increase field size due to increase scatter and decreases with increase energy due to the decrease effect of scatter.

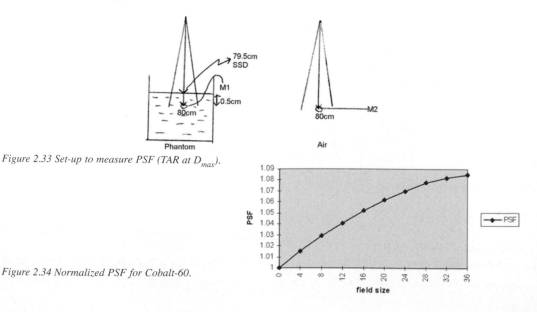

Figure 2.33 Set-up to measure PSF (TAR at D_{max}).

Figure 2.34 Normalized PSF for Cobalt-60.

For high energy treatment units, the air measurement is not a true air measurement because of the increase size of the build-up cap to achieve electronic equilibrium. This increase size of the build-up cap creates scatter which degrades the air measurement. Because of this, the PSF is measured at D_{max} in phantom. The collimator is set to the largest field size and lead blocks are used to cone down to the desired blocked field size. For each measurement, a hundred (100) MU is delivered and a reading is taken using an Ion chamber.

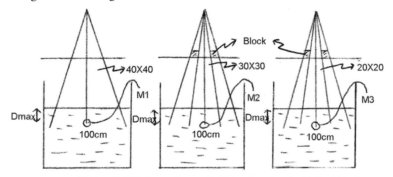

Figure 2.35 Set-up to measure PSF for 15 MV photon beam. Field size is reduced with lead blocks.

Table 2.5 Ion chamber readings* for field size 8 × 8 cm² to 40 × 40 cm².

Field Size(cm²)	Reading	Normalized PSF
40×40	102.87	1.058
36×36	102.87	1.058
32×32	102.87	1.058
28×28	102.77	1.057
24×24	102.48	1.054
20×20	101.99	1.049
16×16	101.22	1.041
12×12	100.44	1.033
8×8	99.47	1.023
0×0	97.25	1.000

*The ion chamber readings are normalized to 0×0 cm² field size.

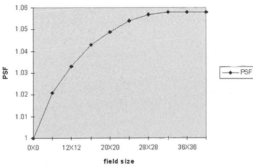

Figure 2.36 Normalized PSF for 15 MV photon beam.

XVIII. TISSUE-MAXIMUM RATIO (TMR)

A. Definition and Measurement

Tissue maximum ratio is defined as the ratio of the dose at a point in phantom to the dose at D_{max}.

TMR replaces TAR for energies higher than Cobalt-60 because the build-up cap necessary to attain electronic equilibrium produces scatter which does not give a true air measurement as required for Tissue-air-ratio.

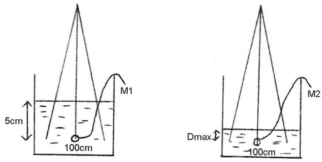

Figure 2.37 Set-up to measure TMR.

TMR is measured by taking an ion chamber reading at D_{max} in a water phantom at 100 cm SAD for a set field size and set exposure. This is repeated with the ion chamber at various depths by increasing the water level keeping the ion chamber at the same point. The whole process is repeated for each change in field size.

$$TMR = \left(\frac{Dose(depth)}{Dose(D_{max})} \right)$$

B. Factors Affecting TMR

The factors affecting TMR are as described for TAR. In addition, TMR increases with beam energy.

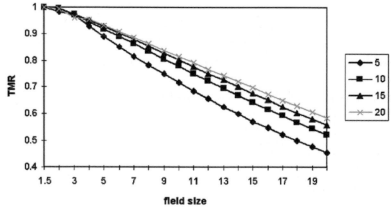

field size

Figure 2.38 TMR change with depth for 5 × 5, 10 × 10, 15×15, and 20 × 20 cm² field for 6 MV photon beam. Increase depth decreases TMR and increase field increases TMR.

Table 2.6. TMR table (6 MV photon).

FS	5(cm)	10	15	20
Depth(cm)				
1.5	1	1	1	1
2	1.01	0.998	0.995	0.994
3	0.971	0.973	0.974	0.974
4	0.928	0.946	0.951	0.953
5	0.889	0.919	0.928	0.932

6	0.852	0.891	0.904	0.909
7	0.816	0.863	0.879	0.886
8	0.782	0.835	0.854	0.863
9	0.749	0.807	0.828	0.839
10	0.717	0.778	0.802	0.815
11	0.686	0.75	0.777	0.791
12	0.656	0.723	0.751	0.767
13	0.628	0.696	0.726	0.744
14	0.600	0.669	0.701	0.720
15	0.573	0.643	0.676	0.697
16	0.548	0.618	0.652	0.674
17	0.524	0.593	0.628	0.651
18	0.5	0.569	0.605	0.629
19	0.478	0.546	0.582	0.607
20	0.456	0.523	0.56	0.585

C. Use of TMR in Calculation

Example:

A patient is treated with a pair of 6 MV photon beam of anterior-posterior fields using a field size of 15×15 cm^2 at 100 cm SAD. The separation of the patient is 20 cm and the daily tumor dose (DTD) to mid depth is 100 cGy from each field. Calculate the MU setting to each field.

Solution:

Daily tumor dose from each field = 100 cGy ♦ Output factor (OF) = 1.038 cGy/MU ♦ TMR (15×15 cm^2, 10 cm depth) = 0.802

$$MU\ Setting \quad \rightarrow MU = \left(\frac{DTD}{OF \times TMR}\right) = \left(\frac{100}{1.038 \times 0.802}\right) = 120$$

Using the data above, calculate the total dose to the cord if the cord is 6 cm from the posterior surface and the total tumor dose at mid-depth is 4000 cGy.

As stated earlier, TMR is dependent on field size and depth. To calculate the cord dose, the TMR at the cord depth must be calculated first.

$$The field\ size\ from\ Anterior\ at\ cord\ depth = \left(\frac{104}{100}\right) \times 15 = 15.6\ cm^2$$

$$TMR(15.6cm^2\ at\ 14cm\ depth) = 0.703$$

$$The\ field\ size\ from\ Posterior\ at\ cord\ depth = \left(\frac{96}{100}\right) \times 15 = 14.4\ cm^2$$

$$TMR(14.4cm^2\ at\ 6cm\ depth) = 0.903$$

$$Dose\ to\ cord\ from\ Anterior = \left(\frac{TTD(ant)}{TMR(10cm\ depth)}\right) \times (TMR(14cm)) \times \left(\frac{SAD}{SSD + cord(depth)}\right) = \left(\frac{2000}{0.802}\right) \times 0.703 \times \left(\frac{100}{104}\right)^2 = 1621cGy$$

$$Dose\ to\ cord\ from\ Posterior = \left(\frac{TTD(post)}{TMR(10cm\ depth)}\right) \times (TMR(6cm)) \times \left(\frac{SAD}{SSD + cord(depth)}\right) = \left(\frac{2000}{0.802}\right) \times 0.903 \times \left(\frac{100}{96}\right)^2 = 2443cGy$$

Therefore, Total Cord Dose = 1621 + 2443 = 4064cGy

D. Relationship of TMR, TAR, and %DD

Since TMR is a ratio of the dose at a point in phantom to the dose at D_{max} at the same point in phantom, the scatter cancels out. Hence, TMR does not include PSF *(Scatter)* unlike TAR which does.

$$MR \ is \ related \ to \ TAR \ by \ TMR = \left(\frac{TAR}{PSF(d)} \right)$$

or $\rightarrow TAR = TMR \times PSF(d)$

where $\rightarrow PSF(d) = PSF$ *for field size at depth d. As given earlier, TAR and %DD are related by,*

$$\%DD = \left(\frac{SSD + D_{max}}{SSD + depth} \right)^2 \times (TAR) \times \left(\frac{1}{PSF(D_{max})} \right) \times 100$$

TMR and %DD are related by,

$$TMR = \left(\frac{SSD + depth}{SSD + D_{max}} \right)^2 \times (\%DD) \times \left(\frac{1}{PSF(depth)} \right) \times (PSF(D_{max})) \times \left(\frac{1}{100} \right)$$

$$\%DD = \left(\frac{SSD + D_{max}}{SSD + depth} \right)^2 \times (TMR) \times ((PSF(depth)) \times \left(\frac{1}{PSF(D_{max})} \right) \times 100$$

E. Calculation of %DD Given TMR

Example:

Point P is at 10 cm depth in a 100 cm SAD set-up with 10 × 10 cm^2 field size at P. If the TMR at P is known, the %DD at P can be calculated.

The field size at p is 10 × 10 cm^2 and the TMR (10 cm depth) = 0.778 ♦ *PSF(d) for 10 × 10 cm^2 = 1.035*

The field size at D_{max} (1.5 cm) = (91.5/100) × 10 cm^2 = 9.15 cm^2 ♦ *PSF (D_{max}) for 9.15 × 9.15 cm^2 = 1.033*

$$\%DD \ at \ P = \left(\frac{SSD + D_{max}}{SSD + depth} \right)^2 \times (TMR) \times ((PSF(depth)) \times \left(\frac{1}{PSF(D_{max})} \right) \times 100$$

$$= \left(\frac{90 + 1.5}{90 + 10} \right)^2 \times (0.778) \times (1.035) \times \left(\frac{1}{1.033} \right) \times 100 = 65.3\%$$

F. Calculation of TMR Given %DD

Example:

Field size at D_{max} = (91.5/100) × 10 cm^2 = 9.15 cm^2 ♦ *PSF 9.15 cm^2 = 1.033* ♦ *PSF for 10 × 10 cm^2 = 1.035*

%DD at 10 cm depth at 100 cm SSD for 9 × 9 cm^2 = 66.0%

$$Corrected \ \%DD = \left(\frac{SSD + D_{max}}{SSD + depth} \right)^2 \times \left(\frac{100 + depth}{100 + D_{max}} \right)^2 \times \%DD = \left(\frac{90 + 1.5}{90 + 10} \right)^2 \times \left(\frac{100 + 10}{100 + 1.5} \right)^2 \times 66\% = 64.9\%$$

$$TMR = \left(\frac{SSD + depth}{SSD + D_{max}} \right)^2 \times (\%DD) \times \left(\frac{1}{PSF(depth)} \right) \times ((PSF(D_{max})) \times \left(\frac{1}{100} \right) = \left(\frac{90 + 10}{90 + 1.5} \right)^2 \times (64.9) \times \left(\frac{1}{1.035} \right) \times$$

$$((1.033)) \times \left(\frac{1}{100} \right) = 0.774$$

The calculated TMR of 0.774 is slightly different from the TMR in the table. This is because the %DD of 64.9% used in the calculation was approximated using the Mayneord Factor.

G. Calculation of %DD at Extended Treatment Distance Using TMR

Example:

i) 120 cm SSD set-up

Point p is at 10 cm depth in a 30 × 45 cm^2 field at 120 cm SSD set-up. By first obtaining the TMR at point P, the %DD can be calculated.

$$Field\ size\ at\ P = \left(\frac{120 + 10}{120}\right) \times 36\ cm^2 = 39.0\ cm^2$$

$$PSF\ for\ 39.0\ cm^2\ field\ from\ table = 1.110$$

$$TMR\ for\ 39.0\ cm^2\ field\ at\ 10cm\ depth\ from\ table = 0.840$$

$$Field\ size\ at\ D_{max} = \left(\frac{120 + 1.5}{120}\right) \times 36\ cm^2 = 36.5\ cm^2$$

$$PSF\left(D_{max}\right)\ for\ 36.5\ cm^2 = 1.097$$

$$Therefore\ \%DD\ at\ P = \left(\frac{120 + 1.5}{120 + 10}\right)^2 \times (0.840) \times (1.110) \times \left(\frac{1}{1.097}\right) \times 100 = 74.2\%$$

XIX. TISSUE-PHANTOM RATIO (TPR)

For energies higher than 10 MV, D_{max} changes with field size becomes significant. Due to this factor, TPR is used instead of TMR because TPR is the ratio of the dose at a point in phantom to the dose at a reference point. The reference point is at a depth beyond the D_{max} region.

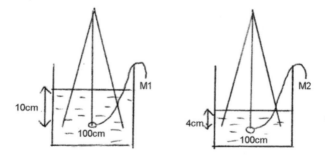

Figure 2.39 Set-up to measure TPR. Normalization at 4 cm.

TPR is measured by taking an ion chamber reading at a reference depth such as 4 cm at 100 cm SAD for a set field size and set exposure. This is repeated with the ion chamber at various depths by increasing the water level keeping the ion chamber at the same point. The whole process is repeated for each change in field size.

$$TPR = \left(\frac{Dose(10cm)}{Dose(ref\,4cm)}\right)$$

The factors affecting TPR are as described for TAR and TMR.

Table 2.7. Tissue-Phantom Ratio (TPR)*(10 MV photons).*

FS(cm²)→	5	10	15	20
Depth(cm)				
3	1	1	1	1
4	0.987	0.988	0.988	0.988
5	0.965	0.968	0.969	0.971
6	0.938	0.945	0.951	0.954
7	0.91	0.923	0.931	0.935
8	0.884	0.9	0.91	0.917
9	0.861	0.881	0.889	0.897
10	0.831	0.854	0.869	0.878
11	0.804	0.83	0.847	0.857
12	0.78	0.808	0.825	0.836
13	0.754	0.786	0.804	0.816
14	0.731	0.764	0.782	0.795
15	0.708	0.743	0.761	0.775
16	0.685	0.719	0.74	0.755
17	0.661	0.695	0.719	0.735
18	0.64	0.675	0.698	0.714
19	0.618	0.655	0.679	0.696
20	0.6	0.633	0.66	0.678

XX. TISSUE-DOSE RATE (TDR) or ABSORBED-DOSE RATE IN TISSUE(cGy/min)

A. Definition and Measurement

Tissue-dose rate is the absorbed-dose rate in tissue. TDR is measured in a water phantom at a reference depth such as 5 cm at 80 cm SSD. A time of one minute plus timer correction is set for the measurement. The true TDR at 0.5 cm depth is calculated using depth dose table. This is repeated for different field sizes.

Table 2.8 Table of TDR for field size 5 × 5 to 15 × 15 cm².

Field Size(cm²)	TDR(d=5cm)	Calculated TDR at 0.5 cm depth
5×5	104.6	140.4*
10×10	114.4	146.3*
15×15	120.9	151.1*

*$TDR = 104.6 \times (100\%/74.5)$

where the %DD at 5 cm is 74.5%, Source to D_{max} distance is 80 + 0.5 cm.

B. Factors Affecting TDR

Tissue dose rate increases with field size due to increase scatter and decreases with distance due to inverse square.

C. Calculation Using TDR

TDR is used in the calculation of treatment time in SSD set-up. If the dose is prescribed to D_{max}, the treatment time is calculating by dividing the D_{max} dose *(given dose)* by the TDR.

$$Treatment\ time = \left(\frac{Given\ dose}{TDR} \right)$$

If the prescription is to a specified depth, the daily given dose is calculated first and then the treatment time is calculated as shown in the example below.

Example:

A patient is treated with a single direct field to the spine at 80 cm SSD. The field size is 6 × 15 cm^2 and the total tumor dose prescribed to the spine at 6 cm depth is 3000 cGy in 20 treatments. Calculate the treatment time for each treatment.

Daily tumor dose (DTD) = 150 cGy ♦ %DD for 10 × 10 cm^2 at 6 cm depth = 72.3% ♦ Timer correction (TC) = +0.02 min ♦ Tissue dose rate (TDR) for 10 × 10 cm^2 at 80 cm SSD = 144.7 cGy/min

$$Daily\ given\ dose(DGD)\ at\ 0.5cm\ at\ 80cm\ SSD = \left(\frac{(DTD) \times 100}{\%DD} \right) = \left(\frac{150 \times 100}{72.3} \right) = 207.5\ cGy$$

$$Treatment\ time = \left(\frac{DGD}{TDR} \right) + timer\ correction = \left(\frac{207.5}{144.7} \right) + 0.02 = 1.45\ min$$

XXI. AIR-DOSE RATE(ADR)(cGy/min)

A. Definition

Air-dose rate is the dose rate in air (free space) with no scatter. In practice, air-dose rate is derived from tissue dose rate by removing the scatter component and correcting for inverse square.

Table 2.0 Table of TDR and ADR.

FS(cm^2)	TDR	ADR
5×5	140.4	139.6
6×6	141.7	141.4
7×7	142.9	141.1
8×8	144.1	141.8
9×9	145.2	142.5
10×10	146.3	143.2
11×11	147.4	143.8
12×12	148.4	144.3
13×13	149.3	144.9
14×14	150.2	145.4
15×15	151.1	145.8
16×16	151.9	146.2
17×17	152.7	146.6
18×18	153.4	147

ADR is used in the calculation of treatment time in SAD set-up. Treatment time is calculated by dividing the daily tumor dose (DTD) by the TAR and the ADR.

$$Treatment\ time = \left(\frac{DTD}{(ADR) \times (TAR)} \right)$$

B. Factors Affecting Air-Dose Rate

Air dose rate increases with field size due to increase collimator scatter and decreases with distance due to inverse square.

C. Calculation Using Air-Dose Rate

Example:

A patient is treated with a single direct field to the spine at 80 cm SAD with a field size of 6 × 15 cm² The total tumor dose (TTD) prescribed is 3000 cGy in 20 treatments to a depth of 6 cm. Calculate the treatment time for each treatment.

Daily tumor dose (DTD) = 150 cGy ◆ TAR (6 × 15 cm², 6 cm depth) = 0.844 ◆ ADR (10 × 10 cm²) = 142.2 cGy/min ◆ Timer correction (TC) = +0.02 min

$$Treatment\ time = \left(\frac{DTD}{(ADR) \times (TAR)} \right) + TC = \left(\frac{150}{142.2 \times 0.844} \right) + 0.02 = 1.27 \quad min$$

XXII. OUTPUT FACTOR (OF) cGy/MU

A. Measurement

High energy linear accelerators are calibrated to give 1 cGy/MU for a 10×10 cm² field at 100 cm SAD. OF for all other fields are normalized to the OF for 10×10 cm².

Output factors are measured in a water phantom at a reference depth at 100 cm SAD. OF is used to calculate MU setting in the same way as ADR is used to calculate treatment time.

Table 2.10 Table of OF for 15 MV photon beam. Normalized to 10×10 cm².

FS(cm²)	OF(cGy/MU)
5×5	0.917
10×10	1
15×15	1.035
20×20	1.047
25×25	1.053
30×30	1.06
35×35	1.068
40×40	1.067

B. Factors Affecting Output Factor (OF)

Output factor increases with field size due to increase scatter from the collimator and phantom and decreases with distance due to inverse square.

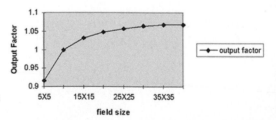

Figure 2.40 Output factor for 15 MV photon beam at 100 cm SAD. Depth of OF measurement is at 4 cm (D_{max}).

C. Calculation Using OF

Example:

A patient is treated with a single direct field at 100 cm SAD with a 15 × 15 cm^2 field size. A total tumor dose (TTD) of 3000 cGy in 20 treatments is prescribed to a point 10 cm depth. Calculate the MU setting for each treatment on the 15 MV photon beam.

Daily tumor dose (DTD) = 150 cGy ◆ *OF for 15 × 15 cm^2 = 1.035 cGy/MU* ◆ *TPR for 15 × 15 cm^2 at 10 cm depth = 0.888*

$$MU\ Setting = \left(\frac{DTD}{(OF) \times (TPR)}\right) = \left(\frac{150}{1.035 \times 0.888}\right) = 163\ MU$$

Note that in the calculation of MU setting, there is no timer correction involved because the MU set is counted by the built in ionization chamber and when the MU set is completed, the radiation ceases.

Since the OF is measured at a reference depth at 100 cm focus to chamber distance, a correction must be made to the OF if the treatment distance is not at 100 cm.

Example:

A patient is treated with a single direct field at 110 cm SSD with a 16.5 × 16.5 cm^2 field size on a 6MV linear accelerator. A total tumor dose (TTD) of 3000 cGy in 20 treatments is prescribed to D$_{max}$. Calculate the MU setting for each treatment. D$_{max}$ is at 1.5 cm.

Daily tumor dose (DTD) = 150 cGy ◆ *Field size at 110 cm = 16.5 cm^2* ◆ *Field size at 100 cm = 15 cm^2* ◆ *OF for 15 × 15 cm^2 at 100 cm = 1.035cGy/MU*

$$OF\ corrected\ to\ 110cm = \left(\frac{100}{111.5}\right)^2 \times 1.035 = 0.833\ cGy\ /\ MU$$

$$MU\ Setting = \left(\frac{DTD}{OF}\right) = \left(\frac{150}{0.833}\right) = 180\ MU$$

XXIII. FILTERS

A. Shielding Tray Filter

Shielding trays are used to mount lead/cerrobend blocks to shield normal tissues and/or vital organs. These trays are usually made of perspex and they are placed in the tray slot at the head of the treatment unit. Tray factors are accounted in the treatment time or monitor unit setting due to their attenuation.

Table 2.11 Table of shielding tray factors for treatment units.

Treatment Unit	Tray Factor
Cobalt-60	0.959
6 MV	0.97
10 MV	0.976
15 MV	0.98

XXIV. TRAY FACTOR IN CALCULATION OF TREATMENT TIME

Daily tumor dose (DTD) = 100 cGy ◆ *Air dose rate (ADR) = 120 cGy/min* ◆ *Tray factor (TF) = 0.959 & TAR = 0.820* ◆ *Timer correction (TC) = +0.02 min*

$$Treatment\ time = \left(\frac{DTD}{(ADR) \times (TAR) \times (TF)}\right) + TC = \left(\frac{100}{120 \times 0.820 \times 0.959}\right) + 0.02 = 1.08\ min$$

B. Wedge Filter

Wedges may be used to compensate for missing tissue or to "bend" isodose curves to fit a desired target volume. They are usually made of lead or steel and are placed in the path of the radiation beam in the wedge slot in the head of the treatment unit. They attenuate radiation and hence their factors must be taken into account in the treatment time or monitor unit setting calculation.

Table 2.12 Table of wedge filter factors for treatment units.

Treatment Unit	30° wedge	45° wedge	60° wedge
Cobalt-60	0.724	0.59	0.424
6 MV	0.681	0.627	0.601
10 MV	0.76	0.621	0.595
15 MV	0.774	0.644	0.604

C. Lead Compensating Filter

Lead compensating filter may be constructed out of lead sheets in the form of step wedge or machined from a solid piece of lead. They are designed to compensate to a desired depth. For compensator construction, see chapter on compensator. Because of their attenuation, the compensator factor must be measured and accounted in the treatment time or monitor unit calculation.

Example:

Daily tumor dose (DTD) = 100 cGy from each side of a parallel opposed field. ◆ Air dose rate (ADR) = 145.8 cGy/min & TAR = 0.717 ◆ Compensator factor (CF) = 0.895 ◆ Timer correction (TC) = +0.02 min

i) Anterior

$$Treatment \ time = \left(\frac{DTD}{(ADR) \times (TAR) \times (CF)} \right) + TC = \left(\frac{100}{145.8 \times 0.717 \times 0.895} \right) + 0.02 = 1.09 \ min$$

ii) Posterior

Since there is no compensator for the posterior field, the compensator factor is not used in the treatment time calculation.

$$Treatment \ time = \left(\frac{DTD}{(ADR) \times (TAR)} \right) + TC = \left(\frac{100}{145.8 \times 0.717} \right) + 0.02 = 0.98 \ min$$

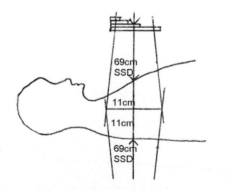

Figure 2.41 Set-up with retracted lead step compensator in place for anterior field.

D. Wax Compensating Filter

Wax compensator is sometimes used instead of lead compensator in some centers. Wax compensators may be made to adhere to the patient's shell (cast) or mounted on a tray retracted from the patient. If it is adhere to the patient's shell, the thickness of the wax is added to the depth in the calculation of treatment time or monitor unit setting. This is not a very good method of missing tissue compensation because skin sparing is lost.

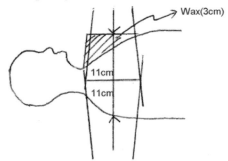

Figure 2.42 Set-up with wax compensator on patient's shell (cast).

i) Anterior

Daily tumor dose (DTD) = 100 cGy ♦ Air dose rate (ADR) = 145.8 cGy/min ♦ TAR (11+3 cm) = 0.620 ♦ Timer correction (TC) = +0.02 min

$$Treatment\ time = \left(\frac{DTD}{(ADR) \times (TAR)} \right) + TC = \left(\frac{100}{145.8 \times 0.620} \right) + 0.02 = 1.13\ \ min$$

ii) Posterior

Daily tumor dose (DTD) = 100 cGy ♦ Air dose rate (ADR) = 145.8 cGy/min ♦ TAR (11cm) = 0.717 ♦ Timer correction (TC) = +0.02 min

$$Treatment\ time = \left(\frac{DTD}{(ADR) \times (TAR)} \right) + TC = \left(\frac{100}{145.8 \times 0.717} \right) + 0.02 = 0.98\ \ min$$

If the wax compensator is mounted on a tray remote from the patient, a transmission factor through the compensator and the tray, is measured and is used in the timer or monitor unit calculation similar to that for the lead compensator.

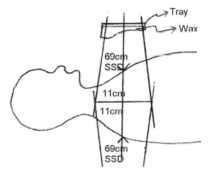

Figure 2.43 Set-up with retracted wax compensator.

E. Film Compensating Filter

This is sometimes used to compensate for uneven contours in the treatment of skin tumors. The film compensator is made up of strips of exposed x-ray film in a step fashion similar to the lead step compensator. The transmission factor is measured and is used in the treatment time calculation.

XXV. PROBLEMS

Problem 2.1

Calculate the equivalent square for a rectangular field measuring 10×18 cm^2.

$$Equivalent\ Square(Eq.Sq.) = 4 \times \left(\frac{A}{P}\right) = 4 \times \left(\frac{10 \times 18}{2(10 + 18)}\right) = 12.9\ cm^2$$

Problem 2.2

Calculate the penumbra if the source size is 2.5 cm, the SSD is 80 cm and the source diaphragm distance is 45 cm.

where SS = 2.5 cm , DSD = 80 -SDD = 80 - 45 = 35 cm, and SDD = 45 cm

$$Penumbra = \frac{Source\ size(SS) \times Diaphragm\ skin\ dist(DSD)}{Source\ diaphragm\ dist(SDD)} = \frac{2.5 \times 35}{45} = 1.9\ cm$$

Problem 2.3

What is the gap on the skin if two fields 25 cm and 22 cm long at 80 cm SSD are matched at cord depth at 5.5 cm?

$$First\ gap = \frac{(1/2)length \times depth}{SSD} = \left(\frac{12.5 \times 5.5}{80}\right) = 0.86\ cm \quad \& \quad Second\ gap = \frac{(1/2)length \times depth}{SSD} = \left(\frac{11 \times 5.5}{80}\right) = 0.76\ cm$$

Total gap = 0.86 + 0.76 = 1.62 cm

Problem 2.4

What is the TAR for a 10×13 cm^2 field size at 8.75 cm depth?

Assuming: $\rightarrow$ *TAR(d=8.5 cm, FS=11 cm^2)= 0.771, TAR(d=8.5 cm, FS=12 cm^2)= 0.781*

TAR(d=9.0 cm, FS=11 cm^2)= 0.753, TAR(d=9.0 cm, FS=12 cm^2)= 0.762

Eq.Sq for 10 × 13 cm^2 =11.3 cm^2

Therefore,

$$TAR(d = 8.5\ cm,\ FS = 11.3\ cm^2) = \left(\frac{0.781 - 0.771}{10}\right) \times 3 + 0.771 = 0.774$$

$$TAR(d = 9.0\ cm,\ FS = 11.3\ cm^2) = \left(\frac{0.762 - 0.753}{10}\right) \times 3 + 0.753 = 0.756$$

Resulting in,

$$TAR(d = 8.75\ cm,\ FS = 11.3\ cm^2) = \left(\frac{0.774 - 0.756}{2}\right) + 0.756 = 0.765$$

Problem 2.5

Calculate the %DD at 12 cm depth for 10×15 cm^2 field at 80 cm SSD (Cobalt-60) using TAR table.

$$\%DD = \left(\frac{SSD + D_{max}}{SSD + d}\right)^2 \times \left(\frac{TAR}{PSF}\right) \times 100$$

$Eq.Sq.(10 \times 15) = 12 \ cm^2 \ at \ 80 \ cm \ SSD$ & $Eq.Sq. \ at \ 12cm \ depth = \left(\frac{92}{80}\right) \times 12 = 13.8 \ cm^2$

$TAR(d = 12 \ cm, \ FS = 13.8 \ cm^2) = 0.673$ & $PSF(12 \ cm^2) = 1.041$

$Therefore \rightarrow \quad \%DD = \left(\frac{80 + 0.5}{80 + 12}\right)^2 \times \left(\frac{0.673}{1.041}\right) \times 100 = 49.5\%$

Problem 2.6

Calculate the TAR at 15 cm depth for 12×16 cm field at 80 cm SSD using %DD table.

$$TAR = \left(\frac{SSD + D}{SSD + D_{max}}\right)^2 \times \left(\frac{\%DD}{100}\right) \times PSF$$

$Eq.Sq (10 \times 15 \ cm^2) = 12 \ cm^2$

$From \ \%DD \ table, \ \%DD \ (12 \ cm^2, \ 12 \ cm \ depth) = 49.44\%, \ and \ PSF = 1.041$

$$TAR = \left(\frac{80 + 12}{80 + 0.5}\right)^2 \times \left(\frac{49.44}{100}\right) \times 1.041 = 0.672$$

Problem 2.7

What is the %DD at 14 cm depth if the field size is 15×15 cm^2 at 90 cm SSD (Cobalt-60).

$\%DD \ (15 \ cm^2, \ 14 \ cm \ depth \ at \ 80 \ cm \ SSD) = 44.8\%$

$Corrected \ \%DD \ at \ 90cm \ SSD = \left(\frac{80 + depth}{80 + D_{max}}\right)^2 \times \left(\frac{SSD + D_{max}}{DDS + depth}\right)^2 \times \%DD = \left(\frac{80 + 14}{80 + 0.5}\right)^2 \times \left(\frac{90 + 0.5}{90 + 14}\right)^2 \times 44.8 = 46.3\%$

Problem 2.8

If 4500 cGy is given to mid depth by parallel opposed fields to a patient with a separation of 18 cm, calculate the cord dose if the cord is 5.5 cm from the posterior surface. Field size is 12×16 cm^2 at 80 cm SSD on a Cobalt-60 unit.

$Tumor \ dose \ (TD) \ from \ each \ field = 2250 \ cGy$

$Eq.Sq \ for \ 12 \times 16 \ cm^2 = 13.7 \ cm^2$

$From \ anterior \ field, \ \%DD \ at \ 9 \ cm \ depth = 61.7\%$

$\%DD \ at \ cord \ depth \ of \ 12.5 \ cm \ (18 \ cm-5.5 \ cm) = 48.8\%$

$$Dose \ to \ cord \ from \ Anterior \ field = \left(\frac{\%DD \ cord}{\%DD \ depth}\right) \times TD = \left(\frac{48.8}{61.7}\right) \times 2250 = 1780 \ cGy$$

$\%DD \ at \ cord \ depth \ of \ 5.5 \ cm = 77.3\%$

$$Dose\ to\ cord\ from\ Posterior\ field = \left(\frac{\%DD\ cord}{\%DD\ depth}\right) \times TD = \left(\frac{77.3}{61.7}\right) \times 2250 = 2819\ cGy$$

Total cord dose = 1780 + 2819 = 4599 cGy

Problem 2.9

Repeat 2.8 if the field size is $12 \times 16\ cm^2$ at 80 cm SAD.

Eq.Sq. for $12 \times 16\ cm^2 = 13.7cm^2$ ♦ *TAR ($13.7\ cm^2$, 9 cm depth) = 0.777* ♦ *Distance to cord depth (AP) = 80 cm + 3.5 = 83.5 cm*

$$Field\ size\ at\ cord\ depth = \left(\frac{83.5}{80}\right) \times 13.7 = 14.3\ cm^2$$

TAR($14.3\ cm^2$, 12.5 cm depth) = 0.661

$$Dose\ to\ cord\ from\ Anterior\ field = \left(\frac{TAR(cord\ depth)}{TAR(depth)}\right) \times \left(\frac{SAD}{SSD + cord\ depth}\right)^2 \times TD = \left(\frac{0.661}{0.777}\right) \times \left(\frac{80}{83.5}\right)^2 \times 2250 = 1757\ cGy$$

Distance to cord depth (PA) = 80 - 3.5 = 76.5 cm

$$Field\ size\ at\ cord\ depth = \left(\frac{83.5}{80}\right) \times 13.7 = 14.3\ cm^2$$

TAR ($13.1\ cm^2$, 5.5 cm depth) = 0.903

$$Dose\ to\ cord\ from\ Posterior\ field = \left(\frac{TAR(cord\ depth)}{TAR(depth)}\right) \times \left(\frac{SAD}{SSD + cord\ depth}\right)^2 \times TD = \left(\frac{0.903}{0.777}\right) \times \left(\frac{80}{76.5}\right)^2 \times 2250 = 2860\ cGy$$

Total cord dose = 1757 + 2860 = 4617 cGy

Problem 2.10

If 4500 cGy in 20 treatments is prescribed to mid-depth for parallel-opposed fields and the field size is $10 \times 12\ cm^2$ at 80 cm SAD on a Cobalt-60 unit, calculate the treatment time if the timer correction is + 0.02 min and the patient's separation is 22 cm.

Total tumor dose (TTD) from each field = 2250 cGy in 20 treatments.

Field size at 80 cm SAD (mid depth) = $10 \times 12\ cm^2$, and Eq. Sq = $10.9\ cm^2$ ♦ *TAR ($10.9\ cm^2$, 11 cm depth) = 0.679* ♦ *Air dose rate (ADR) = 143.7 cGy/min* ♦ *Timer correction (TC) = +0.02 min*

$$Treatment\ time(each\ field) = \left(\frac{TTD}{\#\ of\ fract \times TAR \times ADR}\right) + TC = \left(\frac{2250}{20 \times 0.679 \times 143.7}\right) + 0.02 = 1.17\ min$$

Problem 2.11

Repeat 2.10 if field size is $10 \times 12\ cm^2$ at 80 cm SSD.

i) %DD method

%DD ($10.9\ cm^2$, 11 cm depth) = 52.27%

Total tumor dose (TTD) to each field = 2250 cGy in 20 treatments.

$$Total\ given\ dose(TGD)\ to\ each\ field = \left(\frac{TTD \times 100}{\%DD}\right) = \left(\frac{2250 \times 100}{52.27}\right) = 4305\ cGy$$

Tissue dose rate (TDR) for $10.9\ cm^2$ = 147.3 cGy/min

$$Treatment\ time(each\ field) = \left(\frac{TGD}{\#\ of\ fractions \times TDR}\right) + TC = \left(\frac{4305}{20 \times 147.3}\right) + 0.02 = 1.48\ min$$

ii) TAR method

$$\text{Field size at } 11cm \text{ depth} = \left(\frac{80+11}{80}\right) \times 10.9cm = 12.4 \ cm$$

TAR (12.4 cm², 11cm depth) = 0.694 ♦ *Air dose rate (10.9 cm²) = 143.7 cGy/min* ♦ *TTD to each field = 2250 cGy in 20 fractions*

where → $\quad ISF = \left(\dfrac{80}{91}\right)^2 = 0.773$

$$\text{Treatment time(each field)} = \left(\frac{TTD}{\# \text{ of frac} \times TAR \times ADR \times ISF}\right) + TC = \left(\frac{2250}{20 \times 0.694 \times 143.7 \times 0.773}\right) + 0.02 = 1.48 \ min$$

XXVI. TOTAL TUMOR DOSE(TTD)

This is the total dose prescription to the isocenter or to an isodose level that covers the target volume. If the prescribed dose is to an isodose level, the total tumor dose to isocenter must be calculated in order to calculate the treatment time or MU setting. This is necessary because the isocenter is normalized to 100% and data such as air dose rate(cGy/min), output factor(cGy/MU), TAR, TPR are measured at isocenter.

Example:

A patient is treated with three fields at gantry angles of 0°, 120°, and 240° using 10 × 15 cm² field size. The depths are 12 cm, 15 cm, and 14 cm respectively. The total tumor dose to all three fields are equal. Total tumor dose of 5000 cGy in 25 treatments is prescribed to the 95% isodose line. Calculate the MU setting to each field.

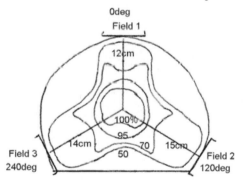

Figure 2.44 Three field plan (isocentric normalized to 100%).

Where,

TTD = 5000 cGy in 25 fractions to the 95% isodose line. Therefore, dose to isocenter (100%)= (100/95) × 5000 = 5263cGy, and Eq.Sq (10 × 15 cm²) = 12 cm² ♦ *Output factor (10 × 15 cm²) = 1.018 cGy/MU* ♦ *TMR (12 cm², 12 cm depth) = 0.736 , TMR (12 cm², 15 cm depth) = 0.658 , and TMR (12 cm², 14 cm depth) = 0.684*

$$\text{TTD to each field} = \left(\frac{5263}{3}\right) = 1754 \ cGy \qquad \& \qquad \text{DTD to each field} = \left(\frac{1754}{25}\right) = 70.2 \ cGy$$

$$\text{MUsetting(field}_1) = \left(\frac{70.2}{1.018 \times 0.736}\right) = 94 \ MU \quad \& \quad \text{MUsetting(field}_2) = \left(\frac{70.2}{1.018 \times 0.658}\right) = 105 \ MU$$

$$\& \quad \text{MUsetting(field}_3) = \left(\frac{70.2}{1.018 \times 0.684}\right) = 101 \ MU$$

XXVII. TOTAL GIVEN DOSE(TGD) OR APPLIED DOSE

This is the total dose to D_{max} that may be on the surface (100 kV SXR) or at the depth of maximum. Given dose is normally used to calculate treatment time or MU setting in SSD set-up.

Example:

A patient is treated with a single direct field using 10×10 cm^2 field size at 80 cm SSD on a Cobalt-60 unit. If a total tumor dose of 2000 cGy in 10 treatments is prescribed to a point 6cm depth, calculate the treatment time.

TTD at 6cm depth = 2000 cGy in 10 treatments.
DTD = 200 cGy
%DD (10×10 cm^2, 6 cm depth) = 73.2%

$$DGD = \left(\frac{100\%}{73.2}\right) \times 200 \;\; cGy = 273 \;\; cGy$$

TDR at 80cm SSD (10×10 cm^2) = 146.3 cGy/min
Timer correction (TC) = +0.02 min

$$Treatment \;\; time = \left(\frac{DGD}{TDR}\right) + TC = \left(\frac{273}{146}\right) + 0.02 = 1.89 \;\; min$$

Repeat the above on a Linear Accelerator unit (6 MV photon beam) at 100 cm SSD.

TTD at 6 cm depth = 2000 cGy in 10 treatments.
DTD = 200 cGy ◆ %DD (10×10 cm^2, 6 cm depth) = 82%

$$DGD = \left(\frac{100\%}{82}\right) \times 200 \;\; cGy = 244 \;\; cGy$$

Output Factor (OF) at 100 cm SSD, 10×10 cm^2 = 1 cGy/MU

$$MU \;\; Setting = \left(\frac{244}{1}\right) = 244 \;\; MU$$

XXVIII. SOURCE SKIN DISTANCE(SSD)

A. Normal SSD

SSD set-up is usually used for single direct field or on a non-isocentric treatment unit. Source skin distance is the distance from the source to the patient's skin. The normal SSD for 100 kV SXR unit is 20 cm, 250 kV DXR unit is 50 cm, Cobalt-60 unit is 80 cm and high energy linear accelerator unit is 100 cm. Collimator setting is calibrated to the field size at the normal SSD for the unit. For example, the Cobalt-60 unit collimator setting is calibrated to give the correct field size at 80 cm SSD. SSD greater than the normal SSD is sometimes necessary for field size larger than the largest field size available for the normal SSD. For example, if the largest field size on a Cobalt-60 unit is 35×35 cm^2 at 80 cm SSD and a field size of 38×38 cm^2 is required, the extended SSD is $38/35 \times 80 = 86.9$ cm^2. If the SSD is retracted or extended from the normal SSD, the field size will be different from the collimator setting. Under these circumstances, the new collimator setting must be used for the output factor and corrected for the new SSD.

Example:

i) The field size required at 90 cm SSD is 8×38 cm^2

The collimator setting to obtain 8×38 cm^2 at 90 cm SSD $= \left(\frac{80}{90}\right) \times (8 \times 38) = 7.1 \times 33.8 \;\; cm^2 = 10.7 \;\; cm^2$

The output factor (TDR) for 10.7 cm^2 at 80 cm SSD = 147.1 cGy/min.

$$Corrected \ TDR \ to \ 90 \ cm \ SSD = \left(\frac{80.5}{90.5}\right)^2 \times 147.1 = 116.4 \ cGy / min$$

(Note: TDR is at 80 + 0.5 cm in phantom)

<u>*ii) The field required at 70 cm SSD is 4 × 8 cm²*</u>

$$The \ collimator \ setting \ to \ obtain \ 4 \times 8 \ cm^2 at \ 70cm \ SSD = \left(\frac{80}{70}\right) \times (4 \times 8) = 4.6 \times 9.1 \ cm^2$$

→ *Eq. Sq. for 4.6 × 9.1 cm^2 = 6.2 cm^2*

TDR for 6.2 cm^2 at 80 cm SSD = 141.9 cGy/min

$$Corrected \ TDR \ to \ 70cm \ SSD = \left(\frac{80.5}{70.5}\right)^2 \times 141.9 = 185 \ cGy / min$$

B. Advantages and Disadvantages of SSD Set-Up

i) Advantages

The advantages are: 1) large fields may be used for extended SSD; 2) treatment unit need not be isocentric; and 3) patient is further away from the collimator thus reducing the scattered radiation reaching the patient. *(In some SAD (80 cm) set-up, the patient may be too close to the collimator especially if the patient is large.)*

ii) Disadvantages

The disadvantages are: 1) in multifield SSD set-up aligning the entrance and exit point is cumbersome compared to SAD isocentric technique; and 2) any change in field depth is more difficult to spot compared to SAD set-up.

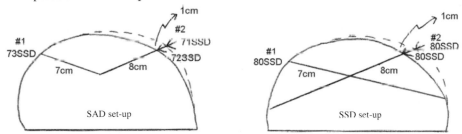

Figure 2.45 SAD and SSD set-up showing depth change for field 2. In the SAD set-up, depth for field 2 changed from 8 cm to 9 cm. The SSD reading changed from 72 cm to 71 cm. In the SSD set-up, depth for field 2 changed from 8 cm to 9 cm but the SSD reading remains at 80 cm.

C. Calculation Using SSD

i) Equal Given Dose

The given dose may be calculated if the tumor dose is known by working back from the percentage depth dose.

Example:

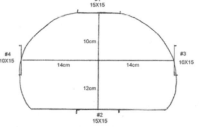

Figure 2.46 Four field box technique on Cobalt-60 at 80 cm SSD.

If TTD of 5000 cGy in 25 treatments is prescribed to x, calculate the (DGD) to each field and the treatment time. Timer correction (TC) = +0.02 min.

Solution:

The %DD for field$_1$ = 58.4%, for field$_2$ = 51.2%, for field$_3$ = 43.0%, and for field$_4$ = 43.0%

Total %DD at x = 195.6% = 5000 cGy. Since the given doses are equal and is equal to 100%, therefore;

$$The\ DGD\ to\ each\ field = \left(\frac{GD\ weight}{Total\%DD\ \times\ \#\ fractions} \right) \times TTD = \left(\frac{100\%}{195.6\%\ \times\ 25} \right) \times 5000 = 102.2\ \ cGy$$

TDR for 15 × 15 cm^2 at 80 cm SSD = 151.1 cGy/min.

$$Treatment\ time(field_1) = \left(\frac{102.2}{151.1} \right) + 0.02 = 0.70\ \ min$$

Treatment time for field 2 is the same as for field$_1$.

$$Treatment\ time(field_3) = \left(\frac{102.2}{148.4} \right) + 0.02 = 0.71\ \ min$$

TDR for 10 × 15 cm^2 at 80 cm SSD = 148.4 cGy/min.

Treatment time for field$_4$ is the same as for field$_3$.

ii) Unequal Given Dose

Using the same data from (i), calculate the DGD and timer setting to each field if the weighting of given dose to field$_1$ is 100%, field$_2$ is 90% and field$_3$ and field$_4$ are 80% each.

Solution:

The %DD for field$_1$ = 58.4% × 1.0 = 58.4%

The %DD for field$_2$ = 51.2% × 0.9 = 46.1%

The %DD for field$_3$ = 43.0% × 0.8 = 34.4%

The %DD for field$_4$ = 43.0% × 0.8 = 34.4%

Total corrected %DD at x = 173.3% = 5000 cGy

$$The\ DGD\ to\ each\ field = \left(\frac{GD\ weight}{Total\%DD\ \times\ \#\ fractions} \right) \times TTD$$

$$DGD(field_1) = \left(\frac{100\%}{173.3\%\ \times\ 25} \right) \times 5000 = 115.4\ \ cGy \quad \& \quad DGD(field_2) = \left(\frac{90}{173.3\%\ \times\ 25} \right) \times 5000 = 103.9\ \ cGy$$

$$DGD(field_3) = \left(\frac{80}{173.3\%\ \times\ 25} \right) \times 5000 = 92.3\ \ cGy$$

DGD to field$_4$ is the same as field$_3$.

TDR for 15 × 15 cm^2 at 80 cm SSD = 151.1 cGy/min.

$$Treatment\ time(field_1) = \left(\frac{115.4}{151.1} \right) + 0.02 = 0.78\ \ min \quad \& \quad Treatment\ time(field_2) = \left(\frac{103.9}{151.1} \right) + 0.02 = 0.71\ \ min$$

TDR for 10 × 15 cm^2 at 80 cm SSD = 148.4 cGy/min

$$Treatment\ time(field_3) = \left(\frac{92.3}{148.4} \right) + 0.02 = 0.64\ \ min$$

Treatment time for field$_4$ is the same as field$_3$.

iii) Equal Tumor Dose

Using the same data from (i), calculate the DGD and treatment time to each field if the TTD to each field are equal.

Solution:

Since the TTD are equal, the TTD to each field = (5000/4) = 1250 cGy

$$DGD \ to \ each \ field = \left(\frac{TTD \ each \ field}{\# \ fractions} \right) \times \left(\frac{weight \ GD}{\% DD} \right)$$

$\%DD$ for field$_1$ = 58.4%   → $DGD \ to \ field_1 = \left(\dfrac{1250}{25} \right) \times \left(\dfrac{100}{58.4} \right) = 85.6 \ \ cGy$

$\%DD$ for field$_2$ = 51.2%   → $DGD \ to \ field_2 = \left(\dfrac{1250}{25} \right) \times \left(\dfrac{100}{51.2} \right) = 97.7 \ \ cGy$

$\%DD$ for field$_3$ = 43.0%   → $DGD \ to \ field_3 = \left(\dfrac{1250}{25} \right) \times \left(\dfrac{100}{43} \right) = 116.3 \ \ cGy$

DGD to field$_4$ is the same as field$_3$

TDR for $15 \times 15 \ cm^2$ at 80 cm SSD = 151.1 cGy/min

$Treatment \ time(field_1) = \left(\dfrac{85.6}{151.1} \right) + 0.02 = 0.59 \ \ min$ & $Treatment \ time(field_2) = \left(\dfrac{97.7}{151.1} \right) + 0.02 = 0.67 \ \ min$

TDR for $10 \times 15 \ cm^2$ at 80 cm SSD = 148.4 cGy/min

$Treatment \ time(field_3) = \left(\dfrac{116.3}{148.4} \right) + 0.02 = 0.80 \ \ min$

Treatment time for field$_4$ is the same as for field$_3$.

iv) Unequal Tumor Dose

Using the same data from (i), calculate the DGD and treatment time to each field if the weighting of tumor dose to field$_1$ is 100%, field$_2$ is 90%, and fields 3 and 4 are 80% each.

Solution:

The total weight at $x = 100 + 90 + 80 + 80 = 350\%$, and TTD at $x = 5000$ cGy

$\%DD$ for field$_1$ = 58.4, $\%DD$ for field$_2$ = 51.2% , and $\%DD$ for field$_3$ = 43.0%.

$$TTD \ to \ each \ field = \left(\frac{weight \ of \ field}{total \ weight} \right) \times TTD$$

$TTD(field_1) = \left(\dfrac{100}{350} \right) \times 5000 = 1428.6 \ \ cGy$ & $TTD(field_2) = \left(\dfrac{90}{350} \right) \times 5000 = 1285.7 \ \ cGy$

$TTD(field_3) = \left(\dfrac{80}{350} \right) \times 5000 = 1142.9 \ \ cGy$

TTD to field$_4$ is the same as for field$_3$.

$$DGD \ to \ each \ field = \left(\frac{TTD \ each \ field}{\# \ fractions} \right) \times \left(\frac{weight \ GD}{\% DD} \right)$$

$DGD(field_1) = \left(\dfrac{1428.6}{25} \right) \times \left(\dfrac{100}{58.4} \right) = 97.8 \ \ cGy$ & $TTD(field_2) = \left(\dfrac{1285.7}{25} \right) \times \left(\dfrac{100}{51.2} \right) = 100.4 \ \ cGy$

$DGD(field_3) = \left(\dfrac{1142.9}{25} \right) \times \left(\dfrac{100}{43} \right) = 106.3 \ \ cGy$

Table 2.13 Table of radii distances and their SAR values for center.

Sector	Radii	SAR	Sector	Radii	SAR
1	5.6	0.169	19	5.7	0.17
2	5.8	0.172	20	5.9	0.174
3	6.2	0.18	21	6.2	0.18
4	6.8	0.192	22	6.9	0.194
5	7.9	0.213	23	8	0.215
6	6.9	0.194	24	6.8	0.192
7	6.2	0.18	25	6.2	0.18
8	5.8	0.172	26	5.8	0.172
9	5.7	0.17	27	5.6	0.168
10	5.7	0.17	28	5.6	0.168
11	5.8	0.172	29	5.8	0.172
12	6.2	0.18	30	6.2	0.18
13	6.8	0.192	31	6.8	0.192
14	7.9	0.192	32	7.8	0.211
15	6.9	0.194	33	6.8	0.192
16	6.2	0.18	34	6.1	0.178
17	5.9	0.174	35	5.8	0.172
18	5.2	0.16	36	5.6	0.168

Average SAR = (6.534/36) = 0.182

TAR at zero field size at 10 cm depth = 0.534

TAR = TAR (zero) +SAR = 0.534 + 0.182 = 0.716

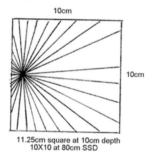

11.25cm square at 10cm depth
10X10 at 80cm SSD

Figure 2.51 Radii at 10° interval to measure distance from off-axis to field edge.

Table 2.14 Table of radii distances and their SAR values for off-axis.

Sector	Radii	SAR	Sector	Radii	SAR
1	5.5	0.176	19	5.7	0.184
2	5.7	0.184	20	4.2	0.14
3	6.1	0.178	21	2.6	0.098
4	6.7	0.19	22	1.9	0.079
5	7.8	0.211	23	1.5	0.069
6	9.6	0.234	24	1.3	0.063
7	11.2	0.252	25	1.2	0.06
8	10.5	0.245	26	1.1	0.058
9	10.2	0.241	27	1.1	0.058
10	10.2	0.241	28	1.1	0.058
11	10.4	0.243	29	1.1	0.058
12	11.2	0.252	30	1.2	0.06

13	9.9	0.238	31	1.3	0.063
14	8	0.215	32	1.5	0.069
15	7	0.195	33	1.9	0.079
16	6.3	0.182	34	2.6	0.098
17	5.9	0.192	35	4.2	0.14
18	5.7	0.184	36	5.5	0.176

Average SAR = (5.463/36) = 0.152

TAR (zero field) at 10 cm depth = 0.534

TAR = 0.534 + 0.152 = 0.686

4000 cGy is given to the center.

The off-axis point receives = (0.686/0716) = 3832 cGy

Table 2.15 Table of TAR zero field size for ^{60}Co.

Depth	TAR	Depth	TAR	Depth	TAR
0	0.377	10	0.534	20	0.277
0.5	1	10.5	0.518	20.5	0.27
1	0.965	11	0.501	21	0.262
1.5	0.935	11.5	0.484	21.5	0.254
2	0.904	12	0.469	22	0.246
2.5	0.875	12.5	0.454	22.5	0.239
3	0.845	13	0.439	23	0.23
3.5	0.819	13.5	0.426	23.5	0.222
4	0.792	14	0.412	24	0.214
4.5	0.767	14.5	0.398	24.5	0.207
5	0.742	15	0.388	25	0.2
5.5	0.718	15.5	0.373	25.5	0.193
6	0.693	16	0.36	26	0.187
6.5	0.672	16.5	0.349	26.5	0.182
7	0.649	17	0.338	27	0.176
7.5	0.629	17.5	0.327	27.5	0.17
8	0.607	18	0.316	28	0.164
8.5	0.589	18.5	0.308	28.5	0.158
9	0.569	19	0.297	29	0.153
9.5	0.552	19.5	0.286	29.5	0.148

Table 2.16 Table of SAR for ^{60}Co.

	Radii(cm)										
	2	4	8	12	16	20	24	28	32	36	40
Depth(cm)											
0	0.004	0.004	0.018	0.035	0.047	0.052	0.053	0.059	0.056	0.056	0.055
1	0.026	0.048	0.078	0.098	0.109	0.118	0.122	0.123	0.123	0.123	0.125
2	0.05	0.08	0.116	0.139	0.152	0.16	0.166	0.168	0.168	0.166	0.167
3	0.07	0.103	0.147	0.172	0.187	0.198	0.204	0.179	0.203	0.205	0.203
4	0.081	0.121	0.17	0.197	0.215	0.228	0.237	0.239	0.239	0.241	0.24
5	0.085	0.134	0.189	0.218	0.24	0.255	0.264	0.266	0.268	0.269	0.27
6	0.089	0.141	0.201	0.234	0.257	0.272	0.282	0.185	0.286	0.288	0.288

7	0.09	0.142	0.209	0.246	0.273	0.29	0.302	0.306	0.308	0.309	0.313
8	0.089	0.142	0.214	0.254	0.285	0.301	0.313	0.317	0.322	0.326	0.328
9	0.086	0.14	0.216	0.26	0.292	0.312	0.324	0.329	0.334	0.337	0.339
10	0.082	0.136	0.215	0.262	0.295	0.318	0.333	0.338	0.343	0.345	0.353
11	0.076	0.132	0.213	0.262	0.296	0.322	0.337	0.343	0.345	0.349	0.355
12	0.074	0.128	0.21	0.261	0.297	0.323	0.34	0.344	0.348	0.353	0.356
13	0.07	0.124	0.207	0.26	0.298	0.325	0.341	0.345	0.353	0.355	0.356
14	0.066	0.12	0.204	0.258	0.297	0.326	0.344	0.352	0.355	0.361	0.369
15	0.062	0.116	0.2	0.255	0.295	0.325	0.344	0.352	0.355	0.361	0.369
16	0.06	0.112	0.196	0.252	0.292	0.322	0.341	0.349	0.355	0.36	0.369
17	0.058	0.108	0.191	0.248	0.288	0.318	0.338	0.343	0.352	0.359	0.364
18	0.056	0.104	0.186	0.244	0.284	0.313	0.334	0.342	0.352	0.359	0.369
19	0.053	0.101	0.181	0.239	0.28	0.309	0.33	0.341	0.35	0.356	0.366
20	0.049	0.097	0.176	0.234	0.275	0.305	0.325	0.334	0.344	0.348	0.356

viii) Extended SSD

Calculation method is basically the same as normal SSD except the %DD is corrected for the extended SSD because %DD increases with increase SSD. As a result, the given dose is reduced to give the same tumor dose but the treatment time is increased due to the reduction in dose rate with increased distance. Using the data from (i), calculate the daily given dose (DGD) and the timer setting to each field if the SSD is increased to 100 cm.

Solution:

a) Field$_1$ $\rightarrow$ *%DD(15 × 15 cm^2, 10 cm) = 58.4%*

$$Corrected\ \%DD\ at\ 100\ cm\ SSD = \left(\frac{SSD + D_{max}}{SSD + d}\right)^2 \times \left(\frac{80 + d}{80 + D_{max}}\right)^2 \times 58.4\% = \left(\frac{100 + 0.5}{100 + 10}\right)^2 \times \left(\frac{80 + 10}{80 + 0.5}\right)^2 \times 58.4\% = 60.9\%$$

b) Field$_2$ $\rightarrow$ *%DD (15 × 15 cm^2, 12 cm) = 51.2%*

$$Corrected\ \%DD\ at\ 100\ cm\ SSD = \left(\frac{SSD + D_{max}}{SSD + d}\right)^2 \times \left(\frac{80 + d}{80 + D_{max}}\right)^2 \times 51.2\% = \left(\frac{100 + 0.5}{100 + 12}\right)^2 \times \left(\frac{80 + 12}{80 + 0.5}\right)^2 \times 51.2\% = 53.8\%$$

c) Field$_3$ and Field$_4$ $\rightarrow$ *%DD (10 × 15, 14cm) = 43.0%*

$$Corrected\ \%DD\ at\ 100\ cm\ SSD = \left(\frac{SSD + D_{max}}{SSD + d}\right)^2 \times \left(\frac{80 + d}{80 + D_{max}}\right)^2 \times 43\% = \left(\frac{100 + 0.5}{100 + 14}\right)^2 \times \left(\frac{80 + 14}{80 + 0.5}\right)^2 \times 43\% = 45.6\%$$

Total %DD at x = 60.9 + 53.8 + 45.6 + 45.6 = 205.9%.

Total tumor dose at x = 5000 cGy to 205.9%.

Since the GD are equal, therefore $\rightarrow$ *The DGD to each field = (100 × 5000)/(205.9 × 25) = 97 cGy*

Field size for fields 1 and 2 is 15 × 15 cm^2 at 100 cm SSD $\rightarrow$ *The collimator setting = (80/100) × 15 cm^2 = 12 cm^2.*

The TDR for 12 cm^2 at 80 cm SSD = 148.4 cGy/min

$$Corrected\ TDR\ to\ 100\ cm\ SSD = \left(\frac{80.5}{100.5}\right)^2 \times 148.4 \times \left(\frac{PSF(d)}{PSF(D_{max})}\right) = \left(\frac{80.5}{100.5}\right)^2 \times 148.4 \times \left(\frac{1.049}{1.042}\right) = 95.9\ cGy\ /\ min$$

where PSF = 1.041 for 12 × 12 cm^2 and PSF = 1.049 for 15 × 15 cm^2.

$$Treatment\ time(field_1\ \&\ field_2) = \left(\frac{DGD}{TDR}\right) + TC = \left(\frac{97}{95.9}\right) + 0.02 = 1.03\ min$$

The field size for fields 3 and 4 is 10×15 cm^2, therefore $\rightarrow$ *Eq.Sq for 10×15 cm^2 at 100 cm SSD = 12 cm^2*

The collimator setting = $(80/100) \times 12$ cm^2 = 9.6 cm^2 & TDR for 9.6 cm^2 at 80 cm SSD = 145.9 cGy/min.

$$\textit{Corrected TDR to } 100cm \text{ } SSD = \left(\frac{80.5}{100.5}\right)^2 \times 145.9 \times \left(\frac{PSF(d)}{PSF(D_{max})}\right) = \left(\frac{80.5}{100.5}\right)^2 \times 145.9 \times \left(\frac{1.041}{1.034}\right) = 94.2 \text{ } cGy \text{ / min}$$

where PSF = 1.034 for 9.6 cm^2 and = PSF = 1.041 for 12 cm^2.

Treatment time (fields 3,4) = (97/94.2) + 0.02 = 1.05 min.

XXIX. SOURCE AXIS DISTANCE (SAD)

A. Normal SAD

Source axis distance is the distance from the source to the axis of the beam (axis of rotation or isocenter of the beam). Therefore, SAD set-up is used only if the treatment unit is an isocentric unit. The normal SAD for Cobalt-60 unit is 80 cm and for high energy linear accelerator it is 100 cm. Collimator setting and output factors are calibrated to the field size at the normal SAD for the unit.

B. Advantages and Disadvantages of SAD Set-Up

i) Advantages
The advantages of SAD set-up are: 1) ease of treatment set-up, once a set-up depth for the fields is determined and set, the other fields are set just by changing the gantry angle and field size, (See section on isocenter.); 2) ability to treat rotational field; and 3) separation change during the course of treatment is easy to spot.

ii) Disadvantages
The disadvantages of SAD set-up are: 1) only isocentric unit may use SAD set-up; 2) fields may not be large enough at the normal SAD set-up; and 3) in some short SAD (80 cm) set-up, the patient may be too close to the collimator especially if the patient is large.

C. Calculation Using SAD

i) Equal Given Dose
The given dose may be calculated if the tumor dose is given by working back from corrected %DD or TAR.

Example:

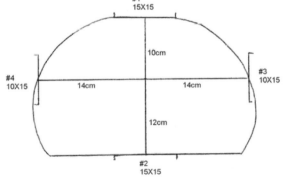

Figure 2.52 Four field box technique on Cobalt-60 at 80 cm SAD.

If total tumor dose of 5000 cGy in 25 treatments is prescribed to isocenter x, calculate the daily given dose to each field and the treatment time. Timer correction = +0.02 min.

Calculation:

$$\%DD \ and \ TAR \ are \ related \ by = \left(\frac{SSD + D_{max}}{SAD}\right)^2 \times \left(\frac{TAR(d)}{PSF}\right) \times GD \ weight$$

$$Field_1 \%DD = \left(\frac{70 + 0.5}{80}\right)^2 \times \left(\frac{0.752}{1.045}\right) \times 100 = 55.9\% \quad \& \quad Field_2 \%DD = \left(\frac{68 + 0.5}{80}\right)^2 \times \left(\frac{0.684}{1.043}\right) \times 100 = 48.1\%$$

$$Field_3 \%DD = \left(\frac{66 + 0.5}{80}\right)^2 \times \left(\frac{0.591}{1.035}\right) \times 100 = 39.5\% \quad \& \quad Field_4 \%DD = 39.5\%$$

Total %DD at isocenter = 183.0% = 5000 cGy.

Note: TAR (d) = TAR at depth for the field size at depth.

PSF (D_{max}) is for the field size at D_{max}.

$$Since \ the \ GD \ are \ equal \ to \ 100\%, \ the \ DGD \ to \ each \ field = \left(\frac{GD \ weight}{Total\%DD}\right) \times \left(\frac{TTD}{\# \ fractions}\right) = \left(\frac{100}{183}\right) \times \left(\frac{5000}{25}\right) = 109.3 \ cGy$$

Field_1 DTD = (55.9/183) × 200 = 61 cGy

$$Treatment \ time = \left(\frac{DTD}{ADR \times TAR}\right) + TC = \left(\frac{61}{145.8 \times 0.752}\right) + 0.02 = 0.58 \ min$$

Field_2 DTD = (48/183) × 200 = 52 cGy

$$Treatment \ time = \left(\frac{DTD}{ADR \times TAR}\right) + TC = \left(\frac{52}{145.8 \times 0.684}\right) + 0.02 = 0.54 \ min$$

Field_3 DTD = (39.5/183) × 200 = 43 cGy

$$Treatment \ time = \left(\frac{DTD}{ADR \times TAR}\right) + TC = \left(\frac{43}{144.3 \times 0.591}\right) + 0.02 = 0.53 \ min$$

Field_4 DTD = 43 cGy

Treatment time for field_4 is the same as for field_3.

ii) Unequal Given Dose

Using the same data from (i), calculate the DGD and timer setting to each field if the weighting of given dose to field_1 is 100%, field_2 is 90% and fields 3 and 4 are 80% each.

Calculation:

$$Field_1 \%DD = \left(\frac{70 + 0.5}{80}\right)^2 \times \left(\frac{0.752}{1.045}\right) \times 100 = 55.9\% \quad \& \quad Field_2 \%DD = \left(\frac{68 + 0.5}{80}\right)^2 \times \left(\frac{0.684}{1.043}\right) \times 90 = 43.3\%$$

$$Field_3 \%DD = \left(\frac{66 + 0.5}{80}\right)^2 \times \left(\frac{0.591}{1.035}\right) \times 80 = 31.6\% \quad \& \quad Field_4 \%DD = 36.1\%$$

Total %DD at isocenter = 162.4%

$$DGD \ to \ each \ field = \left(\frac{GD \ weight}{Total\%DD}\right) \times \left(\frac{TTD}{\# \ fractions}\right)$$

Applying the DGD equation, one could obtain;

$$DGD \ to \ field_1 = \left(\frac{100}{162.4}\right) \times \left(\frac{5000}{25}\right) = 123.2 \ cGy \qquad \& \qquad DGD \ to \ field_2 = \left(\frac{90}{162.4}\right) \times \left(\frac{5000}{25}\right) = 110.8 \ cGy$$

$$DGD \ to \ field_3 = \left(\frac{80}{162.4}\right) \times \left(\frac{5000}{25}\right) = 98.5 \ cGy \qquad \& \qquad DGD \ to \ each \ field_4 = 98.5$$

Field₁ DTD = (55.9/162.4) × 200 = 68.8 cGy

$$Treatment \ time = \left(\frac{DTD}{ADR \times TAR}\right) + TC = \left(\frac{68.8}{145.8 \times 0.752}\right) + 0.02 = 0.65 \ min$$

Field₂ DTD = (43.3/162.4) × 200 = 53.3 cGy

$$Treatment \ time = \left(\frac{DTD}{ADR \times TAR}\right) + TC = \left(\frac{53.3}{145.8 \times 0.684}\right) + 0.02 = 0.55 \ min$$

Field₃ DTD = (31.6/162.4) × 200 = 38.9 cGy

$$Treatment \ time = \left(\frac{DTD}{ADR \times TAR}\right) + TC = \left(\frac{38.9}{144.3 \times 0.591}\right) + 0.02 = 0.48 \ min$$

Field₄ DTD = 38.9 cGy
Treatment time = 0.48 min

iii) Equal Tumor Dose

Using the same data from (i), calculate the DGD and treatment time to each field if the TTD to each field are equal.

Calculation:

Since the TTD are equal, the TTD to each field = (5000/4) = 1250 cGy.

$$DGD \ to \ each \ field = \left(\frac{GD \ weight}{\%DD \ at \ isocenter}\right) \times \left(\frac{TTD \ to \ each \ field}{\# \ fractions}\right)$$

Field₁ DGD = (100/55.9) × (1250/25) = 89.4 cGy

$$Treatment \ time = \left(\frac{DTD}{ADR \times TAR}\right) + TC = \left(\frac{50}{145.8 \times 0.752}\right) + 0.02 = 0.48 \ min$$

Field₂ DGD = (100/48.1) × (1250/25) = 104.0 cGy

$$Treatment \ time = \left(\frac{DTD}{ADR \times TAR}\right) + TC = \left(\frac{50}{145.8 \times 0.684}\right) + 0.02 = 0.52 \ min$$

Field₃ DGD = (100/39.5) × (1250/25) = 126.6 cGy

$$Treatment \ time = \left(\frac{DTD}{ADR \times TAR}\right) + TC = \left(\frac{50}{144.3 \times 0.591}\right) + 0.02 = 0.61 \ min$$

Field₄ DGD = 126.6 cGy.
Treatment time = 0.61 min.

iv) Unequal Tumor Dose

Using the same data from (i), calculate the DGD and treatment time to each field if the weighting of tumor dose to field₁ is 100%, field₂ is 90% and fields 3 and 4 are 80% each.

Calculation:

The total weight at x = 100 + 90 + 80 + 80 = 350%

TTD at x = 5000 cGy

Field₁ TTD = (100/350) × 5000 = 1428.6 cGy

$$Treatment\ time = \left(\frac{DTD}{ADR \times TAR}\right) + TC = \left(\frac{57.1}{145.8 \times 0.752}\right) + 0.02 = 0.54\ \ min$$

Field₂ TTD = (90/350) × 5000 = 1285.7 cGy

$$Treatment\ time = \left(\frac{DTD}{ADR \times TAR}\right) + TC = \left(\frac{51.4}{145.8 \times 0.684}\right) + 0.02 = 0.54\ \ min$$

Field₃ TTD = (80/350) × 5000 = 1142.9 cGy

$$Treatment\ time = \left(\frac{DTD}{ADR \times TAR}\right) + TC = \left(\frac{45.7}{144.3 \times 0.591}\right) + 0.02 = 0.56\ \ min$$

Field₄ TTD = 1142.9 cGy

Treatment time = 0.56 min

$$DGD\ to\ each\ field = \left(\frac{GD\ weight}{\%DD\ at\ isocenter}\right) \times \left(\frac{TTD}{\#\ fractions}\right)$$

Therefore,

Field₁ DTD = (100/55.9) × (1428.6/25) = 102.2 cGy

Field₂ DTD = (100/48.1) × (1285.7/25) = 106.9 cGy

Field₃ DTD = (100/39.5) × (1142.96/25) = 115.7 cGy

DGD to field₄ = 115.7cGy.

v) Cord Dose

Cord dose is calculated by multiplying the tumor dose by the ratio of the TAR at cord to the TAR at isocenter and corrected by inverse square.

Example:

A patient is treated with a pair of parallel-opposed 15 × 15 cm² fields at 80 cm SAD. The anterior depth to isocenter is 10 cm and posterior depth is 12 cm. The cord is situated at 6cm from the posterior surface. Calculate the cord dose if the total tumor dose is 4000 cGy at isocenter (Equal tumor dose.)

Calculation:

The tumor doses are equal for anterior and posterior fields.

The TTD to each field = 2000 cGy.

$$Cord\ dose = \left(\frac{TAR(cord)}{TAR(isocenter)}\right) \times \left(\frac{80}{SSD + cord\ depth}\right)^2 \times TTD(eachfield)$$

$$AP\ field\ size\ at\ cord = \left(\frac{80 + 6}{80}\right) \times 15\ \ cm^2 = 16.1\ \ cm^2$$

TAR (16.1 cm², 16 cm depth) = 0.571

$$PA\ field\ size\ at\ cord = \left(\frac{80 - 6}{80}\right) \times 15\ \ cm^2 = 13.9\ \ cm^2$$

TAR (13.9cm², 6cm depth) = 0.889

Field size at isocenter = 15 cm²

TAR (15 cm², 10 cm depth) – 0.752 & TAR (15 cm², 12 cm depth) = 0.684

$$AP\,cord\,\,dose = \left(\frac{0.571}{0.752}\right) \times \left(\frac{80}{70+16}\right)^2 \times 2000 = 1314 \,\,\,cGy$$

$$PA\,cord\,\,dose = \left(\frac{0.889}{0.684}\right) \times \left(\frac{80}{68+6}\right)^2 \times 2000 = 3038 \,\,\,cGy$$

Therefore, cord dose = 1314 + 3038 = 4352 cGy.

vi) Cord Dose From Multifield SAD Plan

Cord dose from multifield plan may be obtained from the plan by multiplying the prescribed dose by the ratio of the cord isodose line to the prescribed isodose line.

Example:

If 4000 cGy is prescribed to 95% isodose, the cord receives (40/95)× 4000= 1684 cGy.

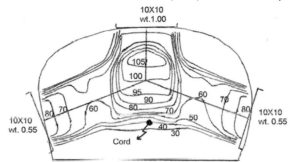

Figure 2.53 Three field 80 cm SAD plan with unequal weights at isocenter. (Normalized to 100% at isocenter)

vii) Dose to Off-Axis

1. Beam profile method

The same procedure applies here as for the SSD set-up except the beam profile is at SAD at the appropriate depth.

2. Isodose chart method

Same procedure as for 80 cm SSD set-up except SAD isodose is used.

3. TAR method

Same procedure as for 80 cm SSD set-up except the field is 10 × 10 cm² at 10 cm depth whereas for the SSD set-up, the field size is 10 × 10 cm² at 80 cm SSD and therefore at 10 cm depth it is 11.25 × 11.25 cm².

XXX. ARC AND ROTATION THERAPY

In arc or rotation therapy, the gantry of the treatment unit rotates around the isocenter a constant set speed. The subscribed arc angle is predetermined.

The choice of arc angle is dependent on the position of the tumor in the patient and position of the support bar of the treatment couch. Attenuation measurement of the support bar must be done if the beam traverses the bar. This must be taken into account in the dose distribution.

Arc or rotation therapy is a good technique to use if the target volume is small and is centrally located in the patient. For large target volume, the integral dose may be too high and coverage of the target volume may not be optimal due to the shape of the volume.

A. Dose Distribution for ARC and Rotation Therapy

Dose distribution for 120°, 240°, 300°, and 360° are shown in Figure 2.54. The hot spot of 130% for the 120° arc open field can be decreased by using 30° wedge for each half of the 120° arc as shown in Figure 2.54(b).

Due to the target volume not being centrally located within the patient for the 240° arc rotation, the dose coverage for the target is asymmetrical. To overcome this, the isocenter is dropped posteriorly from the reference center of the target volume as shown in Figure 2.54 (d). The dose coverage around the target volume is improved. This is sometimes referred to as pass pointing.

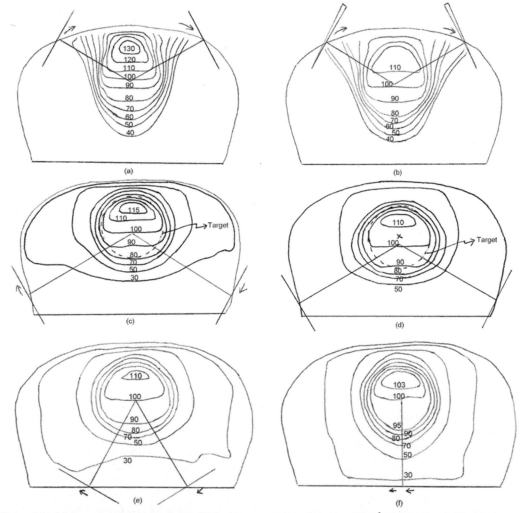

Figure 2.54 **(a)** *Dose distribution for Cobalt-60 for 120° arc (300° to 60°) 10 × 10 cm² at 80 cm SAD.* **(b)** *120° arc with 30° wedge (300° to 60°) 10 ×10 cm² at 80 cm SAD.* **(c)** *240° arc (240°to 120°) 10 × 10 cm² at 80 cm SAD.* **(d)** *240° arc (240° to 120°.) 10 × 10 cm² at 80 cm SAD. The isocenter is dropped posteriorly from the target center to give a better coverage around the target.* **(e)** *300° arc (210° to 150°) 10 × 10 cm² at 80 cm SAD.* **(f)** *360° rotation therapy (180° to 180°) 10 × 10 cm² at 80 cm SAD.*

B. Calculation for 300° ARC Therapy

Referring to Figure 2.54(e) for the 300° arc therapy, calculate the timer and speed setting if 4000 cGy in 20 treatments is prescribed to the 90% isodose line. Timer correction = + 0.02 min.

$DTD = TTD/(\# fractions) = 4000/20 = 200$ cGy to 90% isodose line

DTD to isocenter (100%) = (100/90) × 200 = 222 cGy

$$Treatment\ time = \left(\frac{DTD}{ADR \times TAR(average)} \right) + TC$$

Table 2.17 Table of TAR at 20° Interval.

Gantry	depth	TAR
210	14	0.568/2
230	18.5	0.442
250	18	0.455
270	17	0.481
290	15	0.538
310	11	0.669
330	9	0.742
350	8	0.78
10	8	0.78
30	7	0.742
50	11	0.669
70	14	0.568
90	17	0.481
110	17.5	0.468
130	19	0.43
150	14	0.568/2

Total TAR = 8.813

Averaged TAR = (8.813/15) = 0.588

Note: The TAR for 210° and 150° are halved because at the start and finish of the arc rotation, only half the beam is in treatment.

Therefore treatment time is:

$$Treatment\ time = \left(\frac{DTD}{ADR \times TAR(average)} \right) + TC = \left(\frac{222}{143.2 \times 0.588} \right) + 0.02 = 2.66\ min$$

Since the treatment time is 2.66 min and the arc to complete in this time is 300° and one full rotation is 360°, the rotation speed to set:

$$Rotation\ speed = (300/(2.66 \times 360°) = 0.313\ rpm\ (rev\ per\ min)$$

XXXI. TREATMENT IN A NON VERTICAL PLANE

When the plane of treatment is not vertical and the treatment fields (beams) are applied at angles other than 0° or 90°, there must be a combination of gantry angle, floor angle and collimator angle to reset the fields in order to cover the target volume in three dimensions.

Assume a lateral film is taken with the collimator angled at 12° to encompass the slant of the esophagus. A contour is taken through this plane (12° angle) and a plan generated using a three field technique. The gantry angles are 0°, 120° and 240° to provide good coverage around the target volume.

Calculation:

i) Field$_1$

Floor angle = 90°
Gantry angle = 12°

ii) Field$_2$

$$\text{The new gantry angle} \quad \rightarrow \quad Cos^{-1}\delta = Cos\phi \times Cos\theta = 119.3°$$

Where ϕ is the collimator angle (12°) and θ is the angle of gantry (120°). Gantry angle of 12° is the collimator angle for field$_2$.

$$\text{Floor angle} = Tan\gamma = \left(\frac{Sin\phi}{Tan\theta}\right) = \left(\frac{Sin12°}{Tan120°}\right) \rightarrow \gamma = Tan^{-1}\left(\left(\frac{Sin12°}{Tan120°}\right)\right) = 6.8°$$

$$\text{Collimator angle} = Tan\alpha = \left(\frac{Tan\phi}{Sin\theta}\right) = \left(\frac{Tan12°}{Sin120°}\right) \rightarrow \alpha = Tan^{-1}\left(\left(\frac{Tan12°}{Sin120°}\right)\right) = 13.8°$$

iii) Field$_3$

The angles are reverse of field$_2$.

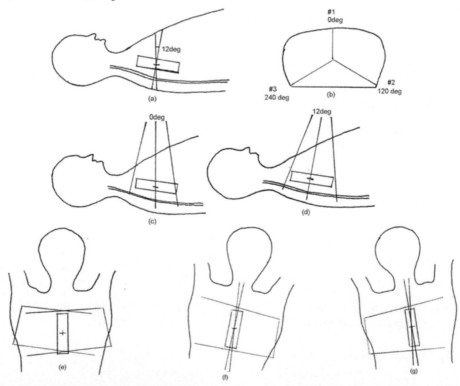

*Figure 2.55 (**a**) Collimator angle from lateral film. (**b**) Gantry angles of 3 field plan. (**c**) No gantry angle for field$_1$. Over-coverage of superior edge of esophagus and undercoverage of inferior edge. (**d**) With 12° gantry angle for field$_1$, good coverage is achieved. (**e**) No floor angle for fields 2 and 3. Undercoverage of inferior edge of esophagus and overcoverage of superior edge. (**f**)&(**g**) With 6.8° floor angle for fields 2 and 3 , good coverage is achieved.*

XXXII. NORMINAL SINGLE DOSE (NSD) AND TIME,DOSE,FRACTIONATION (TDF)

A. NSD

The concept of NSD was introduced by Ellis in 1967. He proposed that the tolerance dose of normal tissues (D cGy) could be related to the number of fractions (N) and the overall treatment time (T days) by:

$$D = (NSD) \times N^{-0.24} \times T^{-0.11}$$

where $NSD = D \times N^{-0.24} \times T^{-0.11}$, and $D = Total\ dose = Dose\ per\ fraction(d) \times Total\ fractions(N)$, *and N = Total fractions, and T = Total days*. Therefore;

$$NSD = (d \times T) \times N^{-0.24} \times T^{-0.11}$$

Example:

Calculate the NSD if 200 cGy per fraction is given for 25 fractions, treating 5 fractions a week.
(d= 200 cGy, N=25, T=33)

$$NSD = (200 \times 25) \times (25^{-0.24}) \times (33^{-0.11}) = 1572\ cGy$$

If the same NSD as above is required treating 3 times a week for 20 fractions, **calculate the dose per fraction** required *(d=?, N = 20, T = 46)*. And the NSD from above is 1572 cGy. Therefore,

$$1572 = (d \times 20) \times 20^{-0.24} \times 46^{-0.11} \quad \rightarrow \quad d = 246\ cGy\ per\ fraction.$$

NSD describes a complete course of fractionated radiation therapy which results in full connective tissue tolerance where tissue tolerance of different organs is different. NSD does not allow for split course radiation therapy.

B. Time DoseFractionation (TDF)

Due to the limitations of NSD, the TDF was introduced in 1972 by Orton. It allows for split course radiation therapy with *"decay factor"*.

$$TDF = n \times d^{1.538} \times x^{-0.169} \times 10^{-3}$$

where n = number of fractions, d = dose per fraction , and x = ratio of treatment days over number of treatments.

$$Decay\ factor : \left(\frac{T}{T+R}\right)^{0.11}$$

where T = overall treatment days *(including weekends)*, and R = rest days *(including weekends)*.

Example:

A patient is treated 5 times a week giving 2000 cGy in 10 fractions. Calculate the TDF. (Assuming; n = 10, d = 200 cGy, and x = 12/10 = 1.2)

Solution:

$$TDF = 10 \times (200)^{1.538} \times (1.2)^{-0.169} \times 10^{-3} = 33.5$$

Following are more examples in TDF calculation.

Example: *(Change in total fraction)*

A patient was planned to be treated to a total tumor dose of 5000 cGy in 25 fractions treating 5 times a week. It was decided later to change the fractions from 25 to 20. Calculate the new daily tumor dose to achieve the same TDF as originally planned.

Original dose per fraction = 200 cGy
Number of fractions = 25
Number of fractions per week = 5
From table 2.22, the TDF = 82

To achieve the same TDF of 82 in 20 fractions, the daily dose would be 230 cGy giving a total dose of 4600 cGy in 20 fractions. (The 230 cGy is obtained from Table 2.22. Go down the 20 fraction column until the TDF of 82. Go across to the left, the dose per fraction is 230 cGy.)

Example: *(Change in number of fractions per week)*

A patient was planned to receive 5000 cGy in 25 fractions treating 5 fractions a week. It was later found that he could make it to treatment only 3 times a week. Calculate the new daily dose to achieve the same TDF as originally planned.

Calculation:

Original dose per fraction = 200 cGy
Number of fractions = 25
Number of fractions per week = 5
From Table 2.22, the TDF = 82

From Table 2.20, go down the 25 fraction column until the TDF of 82 and go across to the left, the dose per fraction is 210 cGy in 25 fractions treating 3 times a week.

Example: *(Change in number of fractions per week during treatment)*

A patient was planned to be treated to a total dose of 5000 cGy in 25 fractions treating 5 times a week. After 10 treatments, he said he could only come once a week. Calculate the remaining dose in the remaining fractions to achieve the same TDF treating once a week.

Calculation:

Original dose per fraction = 200 cGy
Number of fractions = 25
Number of fractions per week = 5
From Table 2.22 the TDF = 82
The patient had 10 treatments, the TDF = 33
Therefore, the remaining TDF = 82 - 33= 49

If the same dose per fraction of 200 cGy is maintained, the number of fractions required to obtain a TDF of 49 is 19 fractions treating once a week.

From Table 2.18, go across to the right from 200 cGy per fraction until TDF of 49 is found. Go up along the column from 49, the number of fraction is 19.

Therefore, the remaining dose= 3800 cGy in 19 fractions treating once a week.

Example: *(Split Course Treatment)*

A patient was planned to receive 6000 cGy in 30 fractions treating 5 times a week. After having 10 treatments, he was sick and was put on a 2 week rest. When he resumes treatment, what is the daily dose if it is to be given in 20 fractions.

Calculation:

Original dose per fraction = 200 cGy ♦ Number of fractions = 30 ♦ *Number of fraction per week* − 5

From Table 2.22, the TDF = 99

The patient had 10 treatments, the TDF = 33

The treatment days (inc.week end) = 12

Rest days (inc.week end) = 16

From Table 2.23, the decay is 0.91.

The effective TDF from the 10 treatments is 33 × 0.91 = 30
The remaining TDF from original plan = 99- 30 = 69

From Table 2.22, go down the column for 20 fractions. The TDF of 69 is between 200 cGy per fraction and 210 cGy per fraction. Daily dose of 200 cGy gives a TDF of 66 and 210 cGy gives a TDF of 71. By interpolation, TDF of 69 gives 206 cGy daily dose. Therefore, the remaining dose is 4120 cGy in 20 fractions.

Table 2.18 TDF factors for one fraction per week. (Orton and Ellis 1973). *(D/f=Dose per Fraction)*

D/f	4	5	6	7	8	9	10	11	12	13	14	15	16	17	18	19	20
20	0	0	0	1	1	1	1	1	1	1	1	1	1	1	1	1	1
40	1	1	1	2	2	2	2	2	3	3	3	3	3	4	4	4	4
60	2	2	2	3	3	4	4	4	5	5	6	6	6	7	7	8	8
80	3	3	4	4	5	6	6	7	8	8	9	9	10	11	11	12	13
100	4	4	5	6	7	8	9	10	11	12	12	13	14	15	16	17	18
110	4	5	6	7	8	9	10	11	12	13	14	15	16	18	19	20	21
120	5	6	7	8	9	11	12	13	14	15	16	18	19	20	21	22	24
130	5	7	8	9	11	12	13	15	16	17	19	20	21	23	24	25	27
140	6	7	9	10	12	13	15	16	18	19	21	22	24	25	27	28	30
150	7	8	10	12	13	15	17	18	20	22	23	25	27	28	30	32	33
160	7	9	11	13	15	17	18	20	22	24	26	28	29	31	33	35	37
170	8	10	12	14	16	18	20	22	24	26	28	30	32	34	36	38	40
180	9	11	13	15	18	20	22	24	26	29	31	33	35	37	40	42	44
190	10	12	14	17	19	22	24	26	29	31	33	36	38	41	43	45	48
200	10	13	16	18	21	23	26	28	31	34	36	39	41	44	47	49	52
210	11	14	17	20	22	25	28	31	33	36	39	42	45	47	50	53	56
220	12	15	18	21	24	27	30	33	36	39	42	45	48	51	54	57	60
230	15	16	19	22	26	29	32	35	38	42	45	48	51	54	58	61	64
240	14	17	21	24	27	31	34	38	41	44	48	51	55	58	62	65	68
250	15	18	22	26	29	33	36	40	44	47	51	55	58	62	66	69	73
260	16	19	23	27	31	35	39	43	46	50	54	58	62	66	70	74	77
270	16	21	25	29	33	37	41	45	49	53	57	62	66	70	74	78	82
280	17	22	26	30	35	39	43	48	52	56	61	65	69	74	78	82	87
290	18	23	27	32	37	41	46	50	55	60	64	69	73	78	82	87	92
300	19	24	29	34	39	43	48	53	58	63	68	72	77	82	87	92	96

Table 2.22 TDF factors for five fractions per week. *(Orton and Ellis 1973) (D/f=Dose per Fraction)*

D/f	Number of fractions																
	4	5	6	8	10	12	14	15	16	18	20	22	24	25	26	28	30
20	0	1	1	1	1	1	1	2	2	2	2	2	2	2	3	3	3
40	1	1	2	2	3	3	4	4	4	5	6	6	7	7	7	8	8
60	2	3	3	4	5	6	7	8	8	9	10	11	12	13	13	15	16
80	3	4	5	6	8	10	11	12	13	15	16	18	19	20	21	23	24
100	5	6	7	9	11	14	16	17	18	20	23	25	27	28	30	32	34
110	5	7	8	11	13	16	18	20	21	24	26	29	32	33	34	37	39
120	6	8	9	12	15	18	21	23	24	27	30	33	36	38	39	42	45
130	7	9	10	14	17	20	24	26	27	31	34	37	41	43	44	48	51
140	8	10	11	15	19	23	27	29	31	34	38	42	46	48	50	53	57
150	9	11	13	17	21	25	30	32	34	38	42	47	51	53	55	59	64
160	9	12	14	19	23	28	33	35	37	42	47	51	56	58	61	66	70
170	10	13	15	21	26	31	36	39	41	46	51	57	62	64	67	72	77
180	11	14	17	22	28	34	39	42	45	50	56	62	67	70	73	79	84
190	12	15	18	24	31	37	43	46	49	55	61	67	73	76	79	85	97
200	13	17	20	26	33	40	46	49	53	59	66	73	79	82	86	92	99
210	14	18	21	28	36	43	50	53	57	64	71	78	85	89	92	99	107
220	15	19	23	31	38	46	53	57	61	69	76	84	92	95	99	107	115
230	16	20	25	33	41	49	57	61	65	74	82	90	98	102	106	114	123
240	17	22	26	35	44	52	61	65	70	79	87	96	105	109	113	122	131
250	19	23	28	37	46	56	65	70	74	84	93	102	112	116	121	130	139
260	20	25	30	40	49	59	69	74	79	89	99	109	118	123	128	138	148
270	21	26	31	42	52	63	73	78	84	94	105	115	126	131	136	146	157
280	22	28	33	44	55	66	77	83	89	100	111	122	133	138	144	155	
290	23	29	35	47	58	70	82	88	93	105	117	128	140	146	152		
300	25	31	37	49	62	74	86	92	98	111	123	135	148	154			

Table 2.23 "Decay factors" for use with TDF with rest breaks.

T(days)	Rest Period (days)											
	5	10	15	20	25	30	35	40	50	60	80	100
5	0.93	0.89	0.86	0.84	0.82	0.81	0.8	0.79	0.77	0.75	0.73	0.72
10	0.96	0.93	0.9	0.89	0.87	0.86	0.85	0.84	0.82	0.81	0.79	0.77
15	0.97	0.95	0.93	0.91	0.9	0.89	0.88	0.87	0.85	0.84	0.82	0.8
20	0.98	0.96	0.94	0.93	0.91	0.9	0.89	0.89	0.87	0.86	0.84	0.82
25	0.98	0.96	0.95	0.94	0.93	0.92	0.92	0.9	0.89	0.87	0.85	0.84
30	0.98	0.97	0.96	0.95	0.94	0.93	0.92	0.91	0.9	0.89	0.87	0.85
35	0.99	0.97	0.96	0.95	0.94	0.93	0.93	0.92	0.91	0.9	0.88	0.86
40	0.99	0.98	0.97	0.96	0.95	0.94	0.93	0.93	0.91	0.9	0.89	0.87
45	0.99	0.98	0.97	0.96	0.95	0.95	0.94	0.93	0.92	0.91	0.89	0.88
50	0.99	0.98	0.97	0.96	0.96	0.95	0.94	0.94	0.93	0.92	0.9	0.89

Problem 2.12

A patient is treated on the (6MV) with three fields gantry angles of 0° (AP), 120° (LPO) and 240° (RPO) using 8×10 cm^2 field size at 100 cm SAD. The depths are 13 cm, 15 cm and 16 cm respectively. The weighting at isocenter to all three fields are equal. Total tumor dose of 5000cGy in 25 treatments is prescribed to the 95% isodose line. Calculate the MU setting to each field.

Answer 2.12

Field size = 8×10 cm^2 → Eq. Sq= 8.9 cm^2 ◆ TMR (8.9 cm^2, 13 cm depth)= 0.687 ◆ TMR (8.9 cm^2, 15 cm depth) = 0.634 ◆ TMR (8.9 cm^2, 16 cm depth) = 0.609 ◆ OF (8×10 cm^2) at 100 cm SAD = 0.989 cGy/MU ◆ TTD to 95% isodose = 5000 cGy in 25 treatments ◆ TTD to 100% isodose = (100/95) × 5000= 5263cGy ◆ TTD to each field = (5263/3) = 1754.3 cGy

Since weights are equal,

$$MU\ setting(AP) = \frac{TTD}{\#\ of\ fractions \times TMR \times OF} = \frac{1754.3}{25 \times 0.687 \times 0.989} = 103\ MU$$

$$MU\ setting(LPO) = \frac{TTD}{\#\ of\ fractions \times TMR \times OF} = \frac{1754.3}{25 \times 0.643 \times 0.989} = 112\ MU$$

$$MU\ setting(RPO) = \frac{TTD}{\#\ of\ fractions \times TMR \times OF} = \frac{1754.3}{25 \times 0.609 \times 0.989} = 117\ MU$$

Problem 2.13

Repeat problem 2.12 if the weightings at isocenter are 100%, 80% and 70% respectively.

Answer 2.13

TTD to 100% = 5263 cGy
Total weights at isocenter = 250%.
TTD to AP field = (100/250) × 5263 = 2105 cGy

$$MU\ setting(AP) = \frac{TTD}{\#\ of\ fractions \times TMR \times OF} = \frac{2105}{25 \times 0.687 \times 0.989} = 124\ MU$$

TTD to LPO field = (80/250) × 5283 = 1684 cGy

$$MU\ setting(LPO) = \frac{TTD}{\#\ of\ fractions \times TMR \times OF} = \frac{1684}{25 \times 0.634 \times 0.989} = 107\ MU$$

TTD to RPO field = (70/250) × 5283 = 1474 cGy

$$MU\ setting(RPO) = \frac{TTD}{\#\ of\ fractions \times TMR \times OF} = \frac{1474}{25 \times 0.609 \times 0.989} = 98\ MU$$

Problem 2.14

Repeat *problem 2.12* if the fields are 8×10 cm^2 at 100 cm SSD and 5000 cGy in 25 treatments is prescribed to the intersection of the three fields. The total given dose to all fields are equal.

Answer 2.14

Field size = 8×10 cm^2 at 100 cm SSD → Eq. Sq = 8.9 cm^2
%DD for AP field (13 cm depth) = 55.8% ◆ %DD for LPO (15 cm depth) = 49.9% ◆ %DD for RPO (16 cm depth) = 47.1%

Total % DD at intersection = 152.8% ♦ TTD = 5000 cGy in 25 treatments to intersection (152.8%).

Since TGD to all fields are equal,

TGD to each field = (100/152.8) × 5000 = 3272cGy

OF for 8 × 10 cm^2 (100 cm SAD) = 0.989 cGy/MU

$$MU \ setting = \frac{TGD}{\# \ of \ fractions \ \times \ OF \ \times \ IS}$$

$$MU \ setting(AP) = \frac{TGD}{\# \ of \ fractions \ \times \ OF \ \times \ IS} = \left(\frac{3272}{25 \times 0.989 \times \left(\frac{100}{101.5}\right)^2} \right) = 136 \ MU$$

$$MU \ setting(LPO) = \frac{TGD}{\# \ of \ fractions \ \times \ OF \ \times \ IS} = \left(\frac{3272}{25 \times 0.989 \times \left(\frac{100}{101.5}\right)^2} \right) = 136 \ MU$$

$$MU \ setting(RPO) = \frac{TGD}{\# \ of \ fractions \ \times \ OF \ \times \ IS} = \left(\frac{3272}{25 \times 0.989 \times \left(\frac{100}{101.5}\right)^2} \right) = 136 \ MU$$

*Note: D_{max} is at 1.5 cm and GD is calculated to this point. Set-up is 100 cm, therefore distance to D_{max} is 101.5 cm. OF used is at 100 cm SAD.

Problem 2.15

Repeat 2.12 if the given doses are weighted 80%, 90% and 100%.

Answer 2.15

%DD for AP = 55.8 × 0.80 = 44.6% ♦ %DD for LPO = 49.9 × 0.90 = 44.9% ♦ %DD for RPO = 47.1 × 1.00 = 47.1%

Total %DD at isocenter = 136.6%

TTD = 5000 cGy in 25 treatments to intersection (136.6%)

Therefore TGD to AP field = (80/136.6) × 5000 = 2928 cGy

$$MU \ setting(AP) = \frac{TGD}{\# \ of \ fractions \ \times \ OF \ \times \ IS} = \left(\frac{2928}{25 \times 0.989 \times \left(\frac{100}{101.5}\right)^2} \right) = 122 \ MU$$

TGD to LPO field = (90/136.6) × 5000 = 3294cGy

$$MU \ setting(AP) = \frac{TGD}{\# \ of \ fractions \ \times \ OF \ \times \ IS} = \left(\frac{2928}{25 \times 0.989 \times \left(\frac{100}{101.5}\right)^2} \right) = 122 \ MU$$

TGD to RPO field = (100/136.6) × 5000 = 3660 cGy

$$MU \ setting(RPO) = \frac{TGD}{\# \ of \ fractions \ \times \ OF \ \times \ IS} = \left(\frac{3660}{25 \times 0.989 \times \left(\frac{100}{101.5}\right)^2} \right) = 152 \ MU$$

Problem 2.16

Calculate the treatment and rotation speed if 4000 cGy in 15 treatments is prescribed to the 95% isodose in a 300° arc rotation treatment using 8 × 8 cm² field size at 80 cm SAD on the Cobalt-60 treatment unit. The arc angles and field depths are given below. *(Timer correction = +0.02 min)*

Angle	depth	Angle	depth
210	13	10	13
230	14	30	14
250	15	50	14
270	16	70	15
290	15.5	90	16
310	15	110	16
330	14	130	15
350	14	150	14

Answer 2.16

TTD = 4000 cGy in 15 treatments to 95% isodose.

TTD to 100% (isocenter) = (100/95) × 4000 = 4211 cGy

DTD = (4211/15) = 280.7 cGy

ADR for 8 × 8 cm² = 141.8 cGy/min

TAR is the averaged TAR for every 20° arc.

Angle	depth	TAR	Angle	depth	TAR
210	13	0.288	10	13	0.576
230	14	0.544	30	14	0.544
250	15	0.513	50	14	0.544
270	16	0.485	70	15	0.513
290	15.5	0.499	90	16	0.485
310	15	0.513	110	16	0.485
330	14	0.544	130	15	0.513
350	14	0.544	150	14	0.272

Note: TAR for 210° & 150° is halved.

Total TAR = 7.862

Averaged TAR = 7.862/15 = 0.524

$$Treatment\ time\ \frac{DTD}{ADR \times TAR} + TC = \frac{280.7}{141.8 \times 0.524} + 0.02 = 3.80\ min$$

Since the treatment time is 3.80 min and the arc to complete in this time is 300° and one full rotation is 360°,

$$Rotations\ peed\ to\ set = \frac{300}{3.8 \times 360} = 0.219\ (rpm)rev\ per\ min$$

Problem 2.17

A patient was planned to receive 5000 cGy in 25 fractions treating 5 fractions a week. After 12 treatments, a rest of 5 days was prescribed. Calculate the daily tumor dose for the remaining 13 treatments to achieve the same TDF.

Answer 2.17

Planned treatment = 5000 cGy in 25 treatments (5 a week). ♦ TDF= 82 ♦ Actual treatment = 200 cGy X 12 ♦ TDF = 40 ♦ Treatment days (including weekend) = 17 days ♦ Rest days (inc.week end) = 7 days ♦ Decay = 0.965 → Therefore actual TDF of 40 is decayed to 40 × 0.965 = 38.6. Remaining TDF = 82-38.6 = 43.4. Daily TD to achieve TDF 43.4 in 13 treatments = 201 cGy.

XXXIII. PUBLICATIONS OF INTERESTS

1. Agarwal SK, Marks RD, Constable WC: Adjacent field separation for homogenous dosage at a given depth for the 8MV(Mevatron 8)linear accelerator. AM J Roentgenol 114: 623, 1972.

2. Almond P, Roosenbeek EV, Browne R, Milcamp J, Williams CB: radiation in the position of the central axis maximum build-up point with field size for high energy photon beams(Letter to the editor) Br J Radiol 43:911, 1970.

3. Armstrong DI, Tait JJ: The matching of adjacent fields in radiotherapy. Radiology 108:419, 1973.

4. Batho HF, Theimer O, Theimer R: A consideration of eq. circle method of calculating depth doses for rectangular X-Ray fields. J Can Assn Radiol 7:51, 1956.

5. Burns JE: Conversion of depth doses from one FSD to another. Br J Radiol 31: 643, 1958.

6. Clarke HC: A contouring device for use in radiation treatment planning. Br J Radiol 42: 858, 1969.

7. Clayton C, Thompson D : An optical apparatus for reproducing surface outlines of body cross sections. Br. J Radiol 43:489, 1970.

8. Cunningham JR, Johns HE, Gupta SK: An exam. of the defination and the magnitude of back scatter factor for Cobalt-60 gamma rays. Br J Radiol 38: 637, 1965.

9. Cunningham JR: Scatter-air ratios. Phys Med Biol 17:42, 1972.

10. Day MJ: A note on the calculation of dose in X-Ray fields. Br J Radiol 23: 368, 1950.

11. Gillin MT, Kline RW: Field separation between lateral and anterior fields on a 6MV linear accelerator. Int J Radiat Oncol Biol Phys 6:233, 1980.

12. Glenn DW, FAW FL, Kagan RA, Johnson RE: Field separation in multiple portal radiation therapy. Am J Roentgenol 102:199, 1968.

13. Gupta SK, Cunningham JR: Measurement of tissue air ratios and scatter functions for large field sizes for Cobalt-60 gamma radiation. Br J Radiol 39:7, 1966.

14. Hendee WR: Radiation Therapy Physics. Chigaco, Year Book Medical Publishers, 1981.

15. Hospital Physicists' Association: Central Axis depth dose data for use in radiotherapy. Br J Radiol (Suppl 11), 1978.

16. International Commission on Radiation Units and Measurements (ICRU): Report 33, Radiation Quantities and Units. Washington, DC, United States National Bureau of Standards, 1980.

17. Johns HE, Bruce WR, Reid WB: the dependence of depth dose on focal skin distance. Br J Radiol 31:254, 1958.

18. Johns HE, Whitmore GF, Watson TA, Umberg FH: A system of dosimetry for rotation therapy with typical rotation distributions. J Can Assn Radiol 4.1, 1953.

19. Johns HE, Cunningham JR: The Physics of Radiology, 4th ed Springfield, IL, Charles C Thomas, 1983

20. Karzmark CJ, Dewbert A, Loevinger R: Tissue phantom ratios-an aid to treatment planning. Br. J Radiol 38: 158,1965.

21. Khan FM: The Physics of Radiation Therapy, Baltimore, Williams and Wilkins, 1984.

22. Khan FM, Levitt SH, Moore VC, Jones TK: Computer and approximation methods of calculating depth dose in irregular shaped fields. Radiology 106: 433, 1973.

23. Khan FM: Computer dosimetry of partially blocked fields in cobalt teletherapy. Radiology 97:405, 1970.

24. Orton CG, Ellis F : A simplification in the use of the NSD concept in practical radiotherapy. Br J Radiol 46: 529, 1973.

25. Orton CG, Seibert JB: The measurement of teletherapy unit timer errors. Phys Med Biol 17:198, 1972

26. Powers WE, Korba A, Purdy JA, et al: Dose profiles in treatment planning. Radiology 121:741-742, 1976.

27. Purdy JA: Relationship between tissue phantom ratio and percentage depth dose. Med Phys 4: 66-67, 1977.

28. Sewchand W, Khan FM, Williamson J: Radiation in depth dose data between open and wedged fields 4 MV x-rays. Radiology 127:789, 1978.

—— *CHAPTER 3* ——

Inhomogeneity Corrections

I. EFFECT OF INHOMOGENEITY

Radiation therapy measurements such as %DD, TAR, TMR, and TPR are measured in a water phantom where the density is similar to that of muscle with a density of one (d = 1 g/cc). When treating a patient, however, the radiation beam traverses tissues of different densities such as lung and bone. Due to their different densities from that of muscle, the dose computation is altered. The degree of alteration is dependent on the tissue type, position of the tissue in the path of the radiation beam and on the energy of the radiation.

In order to deliver the correct dose of radiation to the point of interest, correction in the plan and in the monitor unit (MU) or treatment time must be made to account for the tissue density differences.

There are several ways to correct for the inhomogeneities. Given in this chapter are three methods for lung inhomogeneity correction. They are: (A) Isodose shift, (B) TAR ratio, and (C) Batho-Young *(Power Law)* method.

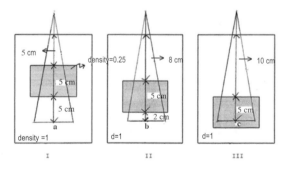

Figure 3.1 Diagrams show lung position in relation to points of interest a, b and c. Dose calculations are made to points a, b and c using each of the three methods of inhomogeneity correction.

II. LUNG INHOMOGENEITY CORRECTION (ON ^{60}Co)

A) Isodose Shift Method
This method calculates the ratio of the effective depth %DD to the real depth %DD. The effective depth %DD is corrected by a shift factor (n).

Point a (Figure 3.1 (I))

TAR for 10 × 10 cm² field size at 15 cm depth = 0.538

Corrected TAR = TAR × CF

$$CF = \frac{\%DD \; effective \; depth}{\%DD \; real \; depth}$$

Real depth = 15 cm, and the %DD at 15 cm depth = 38.71%

Effective depth = real depth + inhomogeneous path length × n = 15 + 5n = 15 + 5 × (-0.4) = 13 cm

Therefore, the percent depth dose (%DD) at 13 cm = 44.72%

Therefore, CF = (44.72/38.1) = 1.155

Therefore, the corrected TAR = 0.538 × 1.155 = 0.621

Inhomogeneity shift factor (n) for ⁶⁰Co & 4 MV photons: → Air: -0.6 ♦ Lung: -0.4 ♦ hard bone: 0.5 ♦ Spongy bone: 0.25

Point b (Figure 3.1 (II)) and Point c (Figure 3.1 (III))

Since the real depth and the lung thickness are the same as in the previous calculation to point a, the corrected TAR is the same, i.e., 0.621.

B) Tissue-Air Ratio Method

This method calculates the ratio of the effective depth TAR to the real depth TAR that is then used to correct the TAR for the real depth. The result is the effective depth TAR.

Point a (Figure 3.1 (I))

TAR for 10 × 10 cm² field size at 15 cm depth = 0.538

Corrected TAR = TAR × CF

$$CF = \frac{TAR \; effective \; depth}{TAR \; real \; depth}$$

Real depth = 15 cm, TAR = 0.538, and e = lung density = 0.25 gm/cc
Effective depth = 5 + (5 × e) + 5 = 5 + (5 × 0.25) + 5 = 11.25 cm
TAR at 11.25 cm depth = 0.660
Therefore, CF = (0.660/0.538) = 1.227
Therefore, the corrected TAR = 0.538 × 1.227 = 0.660

Point b (Figure 3.1 (II))

Real depth = 15 cm , TAR = 0.538
Effective depth = 8 + (5 × e) + 2 = 8 + (5 × 0.25) + 2 = 11.25 cm
TAR at 11.25 cm depth = 0.660
Therefore, CF = (0.660/0.538) = 1.227
Therefore, the corrected → TAR = 0.538 × 1.227 = 0.660

Point c (Figure 3.1 (III))

Real depth = 15 cm , TAR = 0.538
Effective depth = 10 + (5 × e) = 10 + (5 × 0.25) = 11.25 cm
TAR at 11.25 cm depth = 0.660
Therefore, CF = (0.660/0.538) = 1.227
Therefore, the corrected → TAR = 0.538 × 1.227 = 0.660

From the above calculation, it can be seen that the corrected TAR is the TAR for the effective depth.

C) Batho-Young (Power Law) Method

This is the most commonly used method and is the most accurate of the three methods described in this chapter. As will be shown later on in the comparison of the three methods, this method takes into account the distance between the point of interest to the inhomogeneity.

Point a (Fig.3.1 (I))

TAR for 10×10 cm^2 field size at 15 cm depth = 0.538

Corrected TAR = TAR × CF

$$CF = \left(\frac{TAR(z_1)^{\partial_1 - \partial_2}}{TAR(z_2)^{1-\partial_2}} \right) \quad \rightarrow \quad CF = \left(\frac{(0.898)^{1-0.25}}{(0.705)^{1-0.25}} \right) = 1.199$$

Where; z_1 = *distance from point of interest to inner aspect of inhomogeneity*

z_2 = *distance from point of interest to outer aspect of inhomogeneity*

δ_1 = *density at point of interest*

δ_2 = *density of overlying tissue*

Calculate the corrected TAR knowing that:

TAR(z_1 = 5 cm) = 0.898, TAR(z_2 = 10 cm) = 0.705 , δ_1 = 1, and δ_2 = 0.25

$$CF = \left(\frac{(0.898)^{1-0.25}}{(0.705)^{1-0.25}} \right) = 1.199$$

Corrected → *TAR = 0.538 × 1.199 = 0.645*

Point b (Figure 3.1 (II))

For point b → *TAR(z_1 = 2 cm) = 1.002, TAR(z_2 = 7 cm) = 0.819, δ_1 = 1, and δ_2 = 0.25*

$$CF = \left(\frac{(1.002)^{1-0.25}}{(0.819)^{1-0.25}} \right) = 1.163$$

Therefore, Corrected → *TAR = 0.538 × 1.163 = 0.626*

Point c (Figure 3.1 (III))

For point c → *TAR(z_1 = 5 cm) = 0.898, TAR(z_2 = 15 cm) = 0.538, δ_1 = 0.25, and δ_2 = 1.0*

Using the same formula as for point a and b calculation:

$$CF = \left(\frac{(0.898)^{0.25-1}}{(0.539)^{1-1}} \right) = 1.084$$

Therefore, Corrected TAR = 0.538 × 1.084 = 0.583

Table 3.1 Comparison of the three methods of TAR correction to points in tissue.

	point a	point b	point c
Isodose shift	0.62	0.62	0.62
TAR ratio	0.66	0.66	0.66
Batho-Young	0.65	0.63	0.58

The above comparison shows that the isodose shift method and the TAR ratio method does not take into account the distance from the point of interest to the inhomogeneity. The effective attenuation method takes into account the distance from the point of interest to the inhomogeneity but to a limited degree. The Batho-Young method takes into account not only the distance from point of interest to inhomogeneity but also where the point of interest is situated.

Other methods such as the equivalent TAR method and the Monte-Carlo method are being incorporated in treatment planning computer programs. The same methods of correction may be applied to Linear Accelerator by using TMR or TPR instead of TAR.

1) Application of Batho-Young Method in Calculation

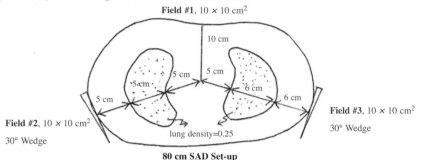

Figure 3.2 *Three fields with the posterior oblique fields through lung.*

In the diagram above, the esophagus is being treated using an anterior field and two posterior oblique fields. The depths are as shown in the diagram. A total tumor dose of 5000 cGy in 25 treatments is prescribed to isocenter with equal tumor dose to each field. Calculate the timer setting for each field for each treatment.

Calculation:

Total tumor dose is 5000 cGy in 25 treatments.

The total tumor dose to each field = 5000/3 = 1666.7 cGy.

The daily tumor dose to each field = (1666.7/25) = 66.7 cGy.

Air dose rate (ADR) for 10 × 10 cm² field size = 143.2 cGy/min

TAR (10 × 10 cm², 5 cm depth) = 0.898 , TAR (10 × 10 cm², 10 cm depth) = 0.705

TAR (10 × 10 cm², 11 cm depth) = 0.669 , TAR (10 × 10 cm², 15 cm depth) = 0.538

TAR (10 × 10 cm², 17 cm depth) = 0.481, Timer Correction = + 0.02 min

Wedge factor (W.F) for 30° wedge = 0.791

<u>**Field 1**</u>

$$Treatment\ time = \frac{DTD}{ADR \times TAR} + TC = \frac{66.7}{143.2 \times 0.705} + 0.02 = 0.68\ \ min$$

<u>**Field 2**</u>

TAR for 10 × 10 cm² field size at 15 cm depth = 0.538

Corrected TAR = TAR × CF

$$CF = \left(\frac{(TAR(5cm))^{\delta_1 - \delta_2}}{(TAR(10cm))^{1-\delta_2}} \right), \quad where; \quad \delta_1 = 1 \quad and \quad \delta_2 = 0.25 \longrightarrow CF = \left(\frac{(0.898)^{1-0.25}}{(0.705)^{1-0.25}} \right) = 1.199$$

Corrected TAR = 0.538 X 1.199 =0.645

Therefore, the treatment time is calculated as follows:

$$Treatment\ time = \frac{DTD}{ADR \times corr.TAR \times WF} + TC = \frac{66.7}{143.2 \times 0.645 \times 0.791} + 0.02 = 0.93\ \ min$$

Field 3

TAR for 10 × 10 cm² field size at 17 cm depth = 0.481
Corrected TAR = TAR × CF

$$CF = \left(\frac{(TAR(5cm))^{\delta_1 - \delta_2}}{(TAR(11cm))^{1-\delta_2}} \right), \quad where; \quad \delta_1 = 1 \quad and \quad \delta_2 = 0.25, \longrightarrow CF = \left(\frac{(0.898)^{1-0.25}}{(0.669)^{1-0.25}} \right) = 1.247$$

Corrected TAR = 0.481 × 1.247 = 0.600

$$Treatment\ time = \frac{DTD}{ADR \times corr.TAR \times WF} + TC = \frac{66.7}{143.2 \times 0.600 \times 0.791} + 0.02 = 1.00 \quad min$$

2) Calculation of Dose to a Point in Lung

(a) Single field

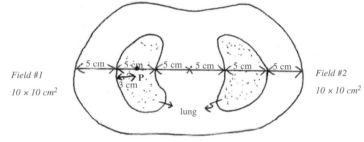

80 cm SAD set-up

Figure 3.3. Point of calculation P in lung (lung density is 0.25 g/cc).

Total tumor dose (T.D) to isocenter field 1 = 1000 cGy

$$Dose\ to\ lung\ at\ point\ P = \left(\frac{TD}{corr.TAR(10 \times 10, 15)} \right) \times corr.TAR(10 \times 10, 8) \times \left(\frac{SAD}{SSD + d} \right)^2$$

$$Corrected\ TAR(10 \times 10,\ 15) = \left(\frac{TAR(5cm)^{\delta_1 - \delta_2}}{TAR(10cm)^{1-\delta_2}} \right) \times TAR(15)$$

Where $\delta_1 = 1.00$ and $\delta_2 = 0.25$
TAR (10 × 10 cm², 15 cm depth) = 0.538, TAR (10 × 10 cm², 5 cm depth) = 0.898, and TAR (10 × 10 cm², 10 cm depth) = 0.705

$$Corrected\ TAR(10 \times 10,\ 15cm\ depth) = \left(\frac{0.898^{1-0.25}}{0.705^{1-0.25}} \right) \times 0.538 = 0.645$$

$$Corrected\ TAR(10 \times 10,\ 8cm\ depth) = \left(\frac{TAR(3cm)^{\delta_1 - \delta_2}}{TAR(8cm)^{1-\delta_2}} \right) \times TAR(8cm)$$

Where → $\delta_1 = 1.00$ and $\delta_2 = 0.25$
TAR (10 × 10 cm², 3 cm depth) = 0.971, TAR (10 × 10 cm², 8 cm depth) = 0.780

$$Corrected\ TAR(10 \times 10,\ 8cm\ depth) = \left(\frac{0.971^{0.25-1}}{0.780^{1-1}} \right) \times 0.780 = 0.797$$

$$Dose\ to\ point\ P\ in\ lung = \left(\frac{1000}{0.645} \right) \times 0.797 \times \left(\frac{80}{73} \right)^2 = 1484 \quad cGy$$

(b) Opposed field

Dose to lung at p from Field #1= 1484 cGy, and TTD from Field #2 at isocenter = 1000 cGy

$$Dose\ to\ point\ P\ in\ lung = \left(\frac{TTD}{corr.TAR(10 \times 10,15)}\right) \times corr.TAR(10.9 \times 10.9cm^2, 20) \times \left(\frac{SAD}{SSD+d}\right)^2$$

Note: Field size at p from Field #1= (87/80) × (10×10)= 10.9 × 10.9 cm²

$$Corrected\ TAR(10 \times 10cm^2,\ 15cm\ depth) = \left(\frac{TAR(5)^{\delta_1-\delta_2}}{TAR(10)^{1-\delta_2}}\right) \times TAR(13)$$

Where → $\delta_1 = 1.00$ *and* $\delta_2 = 0.25$

TAR (10 × 10 cm², 15 cm depth) = 0.538, TAR (10 × 10 cm², 5 cm depth) = 0.898, and TAR (10 × 10 cm², 10cm depth) = 0.705

$$Corrected\ TAR(10 \times 10cm^2,\ 15cm\ depth) = \left(\frac{(0.898)^{0.75}}{(0.705)^{0.75}}\right) \times 0.600 = 0.719$$

$$Corrected\ TAR(10.9 \times 10.9cm^2,\ 20cm\ depth) = \left(\frac{TAR(2)^{\delta_1-\delta_2}}{TAR(7)^{1-\delta_2}}\right) \times \left(\frac{TAR(12)^{\delta_1-\delta_2}}{TAR(17)^{1-\delta_2}}\right) \times TAR(20)$$

Where → $\delta_1 = 0.25$ *and* $\delta_2 = 1.00$ *(for the left bracket)*
Where → $\delta_1 = 1.00$ *and* $\delta_2 = 0.25$ *(for the right bracket)*

TAR (10.9×10.9, 2cm depth) = 1.007, TAR (10.9×10.9, 7cm depth) = 0.829, TAR (10.9×10.9, 12cm depth) = 0.645, TAR (10.9×10.9, 17cm depth) = 0.492, and TAR (10.9×10.9, 20cm depth) = 0.417

$$Corrected\ TAR(10.9 \times 10.9cm^2,\ 20cm\ depth) = \left(\frac{(1.007)^{-0.75}}{(0.829)^{0}}\right) \times \left(\frac{(0.645)^{0.75}}{(0.492)^{0.75}}\right) \times 0.417 = 0.509$$

Therefore, →
$$Dose\ to\ lung\ at\ P = \left(\frac{1000}{0.719}\right) \times 0.509 \times \left(\frac{80}{87}\right)^2 = 599\ cGy$$

Therefore total dose to point P in lung from the two opposed fields = 1484 + 599 = 2083 cGy

Problem 3.1

Using the Batho-Young (Power Law) method, calculate the corrected TAR to isocenter from fields 2 and 3 on the ^{60}Co. (Lung density = 0.30 g/cc)

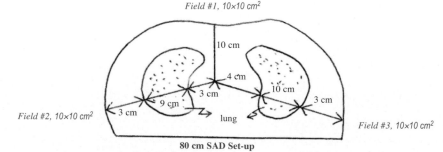

Field #1, 10×10 cm²

10 cm

4 cm

3 cm

9 cm

10 cm

3 cm

3 cm

Field #2, 10×10 cm²

lung

Field #3, 10×10 cm²

80 cm SAD Set-up

Solution:

TAR for Field #2 = TAR (real depth) × (CF)

$$CF = \left(\frac{TAR(3cm)}{TAR(12cm)}\right)^{0.7} = \left(\frac{0.971}{0.634}\right)^{0.7} = 1.348$$

Therefore, → *TAR for Field #2 = 0.538 × 1.348 = 0.725*

TAR for Field #3 = TAR (Real depth) × CF

$$CF = \left(\frac{TAR(4cm)}{TAR(14cm)} \right)^{0.7} = \left(\frac{0.936}{0.568} \right)^{0.7} = 1.419$$

Therefore, → TAR for Field #3 = 0.481 × 1.419 = 0.682

III. PUBLICATIONS OF INTERESTS

1. Batho HF: Lung corrections in cobalt 60 beam therapy. J Can Assn. Radiol 15:79,1964.
2. Fullerton GD, Sewchand W, Payne JT, Levitt SH: CT determination of parameters for inho- mogeneity corrections in radiation therapy of the esophagus. Radiology 124:167, 1978.
3. Greene D, Stewart JR: Isodose curves in non-uniform phantoms. Br J Radiol 38:378,1965.
4. Johns HE, Cunningham JR: The Physics of Radiology, 4th ed. Springfield, Il, Charles C Thomas, 1983, page 391.
5. Khan FM: The Physics of Radiation Therapy, Baltimore, Williams and Wilkins,1984 pages; 254-261
6. Mackie TR, El-Khatib F, Battista J, et al: Lung dose corrections for 6- and 15-MV x rays. Med Phys 12:327-332, 1985.
7. Parker RP, Hobday PA, Cassell KJ: The direct use of CT numbers in radiotherapy dosage calculations for inhomogeneous media. Phys Med Biol 24:802, 1979.
8. Sontag MR, Battista JJ, Bronskill MJ, Cunningham JR: Implications of computed tomography for inho mogeneity corrections in photon beam dose calculations. Radiology 124:143, 1977.
9. Sontag MR, Cunningham JR: The equivalent tissue-air ratio method for making absorbed dose calculations in a heterogenous medium, Radiology 129:787, 1978.
10. Sontag MR, Cunningham JR: Corrections to absorbed dose calculations for tissue inhomogeneities. Med Phys 4:431, 1977.
11. Young MEJ, Gaylord JD: Experimental tests of corrections for tissue inhomogeneity in radiotherapy. Br. J Radiol 43:349, 1970.

—— *CHAPTER 4* ——

Irregular Field Calculation

I. INTRODUCTION

In some treatment set up, part of the field is shielded to protect normal tissues or sensitive organs such as the lens of the eye, kidneys, spinal cord, etc. Due to the shielding, scatter is reduced. This reduction in scatter is reflected in a lower TAR value that in turn changes the treatment time calculation. Due to this change, the new TAR should be calculated. This is accomplished by doing the Clarkson integration that corrects the reduction in scatter and therefore the TAR.

As discussed in Chapter 2, TAR changes with field size and depth. With increase in field size the TAR increases due to increase in scatter. With increase in depth, the TAR decreases due to attenuation. The reverse is true for decrease in field size and decrease in depth. TAR is made up of primary and scatter radiation. TAR is the sum of TAR zero field size *(TAR 0, primary)* and SAR *(scatter)*.

TAR zero field size at a depth is obtained by plotting TAR against field size and then extrapolating back to zero field size. This is repeated for different depths. When the TAR for zero field size is known, the SAR can be calculated by subtracting the TAR zero field size from the TAR for that depth.

II. SCATTER AIR RATIO (SAR)

SAR is defined as the ratio of the scattered dose at a point in phantom to the dose in air at the same point.

SAR is related to TAR by the equation, *TAR = TAR (zero) + SAR*. As discussed, TAR increases with field size due to increase scatter. The increase in TAR is due to the increase in the SAR from increase in scatter.

To obtain SAR, TAR is plotted against field size at a chosen depth. The graph is extrapolated to zero field size to obtain TAR *(zero)*. Knowing TAR and TAR *(zero)*, SAR can be calculated by subtracting TAR *(zero)* from TAR. *SAR = TAR-TAR (zero)*.

SAR is used in the calculation of blocked field TAR using Clarkson's method of SAR integration. Knowing the resulting SAR and the TAR zero field, the TAR for the blocked field can be calculated.

II. IRREGULAR FIELD METHOD

Under the Clarkson's integration method, radii at 10° intervals are drawn from the point of inter-

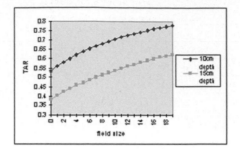

Figure 4.1. TAR graph (^{60}Co). TAR is extrapolated back to yield the TAR zero field.

est to the edge of the field or to the edge of the shield as shown in Figure 4.2. The distance for each radius is measured and the SAR is obtained from the SAR table. For those radii that pass under block the sum of the SAR from the blocked area are subtracted from the sum of the SAR from the unblocked area to arrive at the final SAR.

Example:

a) Calculate the treatment time to deliver 180 cGy to mid depth from parallel-opposed AP-PA 80 cm SAD fields with shielding as shown in Figure 4.2.
b) Calculate the dose to the off axis point.
c) Calculate the dose under the block.

The separation is 20 cm for all three points and the field size is 20 × 16 cm^2. Tray factor (TF) is 0.959. Air dose rate (ADR) is 145.3 cGy/min. Timer correction (TC) is +0.02 min.

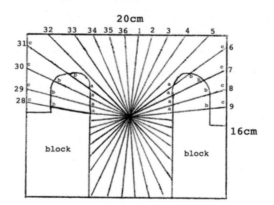

Figure 4.2. Radii at 10° interval to measure distance from center to field edge or block edge.

a) Center

Radius from sector 1 is the distance from the center to the edge of the field. SAR from Table is 0.216 at 10 cm depth. Radius for sector 6a is the distance from the center to the inner block surface. SAR is +0.164.

Radius for sector 6b is the distance from the center to the outer block surface. SAR is -0.205 due to negative scatter under the block. Radius for sector 6c is the distance from the center to the edge of the field. SAR is +0.264.

The net SAR from sector 6 is 0.164 - 0.205+0.264 = 0.223

Total SAR = (4.410 + 4.309) - (0.866 + 0.842) =7.011

Average SAR = 7.011/36 = 0.195

TAR at zero field size at 10 cm depth = 0.534

Corrected TAR = TAR zero field size at 10 cm depth + Average SAR = 0.534 + 0.195 = 0.729

Table 4.1 Table of radii distances and their SAR values for center point. *(SAR taken from Table 4.5)*

Sector	Radii	SAR(+)	SAR(-)	Sector	Radii	SAR(+)	SAR(-)
1	8.1	0.216		19	8	0.215	
2	8.3	0.219		20	8.3	0.219	
3	8.9	0.226		21	8.8	0.225	
4	9.8	0.237		22	6.9	0.193	
5	11.4	0.255		23	5.6	0.168	
6a	5.4	0.164		24	4.8	0.152	
6b	7.5		0.205	25	4.4	0.144	
6c	12.2	0.264		26	4.1	0.138	
7a	4.8	0.152		27	4	0.136	
7b	8.5		0.221	28a	4	0.136	
7c	11	0.25		28b	7.7		0.209
8a	4.5	0.146		28c	10.1	0.24	
8b	8.5		0.221	29a	4.1	0.138	
8c	10.3	0.242		29b	8		0.215
9a	4.4	0.144		29c	10.4	0.243	
9b	8.3		0.219	30a	4.4	0.144	
9c	10	0.239		30b	8.3		0.219
10	4.4	0.144		30c	11.1	0.251	
11	4.5	0.146		31a	4.7	0.15	
12	4.9	0.154		31b	7.2		0.199
13	5.4	0.164		31c	12.2	0.264	
14	6.3	0.182		32	11.4	0.255	
15	7.7	0.209		33	9.8	0.237	
16	8.8	0.225		34	8.9	0.226	
17	8.2	0.217		35	8.3	0.219	
18	8	0.215		36	8.1	0.216	
	Total	**4.41**	**0.866**		**Total**	**4.309**	**0.842**

$$\text{Treatment time} = \frac{DTD}{ADR \times TAR \times TF} + TC = \frac{90}{145.3 \times 0.729 \times 0.959} + 0.02 = 0.91 \quad \text{min}$$

b) Off-axis point

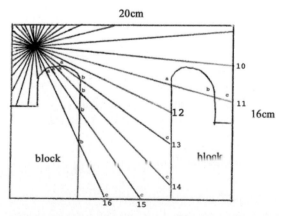

Figure 4.3 Radii at 10° interval to measure distances from off-center to field edge or block edge.

Table 4.2 Table of radii distances and their SAR values for off axis point. *(SAR taken from Table 4.5)*

Sector	Radii	SAR(+)	SAR(-)	Sector	Radii	SAR(+)	SAR(-)
1	2	0.082		16a	2.4	0.093	
2	2.1	0.085		b	9.8		0.237
3	2.2	0.087		c	15.4	0.29	
4	2.5	0.096		17	2.5	0.096	
5	2.9	0.106		18	4.1	0.138	
6	3.5	0.123		19	5.6	0.168	
7	4.8	0.152		20	5.8	0.172	
8	7.7	0.209		21	4.7	0.15	
9	18	0.306		22	3.5	0.123	
10	18.1	0.307		23	2.8	0.104	
11a	13	0.27		24	2.4	0.093	
b	16.9		0.3	25	2.2	0.087	
c	18.7	0.31		26	2	0.082	
12	13.8	0.277		27	2	0.082	
13a	3.1	0.112		28	2	0.082	
b	5.1		0.158	29	2	0.082	
b	15.3	0.289		30	2.2	0.087	
14a	2.7	0.101		31	2.5	0.096	
b	5.9		0.174	32	2.8	0.104	
c	17.7	0.304		33	2.4	0.093	
15a	2.5	0.096		34	2.2	0.087	
b	7.2		0.199	35	2	0.082	
c	17	0.3		36	2	0.082	
TOTAL		**3.612**	**0.831**			**2.473**	**0.237**

SAR = (3.612 + 2.473) - (0.831 + 0.237) = 5.017 ♦ *Average SAR = (5.017)/(36) = 0.139* ♦ *TAR at zero field size at 10 cm depth = 0.534 (Taken from table 4.4)* ♦ *TAR = TAR zero field size at 10 cm depth + Average SAR = 0.534 + 0.139 = 0.673* ♦ *TDR = ADR × TAR × Tray factor = 145.3 × 0.673 × 0.959 = 93.78 cGy/min* ♦ *Center TDR = 145.3 × 0.729 × 0.959 = 101.58 cGy/min*

Therefore, dose at off-axis point = (93.78/101.58) × 180 = 166 cGy

c) Off-center point under block

The dose under the shielding block is made up of the scatter from the unblocked area and transmission (3%) through the block.

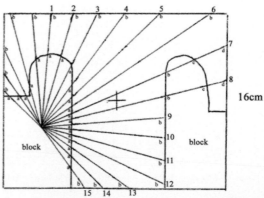

Figure 4.4 Radii at 10° interval to measure distances from off center under block to field edge or block edge.

Table 4.3 Table of radii distances and their SAR values. *(SAR taken from Table 4.5)*

Sector	Radii	SAR(+)	SAR(-)	Sector	Radii	SAR(+)	SAR(-)
1a	6.5		0.186	10a	2.8		0.104
b	10.4	0.243	b		11.2	0.252	
2a	6.6		0.187	11a	2.9		0.106
b	10.7	0.247		b	11.5	0.256	
3a	6.3		0.182	12a	3.1		0.112
b	11.5	0.256		b	12.3	0.264	
4a	4.8		0.152	13a	3.4		0.12
b	12.7	0.268		b	9.7	0.235	
5a	3.9		0.133	14a	4		0.136
b	14.8	0.285		b	8	0.215	
6a	3.4		0.12	15a	5		0.156
b	18.3	0.307		b	7	0.195	
7a	3		0.109	16a	3.9		0.133
b	12.2	0.264		b	4.7	0.15	
c	15.2		0.289	17a	3.3		0.177
d	18.4	0.308		b	7.65.8	0.172	
8a	2.9		0.106	18a	3.53		0.109
b	11.5	0.256		b	10.77.6	0.207	
c	15.5		0.291	19a	6.13.5		0.123
d	17.3	0.302		b	10.410.7	0.247	
9a	2.8		0.104	20a	6.1		0.178
b	11.2	0.252		b	10.4	0.243	
Total		**2.988**	**1.859**			**2.436**	**1.394**

SAR = (2.988+ 2.436) - (1.859 + 1.394) = 2.171

Average SAR = (2.171)/(36) = 0.0603

TAR at zero field size at 10 cm depth = 0.534 (from table 4.4) With 3% transmission through block

TAR at zero field size at 10 cm depth under block = 0.03 × 0.534 = 0.016

Therefore total TAR = TAR under block + Average SAR = 0.016 + 0.0603 = 0.076

TDR = ADR × TAR × Tray factor = 145.3 × 0.076 × 0.959 =10.6 cGy/min

Center TDR = 101.58 cGy/min

Therefore, the dose under the block = (10.6/101.58) × 180 = 19 cGy

Table 4.4 Table of TAR zero field size for ^{60}Co unit.

Depth	TAR	Depth	TAR	Depth	TAR
0	0.377	10	0.534	20	0.277
0.5	1	10.5	0.518	20.5	0.27
1	0.965	11	0.501	21	0.262
1.5	0.935	11.5	0.484	21.5	0.254
2	0.904	12	0.469	22	0.246
2.5	0.875	12.5	0.454	22.5	0.239
3	0.845	13	0.439	23	0.23
3.5	0.819	13.5	0.426	23.5	0.222
4	0.792	14	0.412	24	0.214
4.5	0.767	14.5	0.398	24.5	0.207

5	0.742	15	0.386	25	0.2
5.5	0.718	15.5	0.373	25.5	0.193
6	0.693	16	0.36	26	0.187
6.5	0.672	16.5	0.349	26.5	0.182
7	0.649	17	0.338	27	0.176
7.5	0.629	17.5	0.327	27.5	0.17
8	0.607	18	0.316	28	0.164
8.5	0.589	18.5	0.307	28.5	0.158
9	0.569	19	0.297	29	0.153
9.5	0.552	19.5	0.286	29.5	0.148
				30	0.144

Table 4.5 SAR vaules for ^{60}Co unit.

	Radii									
	2	4	8	12	16	24	28	32	36	40
Depth										
0	0.004	0.004	0.018	0.035	0.047	0.053	0.059	0.056	0.056	0.055
1	0.026	0.048	0.078	0.098	0.109	0.122	0.123	0.123	0.123	0.125
2	0.05	0.08	0.116	0.139	0.152	0.166	0.168	0.168	0.166	0.167
3	0.07	0.103	0.147	0.172	0.187	0.204	0.179	0.203	0.205	0.203
4	0.081	0.121	0.17	0.197	0.215	0.237	0.239	0.239	0.241	0.24
5	0.085	0.134	0.189	0.218	0.24	0.264	0.266	0.268	0.269	0.27
6	0.089	0.141	0.201	0.234	0.257	0.282	0.185	0.286	0.288	0.288
7	0.09	0.143	0.209	0.246	0.273	0.302	0.306	0.308	0.309	0.313
8	0.089	0.142	0.214	0.254	0.285	0.313	0.317	0.322	0.326	0.328
9	0.086	0.14	0.216	0.26	0.292	0.324	0.329	0.334	0.337	0.339
10	0.082	0.136	0.215	0.262	0.295	0.333	0.338	0.343	0.345	0.353
11	0.076	0.132	0.213	0.262	0.296	0.337	0.343	0.346	0.349	0.355
12	0.074	0.128	0.21	0.261	0.297	0.34	0.344	0.348	0.353	0.356
13	0.07	0.124	0.207	0.26	0.298	0.341	0.345	0.352	0.355	0.356
14	0.066	0.12	0.204	0.258	0.297	0.344	0.352	0.355	0.361	0.369
15	0.062	0.116	0.2	0.255	0.295	0.344	0.352	0.355	0.361	0.369
16	0.06	0.112	0.196	0.252	0.292	0.341	0.349	0.355	0.36	0.369
17	0.058	0.108	0.191	0.248	0.288	0.338	0.343	0.352	0.359	0.364
18	0.056	0.104	0.186	0.244	0.284	0.334	0.342	0.352	0.359	0.369
19	0.053	0.101	0.181	0.239	0.28	0.33	0.341	0.35	0.356	0.366
20	0.049	0.097	0.176	0.234	0.275	0.325	0.334	0.344	0.348	0.356

d) A Simple calculation of blocked TAR

For simple shielding, a simple irregular field calculation may be performed by calculating the fraction of the blocked field SAR to the open field SAR.

Example:

TAR zero field size (10 cm depth) = 0.534

TAR (15 × 15 cm², 10 cm depth) = 0.752

SAR = TAR - TAR zero field size = 0.752 - 0.534 = 0.218

Since scatter is only from 3/4 of the field, the net scatter = 0.164.

Therefore the corrected →   *TAR = 0.534 + 0.164 =0.698*

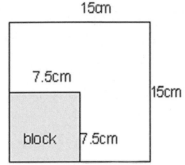

Figure 4.5. 15 × 15 cm² field with 1/4 of the field blocked.

Example:

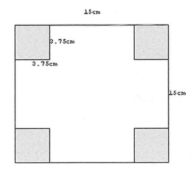

Figure 4.6 15 × 15 cm² field with four corners blocked.

TAR = TAR zero + SAR

TAR zero (10 cm depth) = 0.534

Area of open field = 225 cm²

Area of block = 56.25 cm²

Therefore area of blocked field = 168.75 cm²

Radius for 168.75 cm² → $r^2 = (168.75)/\pi$ → $r = (168.75/\pi)^{1/2} = 7.33$ *cm*

SAR for 7.33 cm at 10 cm depth = 0.202

Therefore, TAR for treated field = 0.534 + 0.202 – 0.736

e) Caculation of dose under block

Example:

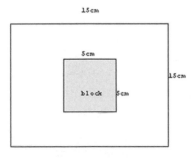

Figure 4.7. 15 × 15 cm² field with the center blocked.

TAR zero field size (10 cm depth) = 0.534

TAR (15 × 15 cm², 10 cm) = 0.752

SAR (15 × 15 cm², 10 cm) = 0.752 - 0.534 = 0.218

SAR for 5 × 5 cm², 10 cm depth = 0.104

Therefore SAR under block = 0.218 - 0.104 = 0.114

TAR zero field size under block assuming 3% transmission (5 HVL) = 0.03 × 0.534 = 0.016

Therefore dose under block = 0.016 + 0.114 × 100% = 13% of open field.

III. SUPERFICIAL X-RAY IRREGULAR FIELD CALCULATION

In the treatment of skin lesions, a lead cut out is often used to shield healthy skin. Due to this shielding, the dose rate is altered from the measured dose rate for a particular applicator. This is due to the reduced scatter from the shielding. Hence, treatment time calculation should take into account of this scatter reduction.

Example a:

A patient is planned for treatment to a skin lesion on the left temple. The diagram below is the outline of the treated area. The applicator is a 5.5 cm circular cone at 20 cm SSD. The treatment unit is the 100 kV 8 mA SXR unit with 1.25 mm AL filter and a HVL of 1.65 mm AL. The prescribed surface dose is 4500 cGy in 15 treatments.

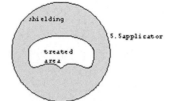

Figure 4.8 Treated area through a 5.5 cm circle applicator.

Use a cm square graph paper to calculate the area of the treated field. The circle is placed over the graph paper and the total square cm covered by the circle is added up. In this example, the treated area is 10.25 cm square. The treated area is converted to diameter to obtain the BSF (back scatter factor) from the BSF table.

Area of a circle = πr^2 = 10.25 cm², where, r = radius
$r^2 = (10.25)/\pi \rightarrow r = (10.25/\pi)^{1/2} = 1.806$ cm
Therefore, the diameter = 2 × 1.806 = 3.612.
From the BSF table, 3.612 cm diameter gives a BSF of 1.115
The air-dose rate for 5.5 cm applicator is 288 cGy/min.
Therefore the corrected surface dose rate = 1.115 × 288 = 321.12 cGy/min.
The timer correction = -0.02 min.
Therefore the timer setting = (4500)/(15 × 321.12)-0.02 = 0.91 min

Example b:

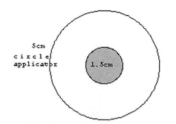

Figure 4.9. Treated area with the center shielded.

Area for 1.5cm circle = 1.77 cm²
Area for 5cm circle = 19.63 cm²
The treated area = 19.63-1.77 = 17.86 cm²
The diameter for 17.86cm square = 4.77 cm
The BSF = 1.141
The air dose rate for 5 cm cone = 287 cGy/min
Therefore corrected surface dose rate = 287 × 1.141 = 327.5 cGy/min

Table 4.6 Table of air dose rate and surface dose rate for Philips RT 100 Superficial treatment unit.

(100 kV 8 mA 1.25 mmAL filter and HVL 1.65 mmAL SSD= 20 cm)

Cone diameter(cm)	Output factor in air	Output factor on tissue surface
1	270	281
1.2	270	282
1.4	271	285
1.6	272	288
1.8	273	291
2	282	302
2.5	283	307
3	283	311
3.5	284	316
4	284	319
4.5	286	325
5	287	329
5.5	288	334
6	292	341
6.5	292	344
7	292	347
7.5	292	349
8	292	350

Table 4.7 Table of BSF for circular cut out on the superficial treatment unit.

Circular cut out	HVL(mmAL)		
	0.82	1.65	6.8
1	1.022	1.039	1.048
1.2	1.028	1.045	1.058
1.4	1.032	1.051	1.067
1.6	1.036	1.058	1.076
1.8	1.041	1.065	1.085
2	1.045	1.071	1.095
2.5	1.057	1.096	1.116
3	1.067	1.099	1.138
3.5	1.076	1.112	1.159
4	1.086	1.124	1.178
4.5	1.096	1.135	1.196
5	1.106	1.147	1.212
5.5	1.114	1.158	1.228
6	1.12	1.168	1.243
6.5	1.124	1.179	1.257
7	1.13	1.187	1.269
7.5	1.135	1.194	1.281
8	1.14	1.2	1.292

Problem 4.1

Calculate the corrected TAR using Clarkson's method given the average SAR = 0.205 and the field size is 20 × 12 cm² at 10 cm depth.

Solution:

TAR = TAR (zero) + SAR, SAR = 0.205, and TAR (zero)(at 10 cm depth) = 0.534

Therefore, → TAR = 0.534 + 0.205 = 0.739

Problem 4.2

Calculate the corrected TAR at 10 cm depth for the blocked field given below.

Solution:

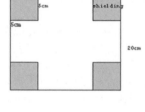

TAR = TAR (zero) + SAR; and TAR (zero)(at 10 cm depth) = 0.534

Area of open field = 400 cm²; and Area of blocked field = 100 cm²

Therefore area of treated field = 300 cm²

Radius for 300 cm² → r = (300/π)^{1/2} = 9.77 cm

SAR for 9.77 cm = 0.236

Therefore, → TAR for treated field = 0.534 + 0.236 = 0.770

Problem 4.3

Calculate the corrected surface dose rate given the blocked field below for 100 kV, 8 mA, 1.25 mm Al filter HVL 1.65 mmAl X-Ray.

Solution:

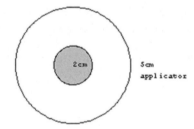

Air dose rate for open field 5 cm circle = 287 cGy/min

Area of a circle = π r²

Area for 2 cm circle = 3.142 cm²

Area for 5 cm circle = 19.63 cm²

Therefore, the treated area = 19.63 - 3.142 = 16.49 cm²

Radius for 16.49 cm² = 2.29 cm

Diameter = 2.29 × 2 = 4.58 cm

BSF for 4.5cm = 1.137

Corrected surface dose rate = 287 × 1.137 = 326.3 cGy/min

IV. PUBLICATIONS OF INTERESTS

1. Clarkson JR: A note on depth doses in fields of irregular shape. Br J Radiol 14:265,1941 Cunningham JR: Scatter-air ratios. Phys Med Biol 17:42, 1972.

2. Johns HE, Cunningham JR: The Physics of Radiology, 4th ed Springfield, IL, Charles C Thomas, 1983 pages 369-376.

3. Khan FM: The Physics of Radiation Therapy, Baltimore, Williams and Wilkins, 1984 pages 178-180.

Principles and Practice of Clinical Physics and Dosimetry
Michael L.F. Lim, CMD, ACT
Advanced Medical Publishing, Inc., USA

—— *CHAPTER 5* ——

Missing and added Tissue Correction

I. INTRODUCTION

In some treatment situations, the incident beam on the treatment site may not be flat due to curved patient contour. The curved surface may be made flat with the use of bolus (added tissue) but this is sometimes not desirable due to high skin dose. Under both of these situations, it may be desirable to calculate the dose to some points in tissue taking into account the missing or added tissue.

Given here are four methods to calculate dose to a point after traversing through missing and added tissue.

I. SHIFT METHOD USING ISODOSE CHART

This method is described in greater detail in later chapter but suffice it here to mention that the iosdose lines are shifted towards the skin surface to correct for the missing and added tissue. The shift is 0.667(2/3) for ^{60}Co unit, 0.64 for 6 MV photons and 0.55 for 15 MV photons. Referring to Figure 5.1, X-Y is the patient contour. The solid lines are the isodose lines for a 10×10 cm^2 ^{60}Co isodose chart. The dotted lines are the shifted isodose lines.

With no shift, the %DD at A(10 cm) = 55.5%, B(8 cm) = 51.0% and C(12 cm) = 51.0%. ♦ *With shift, the %DD at A = 55.5%, B=57% and C= 47%.*

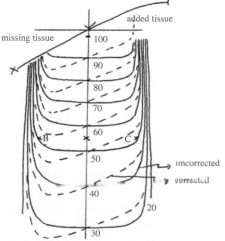

Figure 5.1. Uncorrected and corrected isodose for missing and added tissue.

II. SHIFT METHOD USING %DD TABLE

This method calculates the increased in depth dose through missing tissue and decreased in depth dose through added tissue.

Referring to Figure 5.1 again, point B has an air gap of 2 cm.

Correcting for air gap, the decreased in depth = 2 × (- 0.67) = - 1.34cm.

Therefore, the corrected depth = 10 -1.34= 8.66 cm

The %DD at 8.66cm depth (80cm SSD) = 61%.

Since point B is off-axis and since the beam is not flat, an off axis correction factor should be applied to the %DD calculated above. The off-axis factor is obtained from the beam profile, Figure 5.2. The off axis factor is 0.94.

Therefore, the %DD at B is 61 × 0.94 = 57.3%.

Point C has added tissue of 2 cm.

Correcting for the added tissue, the increase in depth = 2 × (0.67) = 1.34 cm.

Therefore, the corrected depth = 10 + 1.34 = 11.34 cm.

The %DD for 11.34 cm depth (80cm SSD) = 50.4%.

Applying the off axis factor of 0.94, the %DD at C = 50.4 × 0.94 = 47.4%.

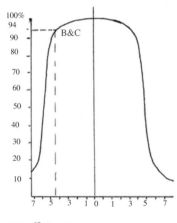

Figure 5.2. Beam profile for 10 × 10 cm^2 field at 80 cm SSD at 10 cm depth for ^{60}Co unit.

III. LINEAR ATTENUATION METHOD

This method calculates the decreased or increased attenuation through the missing and added tissue and corrects the %DD accordingly.

Referring to Fgure 5.1 again, percentage depth dose for A = 55.5%.

Point B has 2 cm of missing tissue.

$$Corrected \ \%DD \ for \ point \ \ B = 55.5 \times \left(1 + \left(\frac{p \times x}{100}\right)\right) = 55.5 \times \left(1 + \left(\frac{5 \times 2}{100}\right)\right) = 61.1\%$$

Corrected for off-axis = 61.1 × 0.94 = 57.4%

p = % correction for missing or added tissue.

x = thickness of missing or added tissue.

Table 5.1 Table of p-values.

unit	*p*
Cobalt-60	5%
6MV	3.5%
10MV	3%
25MV	2%

Point C has 2 cm of added tissue.

$$Corrected \ \%DD \ for \ po\mathrm{int} \ C = 55.5 \times \left(1 - \left(\frac{5 \times 2}{100}\right)\right) = 50\%$$

Corrected for off axis = 50 × 0.94 = 47%.

IV. TISSUE AIR RATIO METHOD

This method calculates the corrected %DD to points B and C by applying the ratio of TAR between central axis and the points of interest.

Percentage depth dose for A = 55.5%.

Field size at A, B and C = 11.25 cm²

TAR for 10 cm depth (A) = 0.718 , TAR for 8 cm depth (B) = 0.793 , and TAR for 12 cm depth (C) = 0.648

$$\%DD \ for \ B = 55.5 \times \left(\frac{0.793}{0.718}\right) = 61.3\%$$

Corrected for off axis = 61.3 X 0.94 = 57.6%.

$$\%DD \ for \ C = 55.5 \times \left(\frac{0.648}{0.718}\right) = 50.1\%$$

Corrected for off axis = 50.1 × 0.94 = 47.1%.

V. COMPARISON OF THE FOUR METHODS OF MISSING AND ADDED TISSUE CORRECTION

Table 5.2 Comparison of correction methods.

	Point A	Point B	Point C
Shift method(isodose chart)	55.5	57.0	47.0
Shift method (%DD)	55.5	57.3	47.4
Linear attenuation method	55.5	57.4	47.0
TAR method	55.5	57.6	47.1

Poblem 5.1

The %DD at A (14.5 cm depth) along central axis for a 10 × 10 cm² field at 80 cm SSD for ^{60}Co is 40.13%. Calculate the %DD to off axis points B and C using the TAR method, if their depths are 12.5 cm (2 cm gap) and 16.5cm (2 cm added tissue) respectively. The off axis factor (OAF) is 0.90.

Solution:

Field size at A, B, C (94.5cm SSD) − 11.8 cm² , TAR for 14.5 cm depth (A) = 0.573 , TAR for 12.5 cm depth (B) = 0.637, and TAR for 16.5 cm depth (C) = 0.515

$$\%DD \ for \ B = \%DD(A) \times \left(\frac{TAR(B)}{TAR(A)}\right) \times OAF$$

$$\%DD \ for \ B = 40.13 \times \left(\frac{0.637}{0.573}\right) \times 0.9 = 40.15\%$$

$$\%DD \ for \ C = \%DD(C) \times \left(\frac{TAR(C)}{TAR(A)}\right) \times OAF$$

$$\%DD \ for \ C = 40.13 \times \left(\frac{0.515}{0.573}\right) \times 0.9 = 32.46\%$$

Problem 5.2

Repeat problem 5.1 using the linear attenuation method.

Solution:

%DD for A = 40.13%

Point B has 2 cm of missing tissue.

$$Corrected\ \%DD\ for\ point\ B = \%DD \times \left(1 + \left(\frac{p \times x}{100}\right)\right) \times OAF = 40.13 \times \left(1 + \left(\frac{5 \times 2}{100}\right)\right) \times 0.9 = 39.7\%$$

$$Corrected\ \%DD\ for\ point\ C = \%DD \times \left(1 + \left(\frac{p \times x}{100}\right)\right) \times OAF = 40.13 \times \left(1 - \left(\frac{5 \times 2}{100}\right)\right) \times 0.9 = 32.51\%$$

VI. PUBLICATIONS OF INTERESTS

1.   Hendee WR: Radiation Therapy Physics. Chicago, Year Book Medical Publishers, 1981.

2.   International Commission on Radiation Units and Measurements (ICRU): Report 24. Determination of

3.   Absorbed Dose in a Patient Irradiated by Beams of X or Gamma Rays in Radiotherapy Procedures. 4. Washington, DC, United States National Bureau of Standards, 1976.

5.   Johns HE, Cunningham JR: The Physics of Radiology, 4th ed. Springfield, IL, Charles C Thomas, 1983.

6.   Khan FM: The Physics of Radiation Therapy, Baltimore, Williams and Wilkins, 1984.

Principles and Practice of Clinical Physics and Dosimetry
Michael L.F. Lim, CMD, ACT
Advanced Medical Publishing, Inc., USA

— CHAPTER 6 —

Compensator

I. INTRODUCTION

Missing tissue results from irregular or sloping surface. The non-uniformity of dose created from the missing tissue may be unacceptable. Due to the non-uniformity of dose, sensitive organs such as the spinal cord may receive excessive dose. One method to overcome the non-uniformity of dose created from the missing tissue is the use of compensator

II. BOLUS BAGS

One of the commonly used compensator is the bolus bag. The bolus bags are made up of tapioca granules or rice grains that have a density close to that of tissue. The bolus bags are placed on the patient to compensate for the missing tissue.

The advantages of using bolus bags are: 1) easy to use, 2) easy to obtain; and 3) ability to compensate in the X-Y planes. The disadvantages are: 1) removes skin sparing for high energy treatment units, 2) may be heavy on the patient, 3) may not be reproducible for each treatment; and 4) may not be easy to hold all the bolus bags in place especially along sloping surface.

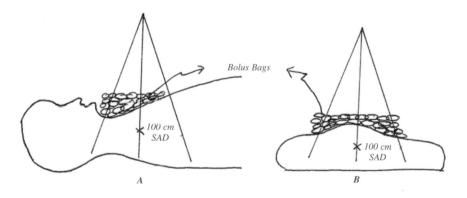

Figure 6.1 (A,B) Bolus bags in place for treatment.

III. WAX BOLUS

The wax bolus compensator is made out of wax that is then fixed on the patient's shell (cast). The wax is made up of an equal mixture of paraffin wax and bees wax and 5% resin with a density close to tissue.

The advantages are: 1) easy to use, 2) easy to obtain, 3) ability to compensate in the X-Y planes; and 4) reproducibility is good. The disadvantages are: 1) may be heavy on the patient, 2) needs a shell (cast) to fix the wax bolus; and 3) removes skin sparing for high energy treatment units.

For both the bolus bag and wax compensator, the thickness of the bolus should be added to the depth of the tissue on the bolus side to be used in the treatment calculation.

IV. EXAMPLE

Separation at the center without bolus is 20 cm. Thickness of wax from the bolus side (anterior) is 4 cm. therefore the anterior depth is 14 cm and the posterior depth is 10 cm.

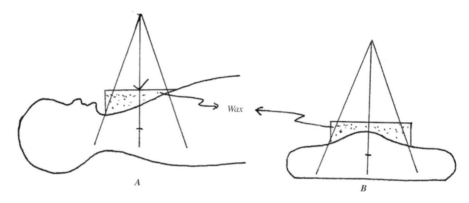

Figure 6.2 (A,B) Wax compensator in place for treatment.

V. RETRACTED WAX COMPENSATOR

An improvement to the wax bolus above is the retracted wax compensator. As the name suggest, the wax compensator sits at a retracted distance from the patient. The fabrication of the retracted wax compensator involves making a reduced wax contour of the patient and mounting in on the bottom of the shielding tray that slides into the head of the treatment unit.

The device for making remote wax compensator is made up of an array of steel rods of a predetermined length. In the case of the 6 MV, the distance from the source to the bottom of the tray is 56.5 cm, therefore the length of the rods are 43.5 cm *(to add up to 100 cm.)* These rods are held in place by inserting them through holes drilled in two support plates. The surface of the patient that needs no compensation is set up at 100 cm SAD. Then the rods are pushed down till they touch the patient's skin or the shell *(cast.)* Softened wax is then molded on the top of the depressed steel rods and the top of the wax is flattened to mount on the bottom of the shielding tray.

The advantages of using remote wax compensator are: 1) skin sparing, 2) accurate daily set-up; and 3) no weight on the patient. The disadvantages are: 1) some loss of %DD especially at shallow depths due to reduced scatter; and 2) need skilled personnel and equipment.

The transmission factor of the finished wax compensator is measured and this factor is used in the calculation of MU setting.

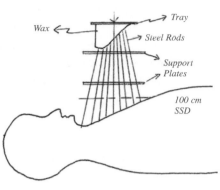

Figure 6.3 Device for fabricating remote wax compensator. (Sagittal view)

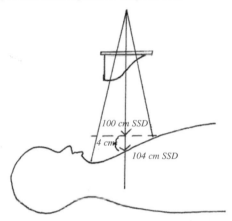

Figure 6.4 Mounted remote wax compensator. (Sagittal view)

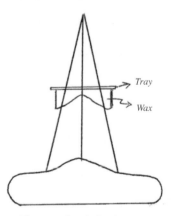

Figure 6.5 Mounted remote wax compensator (Cross sectional view.)

VI. RETRACTED LEAD STEP COMPENSATOR

The lead step compensator is made out of sheets of lead in step form. The finished compensator is mounted on the top of the shielding tray if there is no shielding blocks (cerrobend) or to the bottom of the shielding tray if there is shielding blocks *(cerrobend.)*

The patient is simulated in the treatment position. AP and PA films are taken. Lead wire is taped on the anterior skin surface running sagittally through the center of the field. A lateral film is taken to show the sagittal outline of the patient. *(The spinal cord must be visible if compensation is to the spinal cord.)*

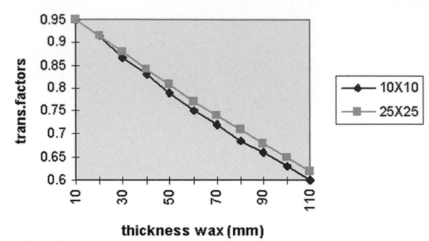

Figure 6.6 Transmission factor for wax compensator.

The sagittal outline of the patient can be traced and de-magnified using a pantograph or via a computer. Once the sagittal outline is obtained, the central axis of the beam is drawn from the source to axis depth. Diverging sagittal lines at one cm apart are drawn from the source to the compensation points.

The diverging lines are numbered from the center to superior and center to inferior. The overlying tissue depths are measured for each line. The TMR is obtained for each depth. The distance from source to compensation point for each fan line is then squared and divided by the TMR of the overlying tissue for that line. These values are then normalized to the point that does not need compensation that is usually the thickest separation of the patient.

Place the transmission factors on the y-axis and the field lengths on the x-axis making sure the center and points superiorly and inferiorly are well labeled. The normalized transmission values are then plotted on the graph. The number of lead sheets required are calculated (this depends on the thickness of the lead sheet used.) and the layers of lead sheets are drawn on the graph.

Since the step compensator is mounted on a tray that slides into the head of the treatment unit, the lead sheets must be de-magnified. In this example, the source tray distance is 55.9 cm. Therefore, the de-magnification factor is 55.9/100 = 0.559. After de-magnification, one cm is added to the superior edge of each lead sheet to ensure there is enough margin beyond the field edge. Similarly the width of the compensator is de-magnified and one cm is added to each side of the compensator. The 0.07 cm thick lead sheets are cut to the size calculated for each sheet. They are glued together, making sure each sheet is off set by the longitudinal distance from the field center as calculated. The field center is drawn on the compensator and this center is aligned to the field center on the tray.

If there are shielding blocks *(cerrobend)*, a few changes are made to the above procedure. The shielding blocks (cerrobend) would be on the tray top and the compensator would be mounted on the bottom of the tray. In this example, the tray thickness is 0.6 cm. Therefore, the distance from the source to bottom of tray is 56.5 cm. Therefore, de-magnification factor is 56.5/100 = 0.565. The compensator is mounted on to the bottom of the tray.

The transmission factor of the compensator is measured and this factor is used in the calculation for the MU setting.

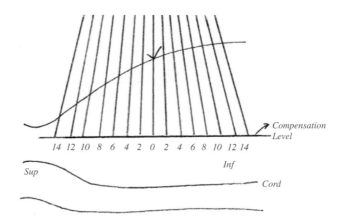

Figure 6.7 Diagram shows diverging sagittal ray lines.

Table 6.1 Transmission curve table.

Distance from Center (cm)	Overlying Tissue Depth (cm)	TMR	Inversed Normalized Transmission
15(sup)	1.7	0.999	0.684
14	2.7	0.980	0.697
13	3.6	0.960	0.711
12	4.8	0.931	0.734
11	5.8	0.906	0.754
10	6.4	0.890	0.767
9	7	0.875	0.781
8	7.6	0.859	0.795
7	8.1	0.846	0.807
6	8.8	0.828	0.825
5	9.4	0.812	0.841
4	9.9	0.799	0.855
3	10.4	0.786	0.869
2	10.8	0.776	0.880
1	11.1	0.767	0.891
0 (center)	11.3	0.762	0.896
1	11.8	0.749	0.912
2	12.2	0.738	0.925
3	12.5	0.731	0.934
4	12.8	0.723	0.945
5	13.1	0.715	0.955
6	13.3	0.710	0.962
7	13.5	0.705	0.969
8	13.7	0.699	0.978
9	13.9	0.695	0.983
10	14	0.692	0.987
11	14.2	0.686	0.996
12	14.3	0.683	1.000
13	14.3	0.683	1.000
14	14.3	0.683	1.000
15(inf)	14.3	0.683	1.000

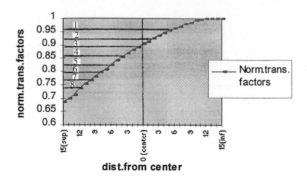

Figure 6.8 Normalized transmission values.

Table 6.2 Actual length lead sheets at tray distance.

Lead Sheet	Length of Strip at 100 cm	Length of Strip at Tray*	Cut**
1	20.5	11.4	12.4
2	16.5	9.2	10.2
3	13.8	7.7	8.7
4	11	6.1	7.1
5	8.8	4.9	5.9
6	6.8	3.8	4.8
7	4.5	2.5	3.5
8	2.9	1.6	2.6

* De-magnify by0.559 (Source tray distance) ** Added 1 cm at superior end.

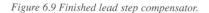

Figure 6.9 Finished lead step compensator.

Table 6.3 Table of point dose factor (No compensator.)
1) Anterior (No Compensator)

Point#	OF × TMR	Point Dose Factor
sup.1	1.028×0.931	0.957
2	1.028×0.875	0.9
3	1.028×0.828	0.851
4	1.028×0.786	0.808
center	1.028×0.762	0.783
inf.1	1.028×0.731	0.751
2	1.028×0.710	0.73
3	1.028×0.695	0.714
4	1.028×0.683	0.702

Point dose factor = Output factor × TMR Output factor for $9 \times 26 \ cm^2 = 1.028 \ cGy/MU$

2) Posterior (No compensator)

Point #	OF × TMR	Point Dose Factor
sup.1	*1.028 × .762*	*0.783*
2	"	"
3	"	"
4	"	"
Center	"	"
Inf.1	"	"
2	"	"
3	"	"
4	"	"

Table 6.4 Table of normalized dose to mid depth for no compensation verses compensation.

1) No compensation

Point #	AP Dose Factor	PA Dose Factor	Total Dose Factor	Normalized to Center	Dose
Sup.1	*0.957*	*0.783*	*1.74*	*111.1*	*4444*
2	*0.9*	"	*1.683*	*107.5*	*4300*
3	*0.851*	"	*1.634*	*104.3*	*4172*
4	*0.808*	"	*1.591*	*101.6*	*4064*
center	*0.783*	"	*1.566*	*100*	*4000*
inf.1	*0.751*	"	*1.534*	*98*	*3920*
2	*0.73*	"	*1.513*	*96.6*	*3864*
3	*0.714*	"	*1.497*	*95.6*	*3824*
4	*0.702*	"	*1.485*	*94.8*	*3792*

2) With compensation

Point #	AP Dose Factor × Comp. Factor	PA Dose Factor	Total Dose Factor	Normalized to Center	Dose
Sup.1	*0.957×0.762=0.729*	*0.783*	*1.51*	*100*	*4000*
2	*0.9×0.792=0.713*	"	*1.5*	*99.3*	*3972*
3	*0.851×0.856=0.728*	"	*1.515*	*100*	*4000*
4	*0.808×0.89=0.719*	"	*1.5*	*99.3*	*3972*
center	*0.783×0.925=0.724*	"	*1.51*	*100*	*4000*
inf.1	*0.751×0.962=0.722*	"	*1.534*	*100*	*4000*
2	*0.73×1=0.73*	"	*1.51*	*100*	*4000*
3	*0.714×1=0.714*	"	*1.5*	*99.3*	*3972*
4	*0.702×1=0.702*	"	*1.49*	*98.7*	*3948*

As can be seen from the tables above, the dose varies from 94.8% to 111.1% when there is no compensation. With compensation, the dose varies from 98.7% to 100%. When plotted on a graph, the dose variation is made more obvious with the high dose at the superior end and low dose at the inferior end when there is no compensation. This is due to missing tissue at the superior end and added tissue at the inferior end. With compensation, the dose variation is small.

The difference between no compensation and compensation can be further illustrated with isodose charts plotted for no compensation verses compensation.

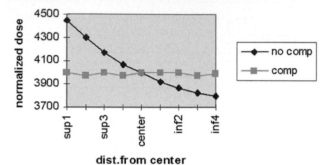

Figure 6.10 Dose at mid depth line with no compensation and with compensation.

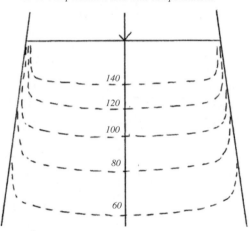

Figure 6.11 Isodose chart for 9 × 26 cm² at 100 cm SAD.

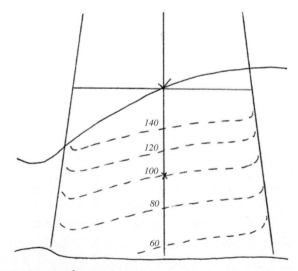

Figure 6.12 Isodose chart for 9 × 26 cm² at 100 cm SAD on patient.

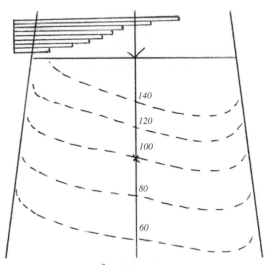

Figure 6.13 *Compensated isodose chart for 9 × 26 cm² at 100 cm SAD.*

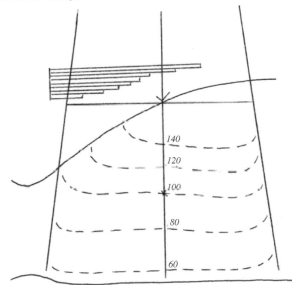

Figure 6.14 *Compensated isodose chart for 9 × 26 cm² at 100 cm SAD on patient.*

VII. FILM COMPENSATOR FOR SUPERFICIAL X-RAY TREATMENT UNIT

Some superficial skin lesions are treated by superficial X-Ray treatment unit *(70 -100 kV)*. Compensation may sometimes be required due to irregular contour such as the nose region. Compensation here is not for missing tissue as was the case with higher energy units. Here the purpose for compensation is for the variation in surface distances from the target of the X-Ray tube. Due to the short treatment distance *(20 cm)*, dose rate varies significantly with small differences in distance.

A lead facemask is fabricated for the patient to shield the surrounding normal tissue. A hole is made in the lead facemask to aligned with the lesion. A hollow wax platform is built on the lead facemask over the treated area. The platform serves as a platform for the treatment applicator and as a platform for the attachment of the film compensator.

Using a formulator, a contour of the treatment site is taken. This is done by placing the formulator on the platform over the treatment site and gently pushing down the fine metal rods until they just touch the skin. A contour is obtained by taking a tracing from the bottom of the rods.

The variations in the SSD to the skin are recorded and the normalized inverse square correction and their reciprocal factors are tabulated as shown in Table 9.7.

On a square graph paper, the transmission factors are labeled on the vertical scale and the field widths are labeled on the horizontal scale. The reciprocal factors are then plotted on the graph. The number of film strips required are calculated and these are drawn on the graph. The film strips are de-magnified to the platform treatment distance where they will be mounted.

The film strips are cut to the size calculated for each strip. They are taped together, making sure each strip is off set by the horizontal distance from the field center as calculated. The field center is drawn on the compensator and this center is aligned to the center of the platform. The compensator is then mounted on the platform. *(The mounting of the compensator to the platform must allow for the removal of the compensator for visualization of the lesion during set up if necessary.)*

The transmission factor of the finished compensator is measured and this factor is used in the calculation for the timer setting for treatment.

Example: *Calculation of timer setting*

Total prescribed dose = 4500 cGy in 15 treatments.
Data: Applicator = 7.5 cm circle, The air dose rate = 292 cGy/min, The PSF for the cut out = 1.124, The stand off = 2.7 cm, Timer correction = -0.02 min , and Transmission factor through film compensator = 0.951

$$Timmer \quad Setting = \left(\frac{4500}{15 \times 292 \times \left(\dfrac{20}{22.7}\right)^2 \times 1.124 \times 0.951} \right) - 0.02 = 1.22 \quad min$$

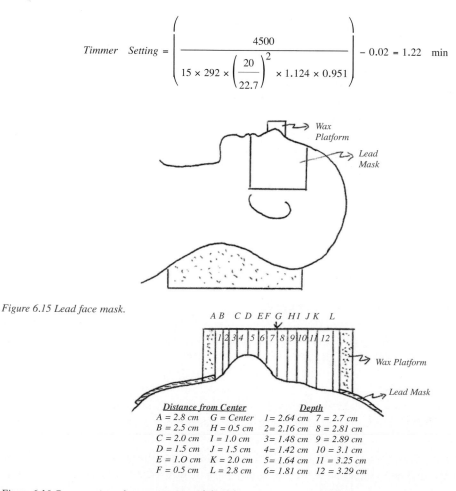

Figure 6.15 Lead face mask.

Distance from Center		Depth	
A = 2.8 cm	G = Center	1= 2.64 cm	7 = 2.7 cm
B = 2.5 cm	H = 0.5 cm	2= 2.16 cm	8 = 2.81 cm
C = 2.0 cm	I = 1.0 cm	3= 1.48 cm	9 = 2.89 cm
D = 1.5 cm	J = 1.5 cm	4= 1.42 cm	10 = 3.1 cm
E = 1.O cm	K = 2.0 cm	5= 1.64 cm	11 = 3.25 cm
F = 0.5 cm	L = 2.8 cm	6= 1.81 cm	12 = 3.29 cm

Figure 6.16 Cross section of treatment site with lead face mask and wax platform.

Table 6.5 Table of normalized inverse square factors.

Distance along Width of Field (cm)	SSD+ Stand Off	Normalized Inverse Square Factor
2.8 (left)	22.64	*0.945
2.5	22.16	0.905
2	21.48	0.85
1.5	21.42	0.846
1	21.64	0.864
0.5	21.81	0.877
0 (center)	22.7	0.95
0.5	22.81	0.959
1	22.89	0.966
1.5	23.1	0.983
2	23.25	0.997
2.8 (right)	23.29	1

$$*\left(\frac{22.64}{23.29}\right)^2 = 0.945$$

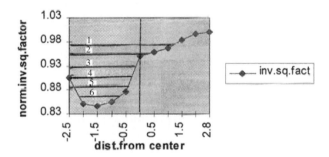

Figure 6.17 Normalized inverse square factors.

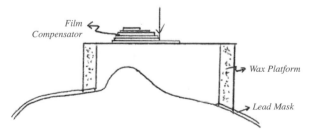

Figure 6.18 Cross section of treatment site with film compensator in place on platform.

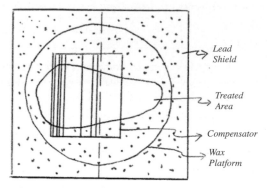

Figure 6.19 Treatment site with cut out and compensator in place.

Table 6.6 Table of actual width of film strips at platform.

Strip #	Width of Strip	De-magnifed Width[*]
1	4.1	3.5
2	2.8	2.4
3	2.5	2.2
4	2.2	1.9
5	1.8	1.6
6	1	0.9

[*]*Film compensator is to be mounted on the wax platform that is 20 cm from source. The greatest compensation distance is 23.29 cm. Therefore the de-magnification factor is 0.86.*

VIII. PUBLICATIONS OF INTERESTS

1. Beck GG, McGonnagle WJ, Sullivan CA: Use of styrofoam block cutter to make tissue-equivalent compensators. Radiology 100:694, 1971

2. Boge RJ, Edland RW, Matthes DC: Tissue compensators for megavoltage radiotherapy fabricated from hollowed styrofoam filled with wax. Radiology 111:193,1974

3. Ellis F, Hall EJ, Oliver R: A compensator for variations in tissue thickness for high energy beam. Br J Radiol 32:421, 1959.

4. Hall EJ, Oliver R : The use of standard isodose distributions with high energy radiation beams- the accuracy of a compensator technique in correcting for body contours. Br J Radiol 34:43,1961

5. Johns HE, Cunningham JR: The Physics of Radiology, 4th ed Springfield, IL, Charles C Thomas, 1983 pages 389-390.

6. Khan FM, Moore VC, Burns DJ: An apparatus for the construction of irregular surface compensators for use in radiotherapy. Radiology 90:593,1968.

7. Khan FM, Moore VC, Burns DJ: The construction of compensators for cobalt teletherapy. Radiology 96:187, 1970.

8. Khan FM, Williamson JF, Sewchand W, Kim TH: Basic data for dosage calculation and compensation. Int J Radiat Oncol Biol Phys 6:745,1980.

9. Khan FM: The Physics of Radiation Therapy, Baltimore, williams and Wilkins, 1984 pages 261-267.

10. Kuchnir FT, Myrianthopoulos LC, Losin E: Computer aided construction and quantitative evaluation of missing tissue compensators. Radiother Oncol 17:239-247, 1990

11. Moyer RF, McElroy WR, O'Brien JE, et al: A surface bolus material for high energy photon and electron therapy. Radiology 146:531, 1983

12. Reinstein LE: New approaches to tissue compensation in radiation oncology. In Purdy JA, ed: Advances in Radiation Oncology Physics: Dosimetry, Treatment Planning, and Brachytherapy. New York, American Institute of Physics, 1992

13. Renner WD: Tissue compensators. J Am Assoc Med Dosim 7:4-8, 1982 Smith RM, Galvin JM, Needhan M, et al: Computer aided design and fabrication of electron and photon compensators [Abstract]. Int J Radiat Oncol Biol Phys 17(Suppl):206, 1989

14. Sewchand W, Bautro N, Scott RM: Basic data of tissue-equivalent compensators for 4MV X-Rays. Int J Radiat Oncol Phys 6:327,1980.

15. Smith RM, Galvin JM, Needhan M, et al: Computer aided design and fabrication of electron and photon compensators [Abstract]. Int J Radiat Oncol Biol Phys 17(Suppl):206, 1989

16. Spicka J, Fleury K, Powers W: Polyethylene-lead tissue compensators for megavoltage radiotherapy. Med Dosim 13:25, 1988

17. Weeks KJ, Fraass BA, Hurchins KM: Gypsum mixtures for compensator construction. Med Phys 15:410, 1988

—— *CHAPTER 7* ——

Isodose Distribution Plans

I. INTRODUCTION

An isodose distribution plan is obtained from a summation of isodose charts placed at optimal positions to achieve the desired dose distribution. The desired dose distribution is a uniform dose around the target volume and minimum dose outside the target volume.

The choice of isodose charts and their optimal placements are dependent on the size, depth and position of the target volume within the patient.

II. ISODOSE CHART

An isodose chart is a chart of isodose lines or isodose curves having the same percent values. These isodose curves are in regular decrements with increase depth and lateral distance from the central axis. The decrease in depth dose with increase depth is due to attenuation and inverse square. The decrease in dose with increase lateral distance from the central axis is due to geometric penumbra and reduced lateral scatter.

The characteristics of isodose charts are altered by several factors. These factors are beam energy, beam type, field size, source to skin distance *(SSD)*, source size and collimation. The depth dose increases with increase in beam energy *(compare the ^{60}Co and 10 MV photon isodose charts.)* With increase in field size, the depth dose increases due to increase in scatter. The depth dose increases with increase in SSD as explained under the section of percentage depth dose. With increase in source size, the geometric penumbra is increased. Finally, the isodoses are altered by different collimation systems and filters placed in the collimator. Filters that alter the isodoses are beam flattening filter, wedge filter, compensating filter and shielding blocks.

Beam type such as the electron beam produces isodoses that are very different from that of photon beam. More on electron beam in the next chapter.

III. NORMALIZATION OF ISODOSE CHART

SSD isodose charts are plotted with the 100% normalized at along central axis. The isodose curves are plotted at regular decrements from D_{max}. These SSD isodose charts are used for generating SSD plans.

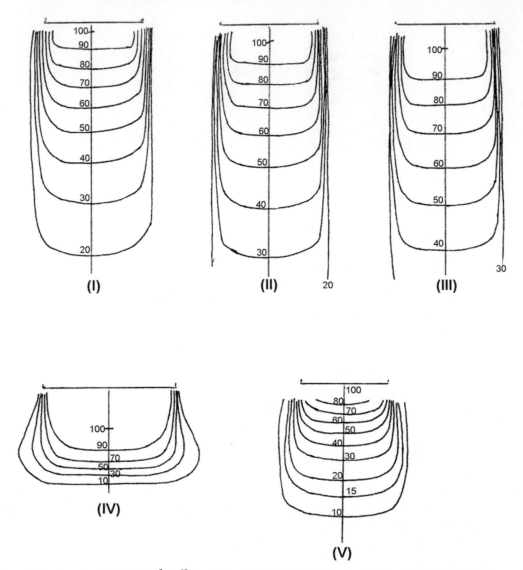

Figure 7.1 Isodose charts 10 × 10 cm² (I) ⁶⁰Co at 80 cm SSD, (II) (6 MV photons) at 100 cm SSD, (III) (10 MV photons) at 100 cm SSD, (IV) 18 MeV electrons at 100 cm SSD, (V) 250kV X-Ray Thoraus Filter at 50 cm SSD.

SAD isodose charts are plotted with the 100% normalized at a chosen depth at isocenter. The isodose curves are at regular decrements from the normalized point with increasing depth and at regular increments from the normalized point with decreasing depth. Due to the normalization at a chosen depth, each beam with a different axis depth requires an isodose chart normalized to that depth.

IV. WEDGED ISODOSE CHART

A wedged isodose chart is a chart of wedged *(tilted)* isodose lines having the same percent values. The tilt of the isodose lines is due to the differential absorption of the radiation through the different thickness of the wedge. The tilt is reflected in the thin end of the wedge having a higher depth dose than the thick end of the wedge. The angle of tilt is dependent on the slope of the wedge filter. This tilt is defined as the wedge angle that is the angle between the 50% isodose line and a line perpendicular to the central axis. Some centers define the wedge angle as the angle between the isodose line at 10 cm depth and a line perpendicular to the central axis.

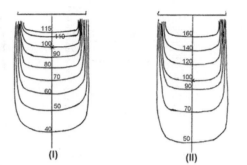

Figure 7.2 Normalized isodose chart from ^{60}Co at 80 cm SAD. (I) Normalized at 5 cm (II) Normalized at 10 cm.

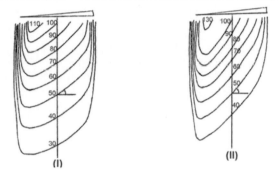

Figure 7.3 Wedged isodose chart from ^{60}Co at 80cm SSD. (I) 30° wedge (II) 45° wedge.

V. NORMALIZATION OF WEDGED ISODOSE CHART

SSD wedged isodose chart may be normalized to 100% at D_{max} at central axis or normalized to 100% times the wedge factor at D_{max} at central axis. If the normalization is of the former, then the wedge factor must be taken into account in the calculation of timer or monitor unit setting. If the normalization is of the latter, the wedge factor is already included in the plan and therefore need not be included in the calculation of treatment time or monitor unit setting.

For SAD wedged isodose chart, the isocenter depth along central axis is normalized to 100% or to 100% times the wedge factor.

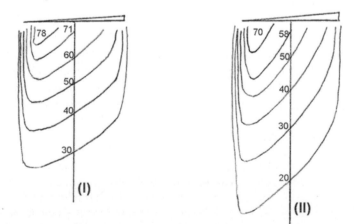

Figure 7.4 Wedged isodose chart from ^{60}Co at 80 cm SSD. (I) Normalized to 30° factor of 71% at D_{max} (wedge factor is 0.714). (II) Normalized to 45° wedge factor of 58% at D_{max} (wedge factor is 0.583).

VI. HINGE ANGLE

The hinge angle is the angle between two wedged fields that would yield the optimum distribution. The optimum wedge to use is calculated from the equation,where ϕ is the hinge angle and θ is the optimum wedge for the given hinge angle.

$$\theta = 90°-(\phi/2)$$

Example:

The hinge angle is 90°. The optimum wedge angle $\theta =90°-(90°/2) = 45°$ wedge. In practice it is more complicated than this. Factors such as missing or added tissue, position and shape of target volume, treatment unit, etc play a major role in the selection of the wedge to be used.

VII. MANUAL PLANNING

Athough all treatment planning departments have computers to generate isodose distribution plans, it is good practice to have some experience with manual planning. Due to its importance, many radiation therapy training centers teach manual planning. It is a drawing of isodose lines, summing the intersecting lines and joining the summed isodose lines for the final plan. Some examples will be given here.

I. SSD Plans

i) Single field

For the single field, the SSD isodose chart is placed on the anterior surface of the skin and the isodose lines are traced within the patient's contour as shown in Figure 7.5 (I).

ii) Opposed fields

For the opposed fields, the anterior field is traced as described for the single field. The posterior field is traced by directing the isodose chart from the posterior skin surface. The anterior and posterior intersecting lines are summed and joined for the final plan as shown in Figure 7.5 (II &III).

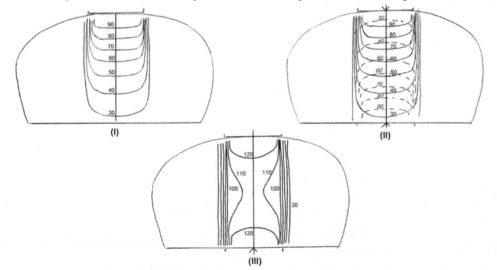

Figure 7.5 Isodose distribution from $^{60}Co 10 \times 10\ cm^2$ open field at 80 cm SSD. (I) single field (II) Anterior-posterior fields superimposed (III) Summed anterior-posterior fields.

iii) Missing and added tissue correction

Missing and added tissue in manual planning is corrected by the isodose shift method as shown in Figure 7.6.

Assume that X-Y is the patient surface and the radiation beam from a ^{60}Co treatment unit 10 × 10 cm^2 field size at 80 cm SSD is incident at point (a). Draw a central line *(central axis)* vertically from point (a) into the contour and a horizontal line H-H1 through point (a). Divergent lines at 1cm apart are drawn on each side of the central axis line. Place the 10 × 10 cm^2 isodose chart beneath the patient contour and lining the central axis of the isodose chart to the central axis incident at point (a) in the patient contour. Line the width of the isodose chart to the line H-H1. Mark the isodose values along the central axis.

For the side of the missing tissue, move the isodose chart towards the patient surface by 2/3 of the gap between the surface and the H-H1 line. Repeat this for every divergent line. For each 2/3 move, mark the isodose values along the respective divergent lines. For the side of the added tissue the reverse is done. The corrected isodose lines are joined to yield the final isodose distribution for the missing and added tissue contour.

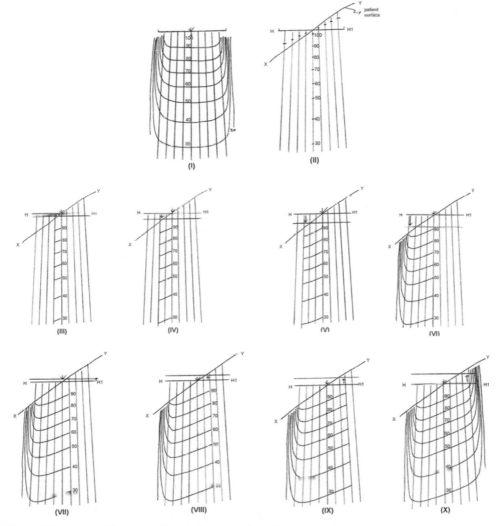

Figure 7.6 Isodose shift method for missing and added tissue correction.

iv) Four fields

The anterior-posterior opposed fields are first joined and summed as described earlier. The same procedure is repeated for the left and right lateral fields making sure the missing or added tissue is corrected as described earlier. The summed anterior-posterior plan is superimposed onto the summed left-right lateral plan and the final four field plan is summed as shown in Figure 7.7.

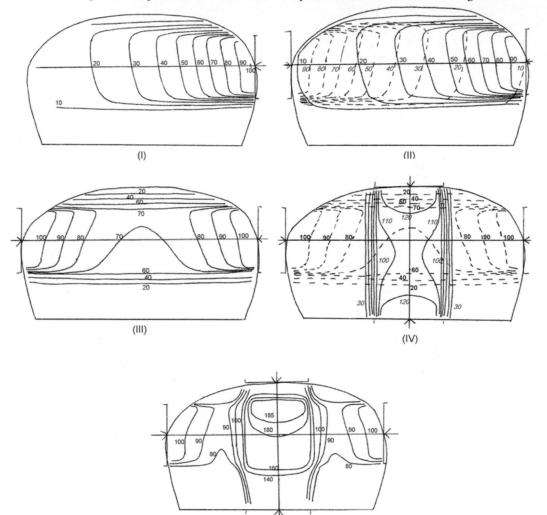

Figure 7.7 Steps in four field summation for a four field plan. (I) Left lateral field using 10 × 10 cm² at 80 cm SSD after correcting for missing and added tissue. (II) Left and right lateral fields superimposed. (III) Summed left-right lateral fields. (IV) Summed anterior-posterior fields superimposed over summed left-right lateral fields. (V) Final four field plan.

v) Three fields

The anterior field is traced as described for the single field. The right posterior oblique or the left posterior oblique field is next traced onto the anterior field using a different pattern line for the isodose lines so that the anterior field and the oblique field isodose lines can be easily recognizable. The other posterior oblique field is traced on using yet another pattern line. The three fields are summed to yield the final three field plan as shown in Figure 7.8.

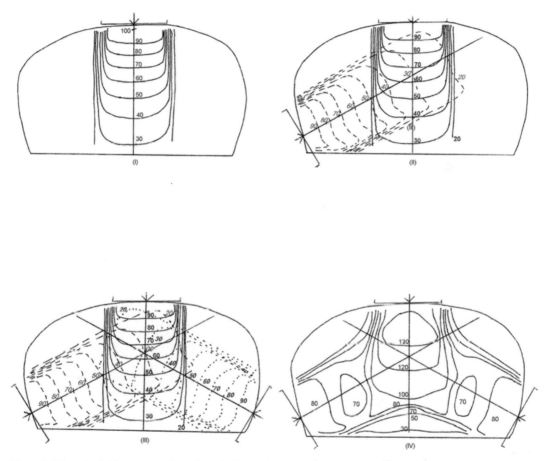

Figure 7.8 Steps in field summation for a three field plan 10 × 10 cm² at 80cm SSD ⁶⁰Co. (I) Anterior field (II) Anterior and right posterior oblique fields superimposed. (III) Anterior, left posterior oblique and right posterior oblique fields superimposed. (IV) Final three field plan.

vi) Wedged fields

For the wedged field plan, the appropriate wedged isodose chart is required. For the example shown here *(parotid tumor)*, the 30° wedge isodose chart is placed over the contour. In order to ensure that the target volume is adequately covered, the field width *(edge)* should be at least 0.5 cm passed the target contour to account for penumbra. The isodose lines are traced after correcting for missing and added tissue. The second field is placed in the manner as shown in the example. The isodose lines are traced as described for the previous field. The fields are summed to yield the final wedged field plan.

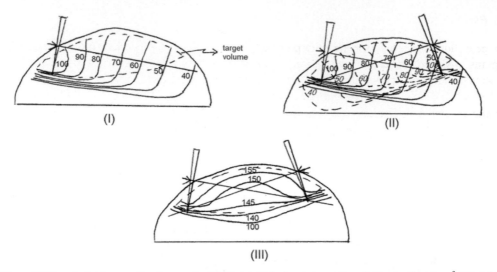

Figure 7.9 Steps in field summation for a wedged field plan.(I) Left anterior oblique field using 7 × 10 cm² 30° right wedge. (II) Left anterior and left posterior oblique fields superimposed. (III) Final wedged field plan.

vii) Weighted fields

For the plans requiring weighting, weighted isodose charts are required. For the example shown here, the weighting is 80% from the anterior field and 100% from the posterior field. For the anterior field, a 80% weighted isodose chart is required. The 80% weighted isodose chart has 80% at D_{max} instead of the normal 100% at D_{max}. The anterior field is traced using the 80% weighted isodose chart. The posterior field is next traced using the 100% weighted isodose chart. The two fields are summed to yield the final weighted plan.

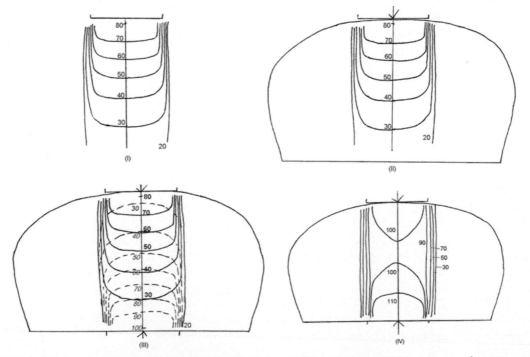

Figure 7.10 Steps in field summation for a weighted field plan. (I) Weighted isodose chart for 10 × 10 cm² at 80 cm SSD ^{60}Co (D_{max} weighted at 80%.) (II) 80% weighted anterior field. (III) 80% weighted anterior field superimposed over 100% weighted posterior field. (IV) Final weighted field plan.

II. SAD Plans

The procedures described for the SSD plans apply to the SAD plans with two differences. For SAD plans, SAD isodose charts are required. For each field with a different depth to isocenter, the corresponding SAD chart normalized to the same depth must be used for that field. The second difference is that the summed plan is normalized to the isocenter being 100%.

For the weighted SAD plans, weighted SAD isodose charts are required. Weighting for SAD isodose charts is at the depth of isocenter and not at D_{max} as for the weighted SSD isodose charts.

i) Opposed fields

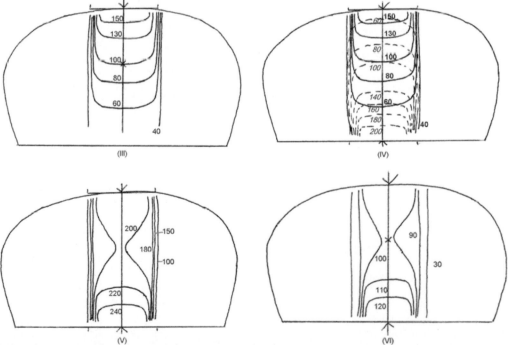

Figure 7.11 Steps in anterior-posterior opposed SAD plan. (I) Normalized isodose chart 10 × 10 cm² at 80 cm SAD at 8 cm depth. (II) Normalized isodose chart 10 × 10 cm² at 80 cm SAD at 12 cm depth. (III) Anterior field at 80 cm SAD at 8 cm depth 10 × 10 cm². (IV) Anterior-posterior SAD fields superimposed. (V) Summed anterior-posterior fields. (VI) Normalized summed anterior-posterior field plan.

ii) Four Field

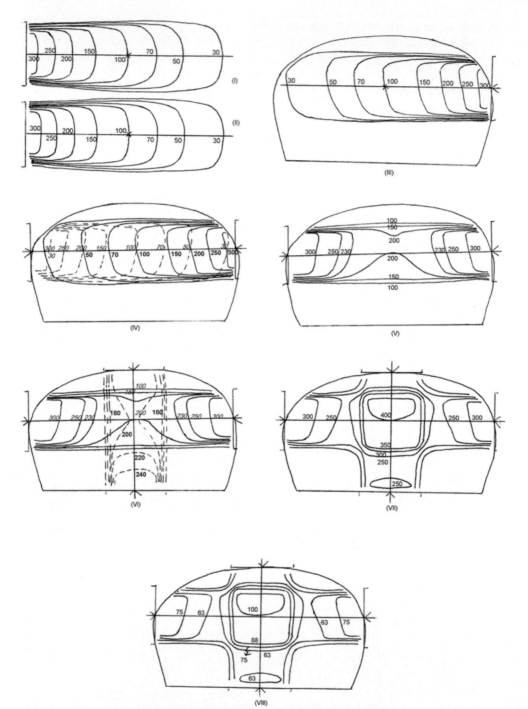

Figure 7.12 Steps in four-field SAD plan. (I) Normalized isodose chart 10 × 10 cm² at 80 cm SAD at 16.5 cm depth. (II) Normalized isodose chart 10 × 10 cm² at 80 cm SAD at 17cm depth. (III) Left lateral field at 80 cm SAD at 16.5 cm depth 10 × 10 cm². (IV) Left and right lateral fields at 80 cm SAD superimposed. (V) Summed left-right SAD fields. (VI) Summed anterior-posterior fields superimposed over left-right fields. (VII) Summed four fields. (VIII) Normalized summed four field plan.

iii) Three fields

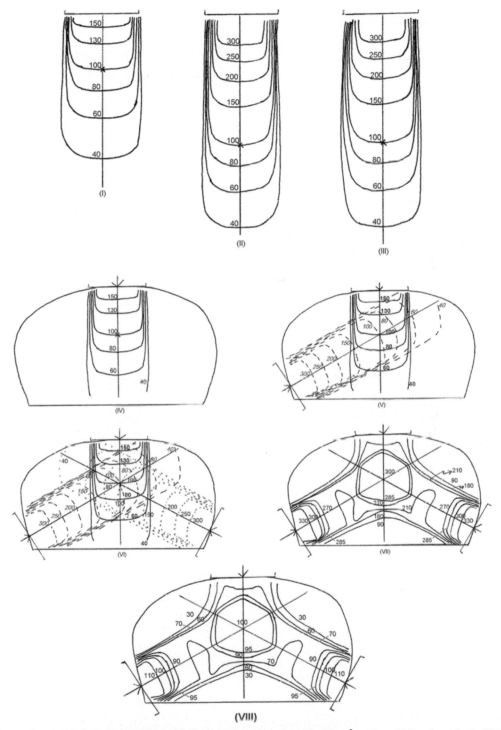

Figure 7.13 Steps in three field SAD plan. (I) Normalized isodose chart 10 × 10 cm² at 80 cm SAD at 8 cm depth. (II) Normalized isodose chart 10 × 10 cm² at 80 cm SAD at 18.5 cm depth.(III) Normalized isodose chart 10 × 10 cm² at 80 cmS SAD at 18 cm depth. (IV) Anterior field at 80 cm SAD at 8 cm depth. (V) Anterior and right posterior oblique SAD fields superimposed. (VI) Anterior, right and left posterior oblique SAD fields superimposed. (VII) Summed three fields. (VIII) Normalized summed three field plan.

iv) Wedged fields

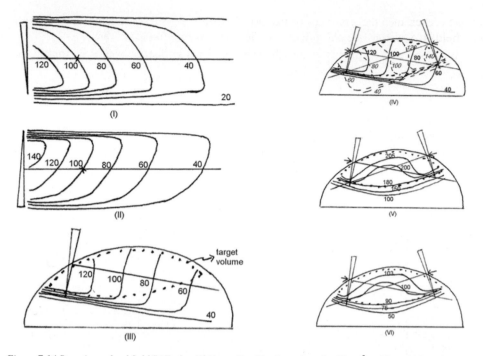

Figure 7.14 Steps in wedged field SAD plan (I) Normalized isodose chart 7×10 cm² at 80 cm SAD at 5 cm depth 30° wedge. (II) Normalized isodose chart 7×10 cm² at 80 cm SAD at 6 cm depth 30° wedge. (III) Left anterior oblique field at 80 cm SAD at 5 cm depth. (IV) Left anterior and left posterior oblique SAD fields superimposed. (V) Summed wedged fields. (VI) Normalized summed wedged field plan.

v) Weighted fields

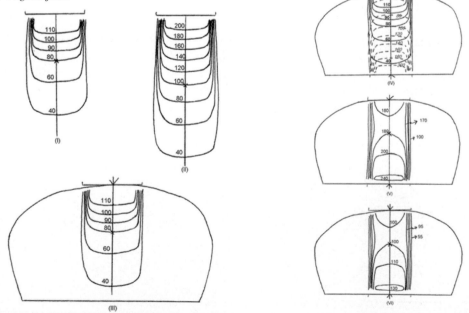

Figure 7.15 Steps in weighted opposed field SAD plan. (I) 80% normalized isodose chart 10×10 cm² at 80 cm SAD at 8 cm depth. (II) 100% normalized isodose chart 10×10 cm² at 80 cm SAD at 12 cm depth. (III) Anterior SAD field at 8 cm depth. (IV) Anterior-posterior SAD fields superimposed. (V) Summed anterior-posterior SAD fields. (VI) Normalized summed anterior-posterior SAD field plan.

VIII. FACTORS AFFECTING ISODOSE DISTRIBUTION

As described earlier, the characteristics of isodose charts are altered by several factors such as beam energy, field size, wedge, etc. As a result, the isodose distribution is altered.

Given in this section are examples to show the resulting isodose distribution plans for changes in beam energy, field size, weighting and wedges.

A. Beam energy

The example here is for a three field plan. One is a ^{60}Co beam plan and the other is a 10 MV photon beam plan. There is very little difference in the target volume coverage but the plan from the ^{60}Co beams deliver higher doses to the left and right posterior oblique fields. This is a result of the lower depth dose from the ^{60}C0 beams verses the 10 MV photon beams. In order to deliver the same tumor dose at isocenter, the given dose or applied dose for the ^{60}Cobeam is higher.

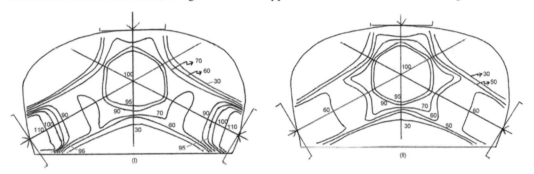

Figure 7.16 Comparison of three field SAD plan from ^{60}Co and 10 MV photon beam). (I) ^{60}Co plan 80 cm SAD. (II) 10 MV photon beam) plan 100 cm SAD.

B. Field size

Success of radiation treatment is due in part to delivering adequate radiation dose to the target volume. To achieve the adequate dose, there must be adequate field coverage. Inadequate coverage results in geographic miss and regeneration of the cancer. Over coverage results in possible over dosage to normal healthy tissue and increases complications.

In this example, the first plan shows inadequate coverage of the target volume due to the inadequate field sizes. In the second plan field sizes increased from *8× 8 cm²* to *10 × 10 cm²*. Coverage of the target volume in the second plan is adequate.

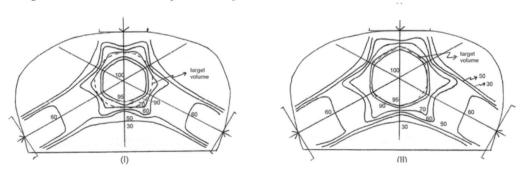

Figure 7.17 Comparison of three field (10 MV photon) 100 cm SAD plan from two different field sizes. (I) Plan from 8× 8 cm² field size.(II) Plan from 10 × 10 cm² field size.

C. Weighting

In the example, the weight reduction for the lateral fields reduces the dose to the lateral tissues from 60% to 50%. In some sites or beam arrangements, the reduction could be more. Coverage of the target volume in both cases is the same.

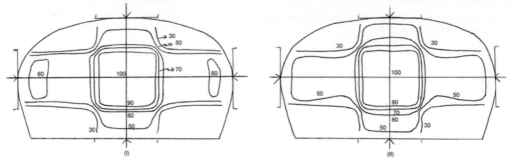

Figure 7.18 Comparison of unweighted and weighted four field plan for 10 MV photon beam at 100 cm SAD 10 × 10 cm². (I) Equal weight. (II) Unequal weight, Anterior-posterior weight of 100% at isocenter and left-right lateral weight of 80% at isocenter.

D. Wedges

For sites where there is severe tissue deficit, wedges may be used to compensate. The purpose here is to provide a uniform dose to the target volume. As shown in the example, the dose variation in the open field plan is severe. The target volume is covered by the 80% isodose line and increases to 115% near the surface where there is greatest tissue deficit. For the wedged plan, the target volume is covered by the 95% isodose line and increases to only 103% near the surface.

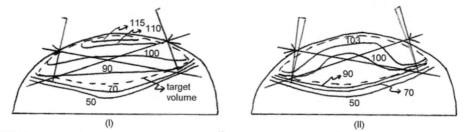

Figure 7.19 Comparison of open and wedged field plan from ⁶⁰Co at 80 cm SAD 7 × 10 cm². (I) open fields. (II) 30° wedged fields.

In some tissue deficit situations, the choice of inappropriate wedges may be too steep for the correction. As shown in the example, lateral opposed open fields result in higher dose to the anterior surface. Lateral opposed 30° wedged fields result in higher dose to the thin end of the wedges. Therefore the 30° wedges are too steep for this situation. To correct for the missing and added tissue in this example, a 15° wedge would be ideal. If 15° wedge is not available, a combination of open and 30° wedge weighted at 50% for each would approximately yield a 15° wedge.

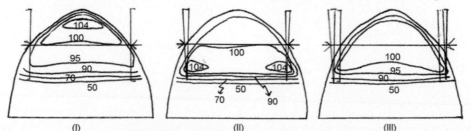

Figure 7.20 Comparison of open, 30° wedge and open and 30° wedge plan for ⁶⁰Co 6 × 6 cm² at 80 cm SAD. (I) Open fields. (II) 30° wedged fields. (III) Open and 30° wedged fields weighted equally to create 15° wedge.

IX. PUBLICATIONS OF INTERESTS

1. Cohen M. Martin SM (eds) : Atlas of Radiation dose distributions, Vol II, Multi-field isodose charts. Vienna, International Atomic Energy Agency, 1966.

2. Khan FM: The Physics of Radiation Therapy, Baltimore, Williams and Wilkins, 1984 chapter 11.

3. Sterling TD, Perry H, Katz L: Automation of radiation treatment planning. IV. Derivation of a mathematical expression for the percent depth dose surface of Cobalt-60 beams and visualization of multiple field dose distribution. Br J Radiol 37:544, 1964.

4. Tapley N: Parallel opposing portal technique. Fletcher GH, (ed): Test book of radiotherapy, 3rd ed. Philadelphia, Lea and Febiger, 1980 page 60.

5. Van de Geijn J: A simple wedge filter technique for Cobalt-60 teletherapy. Br J Radiol 35:710, 1962.

6. Webster EW, Tsien KC (eds): Atlas of radiation dose distributions, vol I, single field isodose charts. Vienna, International Atomic Energy Agency, 1965.

—— *CHAPTER 8* ——

Electron Beam Therapy

I. INTRODUCTION

The most useful characteristic of electron beam is its rapid dose fall off compared to the photon beam. This advantage makes the electron beam useful is treating some shallow tumors such as chest wall, skin tumors, head and neck lymph node boost, etc. The desired tumor dose is delivered to the tumor without excessive dose to underlying normal tissues. The choice of the electron energy depends on the tumor depth.

In the past, electron beams were generated from the Betatron and the Van de Graaff generator. Today, electron beams are generated from Linear Accelerators. The electrons are accelerated in the Linear Accelerator and exit as a pencil beam that scans across a treatment volume or the accelerated electrons are scattered through a scattering foil to produce a broad beam that is then flattened through an electron beam flattening filter.

Collimation of electron beam is achieved via fixed electron cones/applicators or via variable trimmers or jaws. Cerrobend insert/cutout provides for irregular treatment field shape.

II. CHARACTERISTICS OF ELECTRON BEAM

Figures 8.1, 8.2, 8.3, and 8.4 display the characteristics of the electron beam. From the diagrams, one may note the following.

A. *The electron beam depth dose falls rapidly compared to the photon beam depth dose. This is useful clinically in treating shallow tumors to achieve sufficient dose to the tumor without excessive dose to the underlying normal tissues.*

B. *Due to the high surface dose, the electron beam does not have skin sparing property. This property could be an advantage or disadvantage depending on the treatment site.*

C. *The surface dose increases with electron energy. The range of the surface dose is around 75% to 90% of the dose at D_{max}.*

D. *Depth dose increases with increase electron energy.*

E. *Electron beam isodose shows the characteristic isodose "bulge". This is due to side scattering of the electrons in the medium.*

F. *The electron depth dose chart shows "tail" at the lower end of the depth dose. This is due to Bremsstrahlung radiation.*

G. *The depth of the 80% is approximately one third the energy.*

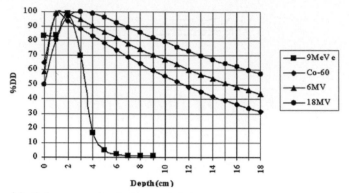

Figure 8.1 Comparison of depth dose curves for electrons and photons.

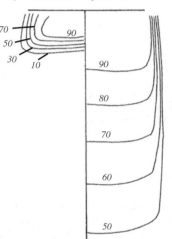

Figure 8.2 Isodose curves for 6 MeV electron and 6 MV photon Beam.

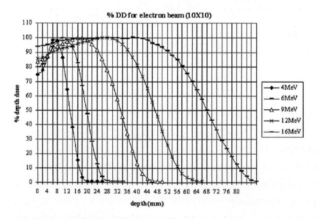

Figure 8.3 Depth dose curves for electron beams 10 × 10 cm^2 cone.

III. ELECTRON OUTPUT FACTORS

The output factors for each cone and for each electron energy must be measured. These output factors are normalized to the output factor for the 10 × 10 cm^2 cone that is set at 1 cGy/MU.

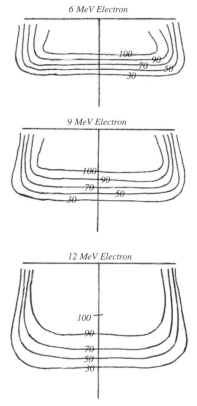

Figure 8.4 Isodose curves for 6, 9, and 12 MeV electron beam.

Table 8.1 Table of electron output factors (cGy/MU) and cone sizes in cm².

MeV	4×4	6×6	10×10	15×15	20×20	25×25
4	0.969	0.976	1	1.021	1.056	1.115
6	0.978	0.998	1	1.004	1.026	1.069
9	0.966	1.03	1	0.921	0.904	0.908
12	0.954	1.012	1	0.958	0.937	0.913
16	1.021	1.057	1	0.919	0.871	0.836

IV. SHIELDING

Irregular treatment fields are sometimes required to protect normal tissues or critical organs near the tumor. Such irregular treatment fields are shaped with lead cutout from layers of lead sheets or fabricated from cerrobend inserts.

For small treatment fields or low electron energies *(below 8 MeV)*, lead cut out is the choice because the cutout better conforms to the body contour. The thickness of lead required is electron energy dependent. If cutouts are used to shield internal structures such as the teeth and gums in the treatment of lip lesions, such cutouts should have a suitable thickness of bolus material such as wax coating or dental compound to cover the shield. The bolus material absorbs the electron backscatter from the lead.

For large treatment fields or higher electron energies, cerrobend inserts are preferred because of the weight of the cutout on the patient and the difficulty of molding the lead to the body contour. These cerrobend inserts are placed inside the appropriate treatment cones for treatment.

If a fifth to a quarter of the field is shielded, the output factor for the lead cutout or cerrobend insert should be measured.

Shielding generally reduces the transmitted dose under the shielding to less than 5%. For high energies, the transmitted dose may be higher due to Bremsstrahlung radiation. The thickness of lead required is approximately 0.5 mm for every 1 MeV

Table 8.2 Table of lead shield thickness for electrons.

4 MeV	2 mm lead	12 MeV	6 mm lead
6 MeV	2 mm lead	16 MeV	8 mm lead
9 MeV	4 mm lead		

V. TREATMENT AT EXTENDED DISTANCES

Occasionally extended treatment distance *(greater than 100 cm SSD)* is necessary due to the proximity of the electron cone to the patient surface. Unlike photon beam output, electron beam output cannot be corrected by simple inverse square correction. Extended distance factors should be measured for the SSD used (Table 8.3). These factors are then incorporated into the MU calculation.

Example:

Total tumor dose = 3000 cGy to the 90% isodose in 15 treatments. (16 MeV electrons)

Therefore the total given dose (applied dose) = (3000 × 100)/90 = 3333 cGy

Data: Collimator setting = 15 × 15 cm², SSD = 110 cm, Output factor = 0.919 cGy/MU, and

Extended distance factor = 0.823, Therefore:

$$MU \; setting \; = \; (3333)/(15 \times 0.919 \times 0.823) = 294 \; MU$$

VI. OBLIQUE INCIDENCE (MISSING TISSUE CORRECTION)

The isodose lines generally follow the contour surface if the surface is not steep. The isodose shift is 1:1 for the air gap. However, if the slope is steep, inverse square and scatter correction must be incorporated in the isodose correction.

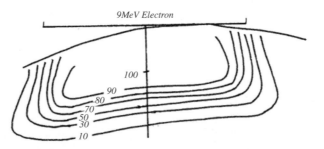

Figure 8.5 Dose distribution for 9 MeV electron corrected for oblique incidence. Note the decrease in deptdose on the side of the air gap.

Table 8.3 Distance correction factors.

Cone(cm²)	SSD(cm)	4 MeV	6 MeV	9 MeV	12 MeV	16 MeV
6×6	100	1	1	1		1
	102	0.945	0.953	0.946	0.956	0.936
	104	0.892	0.905	0.893	0.911	0.892
	106	0.838	0.861	0.847	0.875	0.848
	108	0.784	0.815	0.798	0.832	0.804
	110	0.734	0.776	0.761	0.797	0.766
10×10	100	1	1	1	1	1
	102	0.953	0.952	0.953	0.958	0.959
	104	0.904	0.911	0.914	0.92	0.918
	106	0.866	0.872	0.873	0.883	0.873
	108	0.817	0.832	0.832	0.845	0.845
	110	0.784	0.799	0.801	0.816	0.808
15×15	100	1	1	1	1	1
	102	0.952	0.953	0.955	0.958	0.96
	104	0.903	0.913	0.917	0.921	0.922
	106	0.83	0.873	0.882	0.886	0.889
	108	0.823	0.837	0.847	0.852	0.854
	110	0.783	0.801	0.815	0.82	0.823

VII. BOLUS

Bolus is sometimes used to increase surface dose or decrease the depth dose to a selected area in a treatment volume. The bolus must be tissue equivalent material and must be solid but flexible or malleable to allow it to conform to surface contour. Paraffin wax and "superflab" are two such boluses. Bolus bags stuffed with rice granules or tapioca granules are not suitable due to the air spaces in the bags that make the electron dosimetry unpredictable.

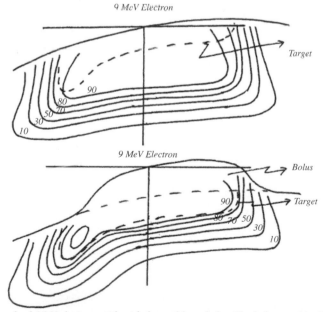

Figure 8.6 Dose distribution for 9 MeV electrons without bolus and 2 cm bolus. The bolus provides better coverage of the target volume by decreasing the depth dose.

VIII. INHOMOGENEITIES

Tissue inhomogeneities affect electron beams more severely than photon beams. The *"coefficient of equivalent thickness" (CET)* is one method that may be used to correct dose distribution for the inhomogeneity. The CET method approximates the effective depth by correcting the real depth accounting for the depth of the inhomogenous tissue. The depth dose for the effective depth is extracted from the depth dose chart/graph for the appropriate electron energy. Therefore;

$$d_e = d_r\text{-}x \times (1\text{-}CET)$$

where, d_e= effective depth, d_r= real depth, x = thickness of inhomogeneity, and CET = electron density.

Example:

Calculate the %DD at point P in tissue after traversing 2 cm of lung tissue with a density of 0.22 gm/cc Point P is 6 cm from the surface and the electron energy is 12 MeV. Subsituting the values:

$$d_e = d_r\text{-}x \times (1\text{-}CET) \ \rightarrow d_e = 6 - 2 \times (1\text{-} 0.22) \ \rightarrow d_e = 4.4 \ cm$$

Therefore the effective depth is 4.4 cm and the depth dose is 45%. Without inhomogeneity correction, the depth is 6 cm and the %DD is 7.5%.

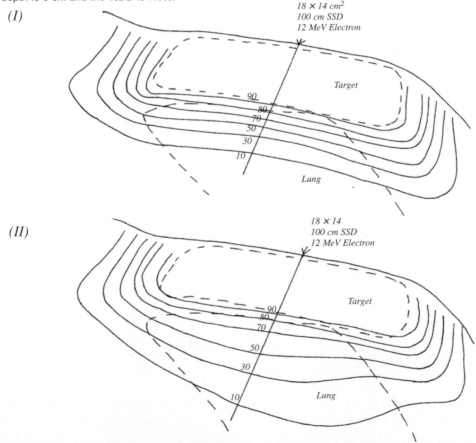

Figure 8.7 Dose distribution from 12 Mev electron beam (I) without inhomogeneity correction and (II) with inhomogeneity correction for lung.

XI. FIELD JUNCTION

Frequently, more than one electron field is required to treat a site due either to the limitation of the field size or steep curvature of the site. For contour with steep curvature, several small fields generate a better dose distribution due to smaller air gaps and field matching is also easier due to smaller divergence of the small fields.

When one field edge is matched to another field edge hot spots are created under the surface due to the bulge of the isodoses. The hot spot and its pattern will vary depending on the energy and on the treatment unit. As the gap between field edges increases, cold spots are created near the surface.

Hot/cold spots may be reduced by moving the junction of the adjoining field. If a variable collimator is used, the width of one field may be increased and the width of the adjoining field may be decreased. The field widths at the opposite ends stay the same. The more frequently the junction is moved, the better the match.

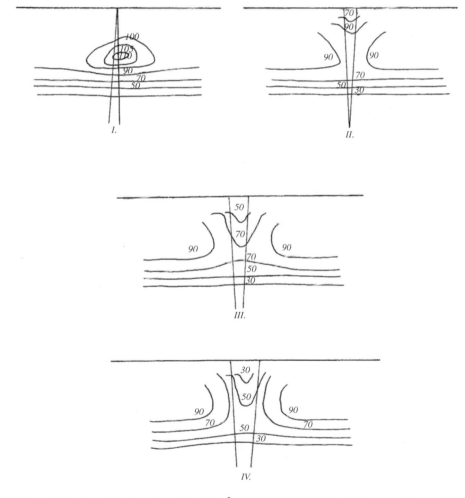

Figure 8.8 Dose distribution at junction of two 12 × 12 cm² (9 MeV) electron fields with (I) no gap between fields, (II) 0.5 cm gap, (III) 1.0 cm gap, and (IV) 1.5 cm gap.

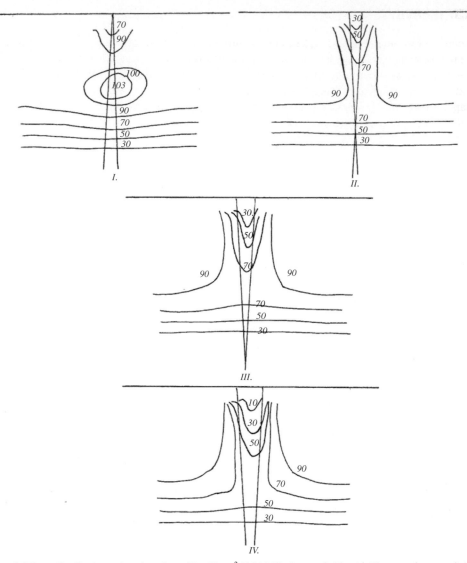

Figure 8.9 Dose distribution at junction of two 12 × 12 cm² (16 MeV) electron fields with (I) no gap between fields, (II) 0.5 cm gap, (III) 1.0 cm gap and (IV) 1.5 cm gap.

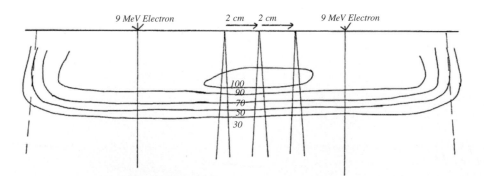

Figure 8.10 Hot/cold spots are prevented at field junction by staggering the junction.

X. ELECTRON ARC THERAPY

As mentioned in the previous section, curved surfaces may be treated with several small fields to reduce the problem of missing tissue *(air gap)* and divergence of the matching fields. Figure 8.11 shows these problems when a curve surface is treated with a single large field, multiple smaller fields and several small fields. Even with several small fields, cold spots appear near the surface due to gaps between adjoining fields. Clinically, it is not practical to treat such a volume with several small fields due to the time required to set up the fields and the problem of reproducibility. The best technique to treat such a large curve surface is electron arc.

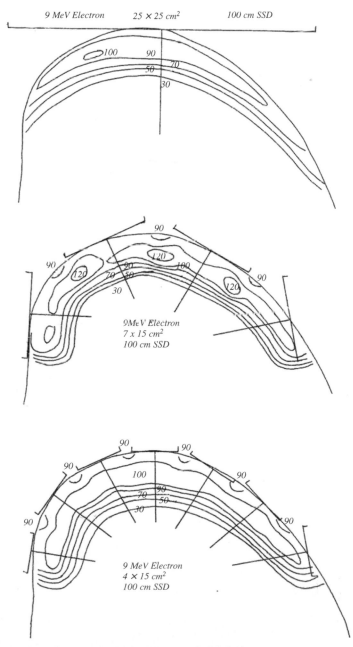

Figure 8.11 (I) Single electron field, (II) four small fields, (III) seven smaller fields.

XI. ELECTRON ARC TREATMENT PLANNING FOR CHEST WALL

The Radiation Oncologist marks the desired treatment volume on the patient. Fabricate an immobilization shell/cast over the treatment site. Place lead sheets all around the edges of the treatment volume to obtain a sharper penumbra. Transfer the patient contour into the treatment planning computer. Determine the thickness of the chest wall from CT or ultrasound so that the appropriate electron beam energy may be chosen to cover the volume to be treated and ensure the underlying lung is not over treated. Bolus over the chest wall may be required if adequate dose to the skin surface is desired. Place the ioscenter at a point at approximately equal distance to the surface treatment volume. Position the start and stop arc angles past the edges of the treatment volume. Select the electron energy to cover the treatment depth and generate the isodose distribution. This is shown in Figure 8.12. The recommended field width for electron arc is 4-6 cm wide that allows for better skin apposition at all the arc angles.

Calculate the MU for treatment by dividing the daily tumor dose by the output factor for the field size used. This output factor must be measured for electron arc at the same isocentric depth for treatment. Calculate the MU per degree by dividing the MU by the total arc angle.

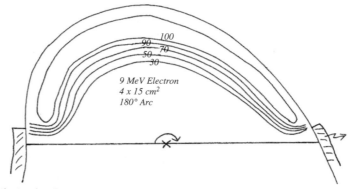

Figure 8.12 Isodose distribution for electron arc therapy.

XII. PUBLICATIONS OF INTERESTS

1.   Dahler A, Baker AS, Laughlin JS: Comprehensive electron beam treatment planning. Ann NY Acad Sci 161:189,1969

2.   Giarratano JC, Duerkes RJ, Almond PR: Lead shielding thickness for dose reduction of 7-28Mev electrons, Med Phys 2:336,1975

3.   Hospital Physicists' Association: A practical guide to electron dosimetry, HPA report series No.4. London, HPA 1971

4.   Kahn FM: The Physics of Radiation Therapy, p 301. Baltimore, Williams & Wilkins, 1984

5.   Laughlin JS: High energy electron treatment planning for inhomogeneities. Br. J Radiol 38:143,1965

6.   Laughlin JS, Lundy A, Phillips R, Chu F, Sattar A: Electron beam treatment planning in inhomogeneous tissue, Radiology 85: 524,1965

7.   Leavitt DD, Peacock LM, Stewart JR. Electron arc therapy: physical measurements and treatment planning techniques. Int.J Radiat Oncol Biol Phys 1985;11:987.

8.   Loevinger R, Karymark CJ, Weissbluth M: Radiation dosimetry with high energy electrons, Radiology 77:906,1961

9.   Mandour MA, Harder D: Systematic optimization of the double scatterer system for electron beam field flattening, Strahlentherapic 154:328,1978

10. Orton CG, Bagne F (eds): Practical aspects of electron beam treatment planning, AAPM publication. New York, American Institute of Physics, 1978 p 80

11. Prasad SC, Bedwinek JM, Gerber RL: Lung dose in electron beam therapy of chest wall. Acta Radiol 22:91,1983

12. Purdy JA: The application of high energy x-rays and electron beams in radiotherapy. IEEE Trans Nucl Sci 26:1833, 1979

13. Sharma SC, Deibel FC, Khan FM: Tissue equivalence of bolus materials for electron beams. Radiology 146:854, 1983

14. Tapley N(ed): Clinical applications of the electron beam. New York, John Wiley & Sons, 1976

—— *CHAPTER 9* ——

Thermoluminescence Dosimeters (TLD)

I. INTRODUCTION

Thermoluminescence dosimeters are made up of lithium fluoride with added activators as impurities. These impurities form "traps" to capture the electrons released by radiation when the TLD is exposed to radiation. When heat is applied to read the TLD, these electrons are given the energy to escape from the "traps" back to the lithium fluoride. When this happens, light is emitted which is proportional to the amount of radiation energy absorbed. The emitted light is read by a photo-multiplier tube that gives out digital reading. This reading is then read off a calibrated value to reveal the dose in cGy absorbed by the TLD.

TLD comes in different forms. The common ones are: i) rods, ii) discs, and iii) crystalline powder. TLD is superior to other kinds of dosimeters for the following reasons: i) they are rugged, ii) they have good response to a wide range of energies, iii) they have low fading over time, iv) they are reproducible, v) they have linearity of dose up to 1000 cGy, vi) they are reusable, and vii) their effective atomic number is close to that of water. The disadvantages of TLD are: i) they are expensive, ii) they do not give instant dose reading, iii) they are inaccurate if some powder is lost or if rods or discs are broken or become dirty, and iv) it is time consuming to anneal, calibrate and read them.

If the TLDs are handled carefully and the annealing, calibration, placement in patient during treatment and reading of the exposed TLDs are correctly executed, accuracy of the TLD is about 3%.

II. ANNEALING

Before TLD are put into clinical use, any electrons still trapped in the impurities must be released and return to its original band. To release these electrons, the TLD must be annealed before calibration for use.

For the annealing, the TLD are placed in a dry and clean pyrex dish and spread out evenly. The dish is placed in an oven at 400° Centigrade for one hour. At the end of the hour, the oven door is opened and the temperature is allowed to drop to 80° centigrade. The dish is placed back into the oven for 24 hours at 80° centigrade. At the end of the 24 hours, the TLD are allowed to cool.

III. GROUPING OF TLD

There are differences between each TLD in any new group. It is advisable to separate the TLDs into groups so that their patient dose measurement may be more accurate.

All the TLDs in the new group are placed in a solid phantom at D_{max} and set up to 100 cm SSD.

The field size is opened to cover all the TLDs, allowing a 2-3 cm margin all around to get away from the field penumbra region. The TLDs are exposed to a dose of 100 cGy.

Each TLD is read and placed in a grid so that they may be easily identified later for grouping. When all the TLDs are read, they are separated into groups where their light readings are plus or minus 2%. Selected TLDs from each of the group are later calibrated. The group should be kept separate for clinical use.

IV. CALIBRATION OF TLD

A few TLDs *(about 5)* from each group are placed in a water equivalent phantom at the appropriate D_{max} for the treatment unit and set up to 100 cm SSD and a 10 × 10 cm² field. They are exposed to a dose of 100 cGy. These TLDs are read and the averaged light reading is used as a reference to calculate the absorbed dose in the future when the TLDs are used to measure dose to patient. For example, 100 cGy yields an average light reading of 5000 units. The TLDs *(2 chips)* are placed in the patient's treatment site during treatment and then read. The average light reading is 400 units. This translates to a dose of 8 cGy.

The calibration should be repeated for each treatment unit in clinical use.

V. OTHER DOSIMETERS

Some of the other dosimeters are: i) calorimeters, ii) Fricke dosimeters, iii) solid state silicon diode dosimeters, iv) free air ionization chambers, and v) film badges.

VI. PUBLICATIONS OF INTERESTS

1.   Cameron JR, Suntharalingham N, Kenney GW: Thermoluminescent Dosimetry. Madison, WI, The University of Wisconsin Press, 1968.

2.   Crosby EH, Almond PR, Shalek RJ: Energy dependence of LiF dosimeters at high energies. Phys Med Biol 11:131, 1966.

3.   Greening JR, Law J, Redpath AT: Mass attenuation and mass energy absorption coefficients for LiF and Li B O for 2 4 7 photons from 1 to 150keV. Ohys Med Biol 17:585,1972 Fundamentals of Radiation Dosimetry. Bristol, Adam Hilger Ltd, 1981,p128.)

4.   Holt JG, Edelstein GR, Clark TE: Energy dependence of the response of lithium fluoride TLD rods in high energy electron fields. Phys Med Biol 20:559, 1975.

5.   Paliwal BR, Almond PR: Application of cavity theories for electrons to LiF dosimeters. Phys Med Biol 20:547, 1975.

6.   Suntharalingham N, Cameron JR: Thermoluminescent response of lithium fluoride to high energy electrons (High Energy Radiation Therapy Dosimetry issue.) Amn NY Acad Sci 161:77, 1969.

7.   Zimmerman DW, Rhyner CR, Cameron JR: Thermal annealing effects on the thermoluminescence of LiF. Health Phys 12:525, 1966.

— *CHAPTER 10* —

Cancer of the Skin

I. INTRODUCTION

Cancer of the skin is the most common of all cancers. Fortunately, for most skin cancers, it is also the most curable due to good visibility and therefore early detection.

The most common cause of skin cancer is long-term exposure to sunlight with no sun shield protection. Fair skin people are more susceptible than dark skin people due to lack of pigmentation to shield the sun's rays. Exposure to ionizing radiation such as those who were treated for acne and early radiation workers, are also more prone to getting skin cancers.

Some of the common skin cancers encountered in radiotherapy are, basal cell carcinoma *(BCC)*, squamous cell carcinoma *(SCC)*, kaposi's sarcoma, mycosis fungoides and melanoma. Benign tumors of the skin such as keloid scars are sometimes treated with ionizing radiation.

Surgery is the treatment of choice for early skin cancers. Radiation therapy is the treatment of choice if: i) the tumor is near the eyelid or nasal labial fold, ii) the tumor is large and infiltrates into muscle; and iii) the patient is elderly and surgery is contra-indicated.

II. BASAL CELL CARCINOMA (BCC) AND SQUAMOUS CELL CARCINOMA (SCC)

Basal cell and squamous cell carcinoma are the commonest of the skin cancers. BCC arise in the basal layer of the epidermis and spreads by infiltration into surrounding tissue. They appear like rodent ulcers with a central depression that erodes, crusts and bleeds but seldom metastasize.

Squamous cell carcinoma arises in the epidermis. They are firm, red and horny in appearance and bleeds easily. They are slow growing and rarely metastasize.

A. Superficial X-ray Therapy

Superficial X-Ray in the 100 kV range at a treatment distance of 20 cm is often used to treat BCC and SCC. The tumor plus 1-2 cm margin is treated to 4500 cGy in 15 treatments. If the shape is irregular, a lead cut out *(1 mm thick)* is made to fit the shape. If the tumor is near the eye, coated lead eye shield is placed under the eyelid to shield the lens and likewise if the tumor is near the nose, coated lead shield is placed in the nostril to protect the nasal septum. If the treatment site is uneven such as near the nose or inner canthus, a lead face mask is fabricated for shielding. A film compensator may be necessary to compensate for the irregular contour.

I. Irregular Field Calculation for SXR Cut Out

Due to the reduction in scatter from the shielding, a new surface dose rate should be calculated before calculating the treatment time. The treated area is calculated and the corresponding BSF is obtained from the BSF table.

Example:

A patient is marked up for treatment to a skin tumor on the cheek. The diagram in Figure 10.1 shows the outline of the treated area. The applicator is a 5.5 cm circular cone at 20 cm treatment distance. The treatment unit is a 100 kV 8 mA SXR unit with 1.25 mm Al filter and a HVL of 1.65 mm Al. The prescribed dose to the surface is 4500 cGy in 15 treatments.

Calculate the treatment time. (Timer correction is -0.02 min.)

Calculation:

The area of the treated shape is 10.25 cm². This area is converted to diameter to obtain the BSF from the BSF table, area of a circle = πr^2, r = 1.806 cm. Therefore diameter = 1.806 × 2 = 3.612 cm.

From the BSF table, 3.612 cm diameter gives a BSF of 1.115.

The air dose rate for 5.5 cm circle applicator = 288 cGy/min.

Therefore the surface dose rate for the treated area = 1.115 × 288 = 321.12 cGy/min.

Prescribed dose = 300 cGy, The treatment time = (300/321.12)-0.02 = 0.9 min.

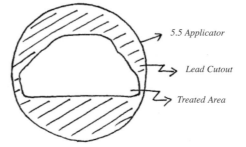

Figure 10.1 Lead cut out for irregular shape treatment.

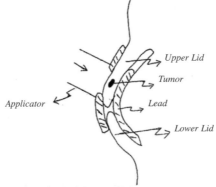

Figure 10.2 Set-up for treatment to the eyelid using SXR.

II. Stand-off correction

Stand off correction *(inverse square correction)* is more important for short treatment distances than for large treatment distances as used in the high energy photon treatment unit. For example, a one cm stand off at 100 cm treatment distance produces a 2% correction factor. For one cm stand off at 20 cm treatment distance, the correction factor is about 10%.

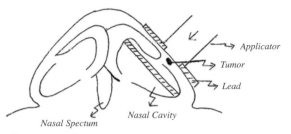

Figure 10.3 Set-up for treatment to skin tumor on the nose.

Example:

A patient with a skin lesion on the left side of the nose is to be treated to a total prescribed dose of 4500 cGy in 15 treatments. The applicator is 2.5 cm circle and the stand off is 1.3 cm. The SXR data is the same as in the previous example.

Calculation:

Air dose rate for 2.5 cm circle applicator = 283 cGy/min., The treated diameter = 2 cm and the BSF = 1.071. Therefore;

$$Treatment\ time = \left(\frac{4500}{15 \times 283 \times \left(\frac{20}{21.3}\right)^2 \times 1.071} \right) - 0.02 = 1.10 \quad min$$

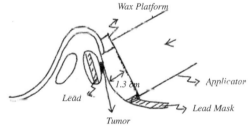

Figure 10.4 Set-up to treat the left side of the nose with lead face mask on and lead shield in left nostril.

III. Film compensator

Due to the uneven surface of the facial contour, compensation may be necessary to even the surface tumor dose. Compensation is with a step compensator fabricated out of exposed X-Ray film. For more details on the construction and calculation, refer to the chapter on compensator.

B. Electron Therapy

Instead of SXR, low energy electrons may be used to treat skin cancers. Due to the rapid decrease of depth dose, it is ideal to treat skin cancers without delivering excessive dose to the underlying structures.

The electron energy chosen is usually in the 3-5 MeV range depending on the depth of the tumor. To ensure a high dose to the surface of the skin, bolus such as 'superflab' may be placed on the skin.

Example:

From the 4 MeV electron depth dose graph, the surface % depth dose is 73% and at 0.5 cm the % depth dose is 87%. If 0.5 cm 'superflab' is placed on the skin, the skin surface receives 87% and 0.5 cm below the skin surface (i.e., 1 cm from the superflab surface) receives 95%.

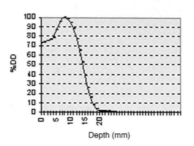

%DD 4 MeV electron 4x4 cm cone

Figure 10.5 Percentage depth dose graph for 4 MeV electron beam at 100 cm SSD (4 × 4 cm² applicator).

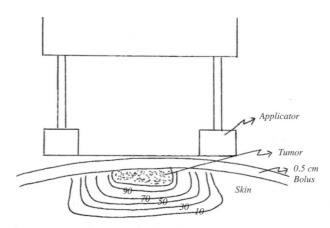

Figure 10.6 Set-up to treat a skin tumor using 5 cm circle applicator at 100 cm SSD (5 MeV electrons).

III. KAPOSI'S SARCOMA

This tumor is more common in the African continent and the Middle East than anywhere else in the world. It appears as a raised pigmented sarcoma of the skin. The tumor can arise anywhere on the body and can metastasize. They are slow growing. Kaposi's sarcoma may also be associated with AIDS. Treatment of choice is localized radiation to the tumor using electron therapy. If the tumor is widespread, the treatment of choice is total skin electron irradiation. Some chemotherapeutic agents have provided some remissions.

IV. MYCOSIS FUNGOIDES

Mycosis fungoides starts as a skin rash, which eventually infiltrates into the subcutaneous tissue and finally turns into a fungating tumor. It can occur in any part of the body. For the early stages, treatment of choice is low energy electron radiation therapy or superficial X-Ray to localized lesions. For massive widespread disease, some centers treat the whole body with low energy electrons. The patient stands on a rotating platform at a large treatment distance from the collimator. The field is set to cover the whole patient. The patient is rotated around to treat the whole body.

Total surface dose is about 3200 cGy in 16 treatments over 8 weeks, treating twice a week.

When the tumor has infiltrated into deep subcutaneous structures, whole body electron therapy may be of minimal benefit.

At the terminal stage, involvement of the lymph nodes, liver and spleen occurs. Some chemotherapeutic agents have provided temporary remission.

V. BENIGN TUMORS OF THE SKIN

i) Keloid Scar

A keloid scar is an overgrowth of collagen fibers. The scar is raised and can cause severe irradiation to the patient. A very thin layer of epidermis covers the scar and this epidermis is easily damaged. Keloid scar is more common in dark complexion people. Surgery to remove the scar followed immediately by radiotherapy using low energy X-Ray (100 kV) is the treatment of choice giving 400 cGy in 4 days. A lead cut out is used to protect the surrounding normal skin.

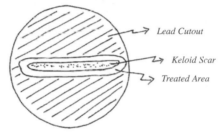

Figure 10.7 Lead cut out to treat keloid scar on the SXR.

VI. CANCER OF THE LIP

Cancer of the lip is more common in men than in women. Lower lip is affected more than upper lip. The causes of lip cancer are the same as for skin cancer. It is commoner with pipe smokers. Radiotherapy is the treatment of choice if· i) the tumor is in the upper lip, ii) involvement of the commissure; and iii) the tumor is more than 2 cm.

A. Superficial X-ray Therapy

The lip may be treated in the same way as described in the treatment of BCC and SCC of the skin. A piece of coated lead shield is placed between the lip and the gum during treatment to protect the gum tissue from radiation.

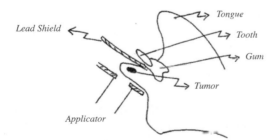

Figure 10.8 Set-up to treat a tumor in the lower lip. A piece of lead is used to protect the gum.

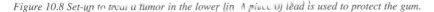

B. Electron Therapy

Very low energy electron (4 MeV) may be used to treat cancer of the lip. Treatment set-up is the same as described for BCC and SCC of the skin.

V. PUBLICATIONS OF INTERESTS

1. Amdur RJ, Kalbaugh KJ, Ewald LM, et al: Radiation therapy for skin cancer near the eye: Kilovolt-age x-rays versus electrons. Int J Radiat Oncol Biol Phys 23:769, 1992

2. Blank AA, Schnyder UW: Soft x-ray therapy in Bowen's disease and erythroplasia of Queyrat. Dermatologica 171:89, 1985

3. Das IJ, Kase KR, Copeland JF, et al: Electron beam modifications for the treatment of superficial malignancies. Int J Radiat Oncol Biol Phys 21:1627, 1991

4. del Regato JA, Vuksanovia M: Radiotherapy of carcinoma of the skin overlying the cartilages of the nose and ear. Radiology 79:203, 1962.

5. Fitzpatrick PJ, Thompson GA, Easterbrook WM et al: Basal and squamous cell carcinoma of the eyelids and their treatment by radiotherapy. Int J Radiat Oncol Biol Phys 10:449,1984.

6. Griep C, Davelaar J, Scholten AN, et al: Electron beam therapy is not inferior to superficial x-ray therapy in the treatment of skin carcinoma. Int J Radiat Oncol Biol Phys 32:1347, 1995

7. McKenna RJ, Macdonald I: Irradiation for cancer of the eyelid California Med 96:184, 1962.

8. Mendenhall NP, Parsons JT, Cassisi NJ, et al: Carcinoma of the nasal vestibule treated with radiation therapy. Laryngoscope 97:626, 1987

9. Perez CA, Lovett RD, Gerber R: Electron beam and x-rays in the treatment of epithelial skin cancer: Dosimetric considerations and clinical results. In Vaeth JM, Meyer JL, eds: Frontiers of Radiation Therapy and Oncology, vol 25, The Role of High Energy Electrons in the Treatment of Cancer, pp 90-106. Basel, Switzerland, Karger, 1991

10. Van Essen CF: Roentgen therapy of the skin and lip carcinoma: Factors influencing success and failure. Am J Roenthenol 83:556,1960.

11. Van Essen CF: Indications for radiation therapy of skin cancer. In: Tumours of the skin Chicago, IL, Year Book Medical Publishers, 1964.

— CHAPTER 11 —

Tumors of the Bone

I. INTRODUCTION

Bone tumors encountered in radiotherapy are primary bone tumor, benign bone tumor and metastatic bone tumors. Examples of primary bone tumors are (i) Oesteogenic sarcoma and (ii) Ewings sarcoma. Examples of benign bone tumors are (i) Osteoblastoma and (ii) Fibroma. By far the most common bone tumors encountered in radiotherapy are the metastatic bone tumors. The common primary sites are (i) breast, (ii) bronchus and (iii) kidney. The most common sites of the metastasis are in the spine and pelvis but they are by no means confined to these sites.

Some of the common presentations of bone tumors are local pain and swelling in the affected area. Pathologic fractures are common with metastatic bone tumors.

II. PRIMARY BONE TUMORS

Diagnosis of bone tumors is by (i) X-Ray of the bone, (ii) CT scan, (iii) Nuclear Medicine bone scan and (iv) needle biopsy. Treatment may be a combination of surgery, radiotherapy and chemotherapy. Radiotherapy is usually by parallel opposed portals using a megavoltage unit such as the 6 MV linear accelerator to maintain skin sparing. Total tumor dose in the region of 7000-8000 cGy in 30 to 35 fractions in 6-7 weeks is common due to the radioresistance of the tumor. It is usual to treat the large field to a dose of 5000 cGy in 20 fractions in 4 weeks and then cone down to a smaller field and give a further 2000 cGy in 10 fractions in 2 weeks. Skin reaction is often fairly severe due to the high dose.

III. BENIGN BONE TUMORS

Radiotherapy does not play an important part in benign bone tumors due to the danger of late malignancy induction in the bones. Also, due to its radioresistance, radiotherapy is not the treatment of choice. Surgery is the treatment of choice. Radiotherapy is considered if surgery is not possible.

IV. METASTATIC BONE TUMORS

As stated earlier, by far the most common bone tumors are of the metastatic type. Pain is usually the most common complaint and the pain gradually gets more severe with the advancement of the disease. Pathological fracture is another end result of metastatic bone tumor.

II. BRAIN

In adults, most CNS tumors are brain tumors. Of these, most are primary astrocytomas and the rest from metastatic lesions from the lung, breast, GI tract and kidney. In children, most CNS tumors arise in the brain stem and cerebellum such as medulloblastoma.

There is no proven cause of CNS cancer though some CNS tumors are associated with genetic factors.

The presentations for brain cancer are headache, nausea, vomiting, seizures, weakness and mental changes. Diagnosis is with the aid of CT, MRI, histopathology, skull X-Ray, ophthalmoscopy, neurologic examinations, brain scan and EEG. Surgery is the treatment of choice if the tumor is small and is situated in a location where it can be safely removed. Radiation therapy is the treatment of choice if the two criteria are not met. Radiation therapy is with a pair of lateral opposed fields to the whole brain followed by a coned down boost.

An immobilization head shell is fabricated for the patient in the supine position for the initial whole brain treatment. The patient is simulated to ensure the treatment field covers the whole brain. Cerrobend blocks are constructed to shield the lens.

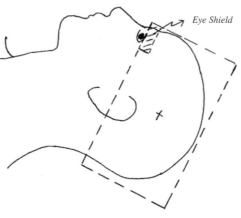

Figure 12.2 Field set-up for lateral opposed fields to the whole brain.

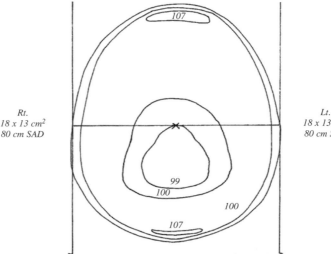

Figure 12.3 Dose distribution from lateral opposed fields to the whole brain. (Cobalt-60)

For the boost field, a new immobilization head shell may be fabricated if the tumor is off set to one side. In this situation, the patient lies on the unaffected side for a new shell to be fabricated. The patient is simulated in the new treatment position. Reference marks are placed on the shell and the patient is CT.

The planning CT images are transferred to the treatment planning computer. Diagnostic CT and diagnostic MRI images are fused to aid in target volume localization on the planning CT images by the RadiationOncologist. A treatment plan is generated for approval by the radiation oncologist before treatment commences.

The patient is re-simulated for plan check. Simulator films are taken for record and the final treatment field marks are marked on the shell.

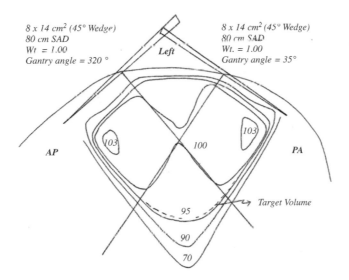

Figure 12.4 Dose distribution from oblique wedged fields to the left side of the brain. (Cobalt-60)

III. SPINAL CORD

Tumors of the spinal cord are gliomas, meningiomas and metastatic lesions. Presentations of spinal cord tumors are pain, muscle weakness and lost of sensations. The area affected is dependent on the site of the tumor in the spinal cord.

Diagnosis is by myelogram, bone scan and CT and the treatment of choice is radiation therapy using a direct posterior field or a pair of oblique wedged fields.

The patient is simulated in the prone position. From the results of the diagnostic studies, the treatment volume is determined at simulation. A direct posterior field or a pair of oblique wedged fields may be used to treat tumors of the spine.

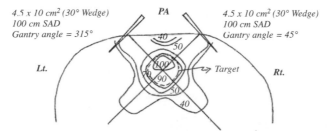

Figure 12.5 Dose distribution for oblique wedged fields to the spinal cord. (6 MV photons)

IV. MEDULLOBLASTOMA

Medulloblastoma often arises in the cerebellum. It is a fast growing tumour and is most common in young children. Spread through the cerebo-spinal fluid is common. Surgery is performed to relieve systems and to confirm diagnosis. Treatment of choice is radiation therapy to the whole brain and the cerebrospinal axis followed with a boost to the primary site.

An immobilization shell is fabricated for the patient in the prone treatment position. The shell/cast serves three purposes: 1) It immobilizes the patient for treatment; 2) It enables reproducible Set-up for treatment each day; and 3) It allows field centers and field marks to be drawn on the shell.

As mentioned earlier, treatment of choice is radiation therapy to the whole brain and the cerebrospinal axis followed with a boost to the posterior fossa. If the patient is a small child, a single direct posterior field may be adequate to cover the whole spine from C2 to S2. If the patient is older, two posterior spinal fields may be required to cover the whole spine.

V. SINGLE SPINAL FIELD

With the gantry at 0°, the spinal field is simulated first by setting the field size to cover the spine from C2 to S2. A typical field size is approximately 6×35 cm^2 at 100 cm SSD. A simulator film is taken and field marks drawn on the shell.

To simulate the right lateral skull field, the gantry is angled to 90°. The field covers the whole brain and inferiorly to the C2 junction. A typical field size is 15×18 cm^2 at 100 cm SAD. In order to match the divergence of the spinal field, the collimator is angled at:

$$Tan\theta = \left(\frac{(1/2) \times 35}{100}\right) \quad \rightarrow \quad \theta = Tan^{-1}\left(\frac{(1/2) \times 35}{100}\right) \quad \rightarrow \quad \theta = 9.9°$$

To match the divergence of the skull field to the spinal field, the floor is angled at:

$$Tan\theta = \left(\frac{(1/2) \times 18}{100}\right) \quad \rightarrow \quad \theta = Tan^{-1}\left(\frac{(1/2) \times 18}{100}\right) \rightarrow \quad \theta = 5.1° \quad See\ Figure\ 12.6$$

A new floor angle is calculated for each junction change. A simulator film is taken and field marks are drawn on the shell. Shielding is indicated on the film by the radiation oncologist. The left lateral skull field is simulated similar to the right lateral skull field with all the angle settings reverse.

During the course of treatment, the junction between the skull fields and the spinal field are moved two to four times. For the brain fields, the superior border remains the same while the inferior border is increased by 1cm at each junction change. The superior border of the spinal field is decreased by 1cm at each junction change but the inferior border remains the same.

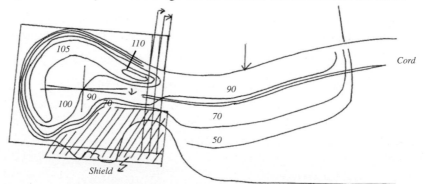

Figure 12.6 Dose distribution for treating the whole brain and spinal cord using single field to cover the whole spinal axis. (6 MV photons)

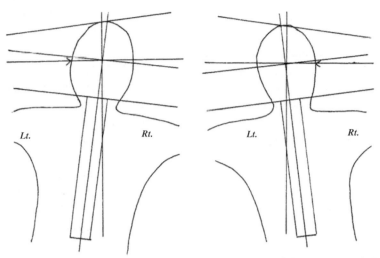

Figure 12.7 Field set-up for treating the whole brain and spinal cord using single field to cover the whole spinal axis (6 MV photons). The floor is angled to match the divergence of the skull field to the spinal field.

VI. TWO SPINAL FIELDS

With the gantry at 0° and the floor at 90°, the superior spinal field is simulated first by setting the field size to cover the spine from C2 to T10. A typical field size is approximately 6 × 24 cm² at 100 cm SSD. A simulator film is taken and field marks drawn on the shell.

The inferior spinal field is simulated to cover the spine from T10 to S2. A typical field size is approximately 6 × 24 cm² at 100 cm SSD. To prevent the overlap of the divergence of the spinal fields, the superior and inferior spinal fields are abutted at their junction at T10. To abut the fields, the superior edge of the inferior field is matched to the inferior edge of the superior field. The inferior field is angled inferiorly to the total divergence of the two spinal fields. The total divergence of the two fields is:

$$Tan\theta_1 = \left(\frac{(1/2) \times 24}{100}\right) \quad \& \quad Tan\theta_2 = \left(\frac{(1/2) \times 24}{100}\right)$$

Therefore,

$$\theta = \theta_1 + \theta_2 = Tan^{-1}\left(\frac{(1/2) \times 24}{100}\right) + Tan^{-1}\left(\frac{(1/2) \times 24}{100}\right) = 13.7^\circ$$

The gantry is angled to read 346.3°. A film is taken and field marks drawn on the shell.

For the lateral skull fields, the floor is angled back to 0 degree and the lateral skull fields are simulated the same way as discussed under single spinal field. A new floor angle is calculated for each junction change.

During the course of treatment, the junction between the skull fields and the spinal field are moved two to four times. For the brain fields, the superior border remains the same while the inferior border is increased by 1cm at each junction change. The superior border of the superior spinal field is decreased by 1cm at each junction change and the inferior border is decreased by 1cm. The superior border of the inferior spinal field is increased by 1cm but the inferior border stays the same.

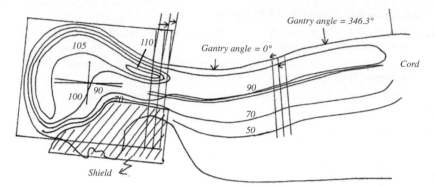

Figure 12.8 Dose distribution for treating whole brain and spinal axis using two spinal fields. (6 MV Photons)

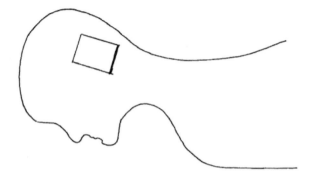

Figure 12.9 Field set-up to treat boost area.

VII. PUBLICATIONS OF INTERESTS

1. Bleehan NM: The central nervous system. Chapter 19. In Bleehan NM, Glatstein E, Haybittle JL (eds): Radiation Therapy Planning, pp 607-615, New York, Marcel Dekker,1983.

2. Bloom HJG, Wallace ENK, Hank JM: The treatment and prognosis of medulloblastoma in children. Am J Roentgenol Radiat Ther Nucl Med 105:43,1969.

3. Bouchard J: Central nervous system. In Fletcher GH(ed): Textbook of Radiotherapy, pp 444-498. Philadel[hia, Lea and Febiger, 1980.

4. Farwell JR, Dohrmann GJ, Flannery JT: Medulloblastoma in childhood: An epidermiological study. J Neurosurg 61:657,1984.

5. Greitz T, Lax I, Bergstrom M, et al: Stereotactic radiotherapy of intracranial lesions-methodological aspects. Acta Radiol (Oncol) 25:81,1986.

6. Gutin PH, Bernstein M: Stereotactic intestitial brachytherapy for malignant brain tumours. In Homburger F (ed): Progress in experimental tumour research, vol 28, pp 166-182, Karger, Basel, 1984.

7. Hochberg FH, Pruitt A: Assumptions in the radiotherapy of glioblastoma. Neurology 30 : 907,1980.

8. Jenkin RDT: Medulloblastoma in childhood radiation therapy. Can Med Assoc J 100:51,1969.

9. Jenkin D: The radiation treatment of medulloblastoma. J Neurooncol 29:45-54, 1996

10. Karlsson UL, Micaily B, Kraus D, et al: Reproducible and anatomically correct positioning of the head for radiation therapy and diagnostic procedures. Personal communication, 1985.

11. Kornblith PL: Increased intracranial pressure. In De Vita VT, Hellman S, Rosenberg SA(eds): Cancer: Principles and Practice of Oncology,pp 1586-1588. Philadelphia, JB Lippincott, 1982.

12. Kramer S, Lee KF: Complication of radiation therapy: The central nervous system. Semin Roentgenol IX:75,1974.

13. Lampert PW, Davis RL: Delayed effects of radiation in the human central nervous system: "Early" and

"late" delayed reactions. Neurology 14:912,1964.

14. Marsa GW, Goffinet DR, Rubinstein LJ, et al: Megavoltage irradiation in the treatment of gliomas of the brain and soinal cord. Br J Radiol 42:198,1969.

15. Michael L.F.Lim, A Study of Four Methods of Junction Change in the Treatment of Medulloblastoma, Medical Dosimetry, January 1985, vol.16, No.1, page 8-13

16. Michael L.F.Lim, Evolution of Medulloblastoma Techniques. Medical Dosimetry, Dec 1986, vol. XI, No.4, page 25-36

17. Sheline GE, Boldreu E, Karlsberg P, et al: Therapeutic considerations in tumours affecting the CNS. Radiology 82:84,1967.

18. Shin KH, Mullen PJ, Greggie PH: Superfractionation radiation therapy in the treatment of malignant astrocytoma. Cancer 52:2040, 1983.

19. Wallner KE: Radiation treatment planning for malignant astrocytomas. Semin Radiat Oncol 1:17-22, 1991

Principles and Practice of Clinical Physics and Dosimetry
Michael L.F. Lim, GMD, ACT
Advanced Medical Publishing, Inc., USA

—— *CHAPTER 13* ——

Cancer of the Ear

I. INTRODUCTION

The ear is made up of the external, middle and inner ear. The external ear consists of the pinna and the external auditory meatus. The pinna is a plate of elastic cartilage covered with skin. The external auditory meatus is the canal that connects the tympanic membrane to the exterior and measures about 2.5 cm long. The canal is made up of cartilage and bone and is lined by skin and contains hair and ceruminous glands that secrete the ear wax. The middle ear consists of the tympanic membrane and the ossicles that are the malleus, incus and stapes. The middle ear is connected to the pharynx through the Eustachian tube.

The inner ear consists of the bony labyrinth and the membranous labyrinth. Within the membranous labyrinth is the organ of hearing. Presentations of tumor arising on the pinna are similar to skin cancer. Presentations of tumor arising in the external auditory meatus and middle ear are pruritus, pain, swelling and decreased hearing.

Diagnosis is by physical examination, otoscopy, biopsy and CT.

Tumors arising on the pinna are similar to skin cancer and are treated as such. Tumors arising in the external auditory meatus and middle ear are treated by surgery and radiation therapy.

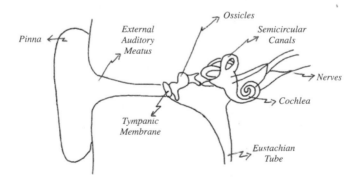

Figure 13.1 Diagram shows structures of the ear.

II. LOCALIZATION

The patient lies on the unaffected side with the head resting on a comfortable headrest. The shoulder is pulled inferiorly to allow for more room for treatment Set-up. The chin is hyper-extended so that the treatment fields would avoid the eyes. A plastic immobilization shell is fabricated for the patient in this position.

The patient is simulated and anterior and lateral films are taken. Field centers are drawn on the shell for referencing. Radio-opaque markers are taped on the field centers on the shell. The radio-opaque markers would show up on CT for centering at the time of planning. The patient is CT. After exporting the CT images to the planning computer, the radiation oncologist delineates the target volume and the organs at risk. Results from the physical examination, otoscopy study and diagnostic CT aid to localize the GTV. Margins are created to form the CTV/PTV.

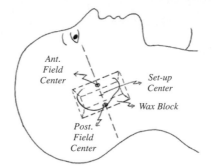

Figure 13.2 Field Set-up to treat cancer of the ear.

III. TREATMENT PLANNING

The intersection of the AP and lateral CT marks on the central CT slice are localized and centered for referencing. Coverage of the target volume is achieved with a pair of wedged fields. After plan approval by the radiation oncologist, the plan isocenter with reference to the original center is documented on the plan. This plan isocenter is set-up at simulation for plan check. The plan fields are simulated as per plan and films are taken for documentation. The new field centers are marked on the shell for treatment set-up.

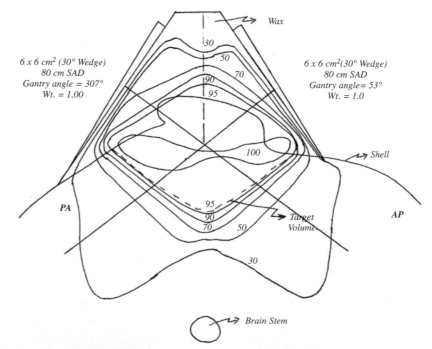

Figure 13.3 Dose distribution of wedged fields in the treatment of cancer of the ear. (Cobalt-60)

IV. PUBLICATIONS OF INTERESTS

1.   Avila J. Bosch A. Aristizabal S, ct al. Carcinoma of the pinna. Cancer 40:2891, 1977

2.   Conley J, Schuller DE: Malignancies of the ear. Laryngoscope 86:1147.1976.

3.   Crabtree JA, Britton BH, Pierce MK: Cancer of the external auditory canal. Laryngoscope 86:405,1976.

4.   Hahn SS, Kim JA, Goodchild N et al: Carcinoma of the middle ear and external auditory canal. Int J Radiat Oncol Biol Phys 9:1003,1983.

5.   Lederman M: Malignant tumours of the ear. J Laryngol Otol 79:85,1965.

6.   Wang CC: Radiation therapy in the management of carcinoma of the external auditory canal, middle ear or mastoid. Radiology 116:713,1975.

Principles and Practice of Clinical Physics and Dosimetry
Michael L.F Lim, CMD,ACT
Advanced Medical Publishing, Inc., USA

—— *CHAPTER 14* ——

Tumors of the Eye

I. INTRODUCTION

The eye is made up of the globe and appendages such as the eyelids, conjunctiva and lachrymal system. The eyelids are two movable folds consisting of an upper eyelid and a lower eyelid. The eyelids form a protective barrier for the cornea. The conjunctiva is the membrane on the inside surface of the eyelids. Over the eyeball *(globe)*, it is loosely connected to the sclera. The lacrimal ducts open into the conjunctiva sac. The lacrimal system is made up of the lacrimal glands, lacrimal sac and lacrimal ducts. Tears are produced in the gland and store in the sac. When needed, the tears are emptied onto the eye via the lacrimal ducts.

The globe or eyeball is spherical and sits in the orbit of the skull. The eyeball is made up of three coats enclosing three refractive media. The first coat is fibrous and is made up of the sclera and the cornea. The second coat is vascular and pigmented and is made up of the choroid, ciliary body and iris. The third coat is the retina that is made up of light sensitive rods and cones.

The three refractive media are the aqueous humour, vitreous body and the lens. The iris is the coloured membrane suspended in the aqueous humour behind the cornea and in front of the lens. The opening in the middle of the iris is the pupil.

The lens is transparent and biconvex enclosed by the lens capsule. Posteriorly is the vitreous body and anteriorly is the iris. With the exception of skin cancers of the eyelid, eye tumors are rare. The skin cancers of the eyelid are treated similar to skin cancers. Benign tumors such as pterygium are occasionally treated by radiotherapy giving low doses. The most common eye tumor is retinoblastoma.

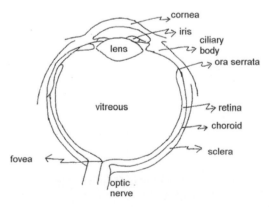

Figure 14.1 Anatomy of the eye.

II. RETINOBLASTOMA

Retinoblastoma is the most common eye tumor in children. It is usually manifested by 2 years of age. The most common presentation is a white pupil due to the mass in the retina.

Diagnostic procedures such as ophthalmic examination, ultra sound and CT are used to diagnose the disease.

Surgery is the treatment of choice if there is permanent loss of vision. The globe is enucleated and if there is any chance of residue disease, radiotherapy should be given to the socket *(orbit)*. A tumor dose of 4000 cGy in 20 fractions in 4 weeks to the mid socket is usually sufficient.

When the globe has been enucleated, a plastic eye is worn by the patient during radiotherapy to prevent socket contraction. A prosthesis may be fitted later when healing is complete.

Radiotherapy is the treatment of choice if there is no permanent loss of vision and if the tumor is small and behind the equator. Due to the high risk of cataract formation, the beam direction must be very precise. Most of the patients presenting with retinoblastoma are children between 1-2 years old. Children who cannot lie still during simulation and treatment may be sedated or anaesthetized.

III. LOCALIZATION

A head shell/cast is fabricated to immobilize the patient and to allow treatment fields to be marked on the shell. The patient is simulated and anterior and lateral films are taken. Field centers are drawn on the shell for referencing. Radio-opaque markers are taped on the field centers on the shell. The radio-opaque markers would show up on CT for centering at the time of planning. The patient is CT at 0.25 cm spacing. After exporting the CT images to the planning computer, the radiation oncologist delineates the GTV and the organs at risk.

IV. TREATMENT PLANNING

A. Localized tumor

I) Direct photon beam

The intersection of the AP and lateral CT marks on the central CT slice are localized and centered for referencing. Coverage of the target volume is achieved with a single direct FAD(SAD) assymetric field 4×4 cm^2 angled 3 degree anteriorly from horizontal to avoid the opposite lens. After plan approval by the radiation oncologist, the plan isocenter with reference to the original center is documented on the plan. This plan isocenter is set up at simulation for plan check. The plan field is simulated as per plan and films are taken for documentation. The new field center is marked on the shell for treatment set-up.

II) Iodine-125 (125I) Eye Plaque

Localized tumor has successfully been treated with Iodine-125 (^{125}I) eye plaque giving a dose of 4000 cGy in 2-3 days. The eye plaques come in different sizes. A suitable one is chosen for the patient based on the size and depth of the tumor. From the size chosen, dosimetry is done to deliver the desired dose in 2-3 days. The activity of the sources as per plan are ordered. A couple of days before the implantation of the plaque, the sources are positioned in the silicon plaque and a gold cap is placed on the back side of the sources to shield the normal tissue behind the globe. The finished plaque is sterilized before delivery to the operating room for the ophthalmologist to suture it at the tumor location. The plaque is left in for the planned time and removed.

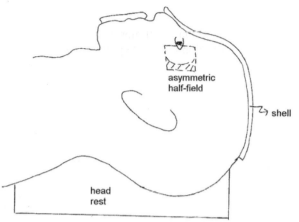

Figure 14.2 Position of the lateral field with asymmetric half-field blocking anteriorly on 6 MV photons.

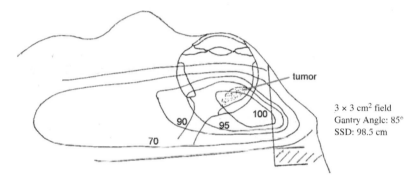

3 × 3 cm² field
Gantry Angle: 85°
SSD: 98.5 cm

Figure 14.3 Dose distribution of asymmetric field in the treatment of retinoblastoma (6 MV photons). Point of normalization is at 3 cm depth in the center of the treated field.

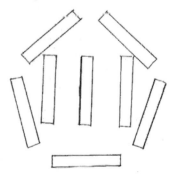

Figure 14.4 Iodine-125 (¹²⁵I) Source positions for the 10 mm diameter eye plaque.

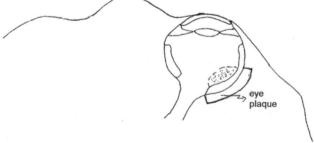

Figure 14.5 Position of the plaque on the sclera.

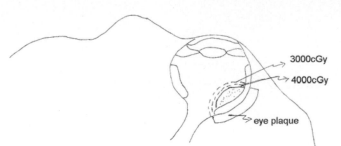

Figure 14.6. Dose distribution of the 10 mm eye plaque giving a dose of 4000 cGy to 5 mm from the outside scleral wall.

B. Multifocal tumor

If the disease is multifocal, the whole retina up to the ora serata should be treated. A simple lateral field behind the lens does not provide adequate coverage. If the lateral field includes the ora serata, the lens and cornea dose are high. In the following techniques described below, the dose to the lens would cause cataract formation but removal of the cataract is an easy procedure but care must be taken to reduce the dose to the cornea to prevent damage to the cornea.

I) Electron pair

A pair of electron fields 3×5 cm^2 (9 MeV) at 100 cm SSD provide good coverage of the GTV. Plan verification is as described for (a) above.

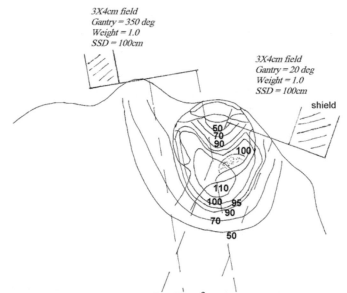

Figure 14.7 Dose distribution of two 9 MeV 3×5 cm^2 electron fields.

II) Anterior/lateral wedge pair

Anterior/lateral wedge pair using 6 MV photons with the isocenter just behind the lens and weighted 1.5 : 0.5 biased to the anterior also provides good coverage to the GTV. Plan verification is as described in subsection (a) above.

III) Superior/inferior oblique 6 MV photon fields

A superior/inferior oblique 6 MV photon fields provide good coverage of the GTV and reduces the exit dose to the opposite lens. Plan verification is as described subsection (a) above.

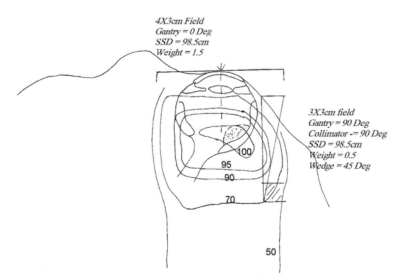

4X3cm Field
Gantry = 0 Deg
SSD = 98.5cm
Weight = 1.5

3X3cm field
Gantry = 90 Deg
Collimator -= 90 Deg
SSD = 98.5cm
Weight = 0.5
Wedge = 45 Deg

100
95
90
70
50

Figure 14.8 Dose distribution of Anterior/Lateral wedge pair using 6 MV photons.

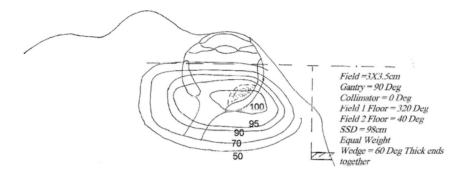

Field =3X3.5cm
Gantry = 90 Deg
Collimator = 0 Deg
Field 1 Floor = 320 Deg
Field 2 Floor = 40 Deg
SSD = 98cm
Equal Weight
Wedge = 60 Deg Thick ends
together

100
95
90
70
50

Figure 14.9 Dose distribution of superior/inferior wedged pair using 6 MV photons.

IV) 6 MV Photon split arc

Two split arc fields with central shielding for the lens provide good coverage of the GTV.

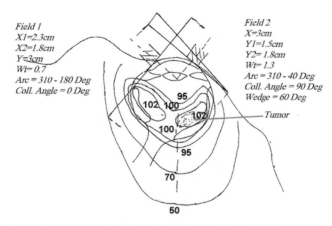

Field 1
X1=2.3cm
X2=1.8cm
Y=3cm
Wt= 0.7
Arc = 310 - 180 Deg
Coll. Angle = 0 Deg

Field 2
X=3cm
Y1=1.5cm
Y2= 1.8cm
Wt= 1.3
Arc = 310 - 40 Deg
Coll. Angle = 90 Deg
Wedge = 60 Deg

— Tumor

102 100
95
102
100
95
70
50

Figure 14.10 Dose distribution of split arc on 6 MV photon using a central lens shield.

V. PUBLICATIONS OF INTERESTS

1. Armstrong DI: the use of 4-6 MeV electrons for the conservative treatment of retinoblastoma. Br J Radiol 47:326,1974.

2. Donaldson SS, Smith LA: Retinoblastoma: Biology, presentation and current management. Oncology 3:45, 1989.

3. Foote RL, Garretson BR, Schomberg PJ, et al: External-beam irradiation for retinoblastoma: Patterns of failure and dose-response analysis. Int J Radiat Oncol Biol Phys 16:823, 1989.

4. Halnan KS: Tumours ofthe eye treated by radiotherapy. Clin Radiol 13:19, 1962.

5. Hernandez JC, Brady LW, Shields CL, et al: Conservative treatment of retinoblastoma: The use of plaque brachytherapy. Am J Clin Oncol 16:397-401, 1993.

6. Hilgers JHC: Strontium-90 beta irradiation, cataractongenicity and pterygium recurrence. Arch Ophthalmol 76:329,1966.

7. Hungerford JL, Toma NMG, Plowman PN, et al: External beam radiotherapy for retinoblastoma. I. Whole eye technique. Br J Ophthalmol 79:109-111, 1995.

8. Lederman M: Radiotherapy in treatment of orbital tumours. Br J Ophthalmol 40:592, 1956.

9. Lentino W, Zaret MM, Rossignol B, et al : Treatment of pterygium by surgery followed by beta irradiation. Am J Roentgenol 81: 93,1949.

10. Markoe AM, Brady LW, Shields JA, et al: Radioactive eye-plaque therapy versus enucleation for the treatment of posterior uveal malignant melanoma. Radiology 156:801, 1985.

11. McCormick B, Ellsworth R, Abramson D, et al: Radiation therapy for retinoblastoma: Comparison of results with lens-sparing versus lateral beam techniques. Int J Radiat Oncol Biol Phys 15:567, 1988

12. Packer S, Stoller S, Lesser ML, et al: Long term results of Iodine 125 irradiation of uveal melanoma. Ophthalmology 99:767-774, 1992.

13. Schipper J: An accurate and simple method for megavoltage radiation therapy of retinoblastoma. Radiother Oncol 1:31,1983.

14. Schipper J, Tan KEWP, van Peperzeel HA: Treatment of retinoblastoma by precision megavoltage radiation therapy. Radiother Oncol 3:117, 1985.

15. Shields JA, Angsburger JJ: Current approaches to the diadnosis and management of retinoblastoma. Surv Ophthalmol 25:347,1981.

15. Shields CL, Shields JA, DePotter P, et al: Plaque radiotherapy in the management of retinoblastoma: Use as a primary and secondary treatment. Ophthalmology 100:216-224, 1993.

16. Shields JA, Giblin ME, Shields CL, et al: Episcleral plaque radiotherapy for retinoblastoma. Ophthalmology 96:530, 1989.

17. Stallard HB: the conversative treatment of retinoblastoma. Trans Ophthalmol Soc UK 82:473,1962.

18. Toma NMG, Hungerford JL, Plowman PN, et al: External beam radiotherapy for retinoblastoma. II. Lens sparing technique. Br J Ophthalmol 79:112-117, 1995.

19. Weiss DR, Cassady JR, Petersen R: Retinoblastoma: A modification in radiation therapy technique. Radiology 114:705,1975.

— *CHAPTER 15* —

Cancer of the Larynx

I. INTRODUCTION

The larynx is made up of the supraglottis, the glottis and the subglottis. The supraglottis includes the false cords, epiglottis, aryepiglottic folds, ventricles and the arytenoids. The glottis is the true vocal cords and the subglottis includes the undersurface of the vocal cords and the area of the angle with the trachea.

Of the three glottic areas, supraglottic tumors have the highest tendency to spread to the lymphatics due to the rich supply of lymphatics in the area. Next is the subglottis. The glottic tumor almost never spread due to its absence of lymphatics.

Men are afflicted with cancer of the larynx much more than women. The possible leading causes of laryngeal cancer are tobacco and alcohol.

Diagnosis is by indirect and/or direct laryngoscopy.

Treatment of choice is by radiotherapy due to a high cure rate for early tumors and preservation of the larynx. Surgery is the choice for treatment of recurrent tumors and large tumors.

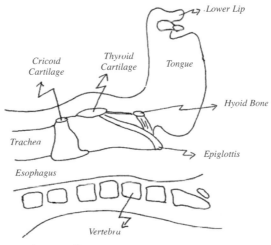

Figure 15.1 Diagram shows larynx and surrounding structures.

II. LOCALIZATION

Radiological examinations such as contrast laryngography and CT scans are useful tools in the tumor localization.

— *CHAPTER 16* —

Cancer of the Maxillary Antrum

I. INTRODUCTION

The maxilla forms much of the face below the orbits and above the jawbone. The maxilla *(with the ethmoid, frontal, and zygomatic bones)* also forms much of the lateral walls of the nasal cavity, the orbital cavity, and part of the cheek. The top row of teeth are set on the maxilla. The roof of the mouth is formed by the palatine bone, which is attached to the maxilla just behind the teeth.

Some of the suggested causes of maxillary antrum tumours are long term sinusitis and exposure to radioactive thorium. The presentations are sinusitis, nasal obstruction, bloody discharge and tenderness in the cheek. Diagnosis is by a series of sinus X-Rays and CT scans. Treatment of choice in the early stage is by surgery and radiation therapy. However, in the late stage, radiation therapy is the treatment of choice due to the large area of involvement.

II. LOCALIZATION

An immobilization shell is fabricated to immobilize the head and neck for simulation and treatment. The chin is hyper-extended so that the superior border of the anterior field passes just inferior to the eyeball to avoid the lens. The patient is simulated and anterior and lateral films are taken. Field centers are drawn on the shell for referencing. Radio-opaque markers are taped on the field centers on the shell. The radio-opaque markers would show up on CT for centering at the time of planning. The patient is CT. After exporting the CT images to the planning computer, the radiation oncologist delineates the GTV and the organs at risk. Margins are created to form the CTV/PTV.

III. TREATMENT PLANNING

The intersection of the AP and lateral CT marks on the central CT slice are localized and centered for referencing. A plan is generated using an anterior wedged field and a lateral oblique wedged field as shown in Figure 16.2. After plan approval by the radiation oncologist, the plan isocenter with reference to the original center is documented on the plan. This plan isocenter is set up at simulation for plan check. The plan fields are simulated as per plan and films are taken for documentation. The new field centers are marked on the shell for treatment set up.

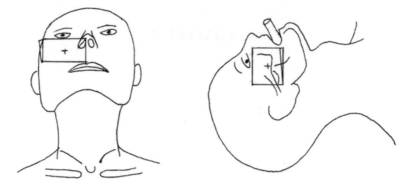

Figure 16.1 Field set up for treating maxillary antrum tumour.

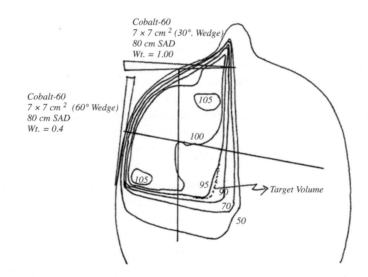

Figure 16.2 Dose distribution for maxillary antrum tumor.

IV. PUBLICATIONS OF INTERESTS

1. Bataini JP, Ennuyer A: Advanced carcinoma of the maxillary antrum treated by cobalt teletherapy and electron beam irradiation. Br J Radiol 44:590,1971.

2. Frich JC Jr: Treatment of advanced squamous carcinoma of the maxillary sinus by irradiation. Int J Radiat Oncol Biol Phys 8:1453-1459, 1982.

3. Lee F, Ogura JH: Maxillary sinus carcinoma. laryngoscope 91:133-139,1981.

4. Pearlman AW, Abadir R: Carcinoma of the maxillary antrum: the role of preoperative irradiation. Laryngoscope 84:400- 409,1974.

5. Trimas SJ, Stringer SP: The use of nasal endoscopes in the diagnosis of nasal and paranasal sinus masses. Am J Rhinol 8:1-5, 1994.

Principles and Practice of Clinical Physics and Dosimetry
Michael L.F. Lim, CMD, ACT
Advanced Medical Publishing, Inc., USA

— *CHAPTER 17* —

Cancer of the Nasopharynx

I. INTRODUCTION

The nasopharynx is situated behind the nasal cavity bordered by the sphenoid bone superiorly, soft palate inferiorly, choanae anteriorly and cervical vertebrae posteriorly. Due its location, the disease has usually spread by the time the patient notices any signs or symptoms. Most patients present with neck nodes at time of diagnosis.

This disease is rare among Caucasian but the incidence is high among the Chinese in Southern China. Some of the possible causes of this disease are genetics, environmental factors such as smoke and diet. The Epstein-Barr Virus (EBV) has been detected in patients with nasopharyngeal cancer.

The presentations are enlarge neck nodes, epistaxis, headache and decrease in hearing. Diagnosis is by nasopharyngoscopy using fiber optics, biopsy, skull films and anti-EBV antibodies. Radiation therapy is the treatment of choice because of the inaccessibility of the nasopharynx, proximity to base of skull and nodal involvement.

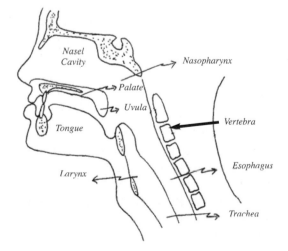

Figure 17.1 Diagram shows the nasopharynx and surrounding structures.

II. LARGE FIELD

a) Localization

The patient lies in a supine position with the chin hyper-extended. An immobilization shell is fabricated for the patient in this position. The lateral nasopharygeal field is simulated and a film is taken. The field edges are: (i) superiorly just past the superior orbital margin; (ii) inferiorly just inferior to the hyoid; (iii) anteriorly to cover the posterior half of the nasal cavity; and (iv) posteriorly to cover the cervical neck nodes. Shielding is drawn on the film. Point of prescription is at the center of the treated field.

The gantry is angled to zero degree to simulate the AP supraclavicular field. The field is adjusted to cover both supraclav and the superior border of the field matches the inferior borders of the nasopharyngeal fields. Point of prescription is at the supraclav.

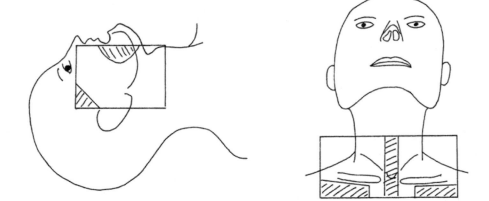

Figure 17.2 Field set-up for treatment of nasapharyngeal tumor.

b) Treatment Planning

The patient is planned for the 6 MV unit. Irregular field calculation is computed to take into account of the reduction in dose rate due to the reduction in scatter.

A total tumor dose of 4000 cGy in 20 fractions in 4 weeks is prescribed to mid depth for the nasopharygeal fields and to 1.5 cm depth for the supraclavicular field.

III. BOOST FIELD

a) Localization

The nasopharyngeal fields are reduced to the primary site. The posterior field border is reduced off the cord. This area is supplemented with electron field in order not to overdose the cervical cord. A new set of simulation film is taken for the lateral nasopharynx and the AP supraclav.

Planning CT may is done for the nasopharyngeal boost field. Target volume is delineated on each CT slice by the radiation oncologist.

b) Treatment Plannin

The CT slices are transferred to the treatment planning computer. The nasopharyngeal boost is planned with a three field technique using lateral opposed fields and an anterior field. Shielding blocks are constructed from BEV. The new field centers are transferred from the plan to the patient's shell for plan check at simulation. The total tumor dose for the boost is 2600 cGy in 13 fractions to the isocenter. As mentioned above, the cervical nodes are boosted with electron field giving 2000 cGy at D_{max}.

The supraclav is treated with a direct anterior field. The total tumor dose to the supraclav at 1.5 cm depth is 2000 cGy in 10 fractions.

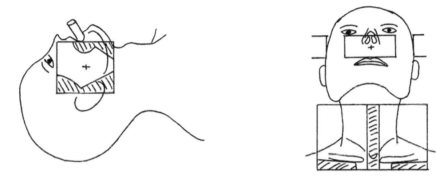

Figure 17.3 Field set-up for treatment of nasapharyngeal boost.

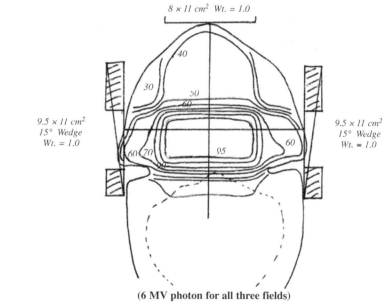

(6 MV photon for all three fields)

Figure 17.4 Dose distribution of nasopharyngeal boost. (6 MV photons)

Brachytherapy is sometimes used to boost residure disease.

IV. PUBLICATIONS OF INTERESTS

1.   Baker SR, Wolfe RA:Prognostic factors of nasopharyngeal malignancy. Cancer 49:163,1982.

2.   Buell P:Nasopharyngeal cancer in Chinese of California. Br J Cancer 19:459,1965.

3.   Chen KY, Fletcher GH:Malignant tumours of the nasopharynx. Radiology 99:165,1971.

4.   Henderson BE, Louie E, Jing JSH, et al: Risk factors associated with nasopharyngeal carcinoma. N Engl J Med 295:1101,1976.

5.   Henle W, Henle G: Evidence for an etiologic relation of the Epstein-Barr Virus to human malignancies.

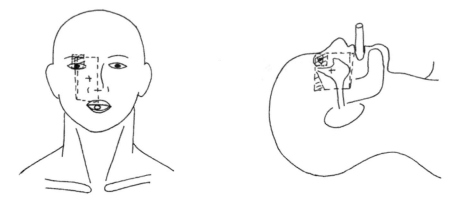

Figure 18.1 Field set-up for treating unilateral ethmoid and nasal cavity tumors.

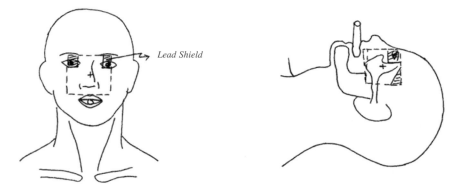

Lead Shield

Figure 18.2 Field set-up for treating bilateral ethmoid and nasal cavity tumors.

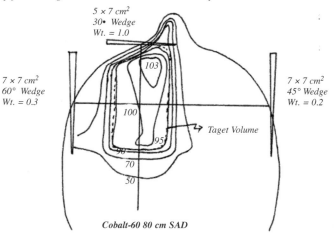

5 × 7 cm²
30• Wedge
Wt. = 1.0

7 × 7 cm²
60° Wedge
Wt. = 0.3

7 × 7 cm²
45° Wedge
Wt. = 0.2

103

100

95

90

70

50

Taget Volume

Cobalt-60 80 cm SAD

Figure 18.3 Dose distribution for unilateral ethmoid and nasal cavity tumors.

b) *Bilateral nasal cavity and ethmoid*

A plan is generated using an anterior field and two lateral opposed wedged field as shown in fig-ure.18.4. After plan approval by the radiation oncologist, the plan isocenter with reference to the original center is documented on the plan. This plan isocenter is set-up at simulation for plan check. The plan fields are simulated as per plan and films are taken for documentation. The new field cen-ters are marked on the shell for treatment set-up.

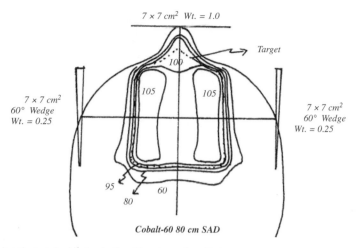

Figure 18.4 Dose distribution for bilateral ethmoid and nasal cavity tumors.

IV. PUBLICATIONS OF INTERESTS

1.	Acheson ED, Cowdell RH, Hadfield EH, et al: Nasal cancer in woodworkers in the furniture industry. Br Med J 2:587,1968.

2.	Ang KK, Jiang G-L, Frankenthaler RA, et al: Carcinomas of the nasal cavity. Radiother Oncol 24:163-168, 1992

3.	Boone ML, Harle TS, Highott HW, et al: Malignant disease of the paranasal sinuses and nasal cavity: Importance of precise localization of extent of disease. Am J Roentgenol

4.	Radium Ther Nucl Med 102:627,1968.

5.	Bosch A, Wallecillo L, Frias Z: Cancer of the nasal cavity. Cancer 37:1458,1976.

6.	Ellingwood KE, Million RR:Cancer of the nasal cavity and ethmoid/sphenoid sinuses. Cancer 43:1517,1979.

7.	Frazell EL, Lewis JS· Cancer of the nasal cavity and accessary sinuses. A report of the management of 416 patients. Cancer 16:1293-1301, 1963.

8.	Guedea F, Mendenhall WM, Parsons JT, et al: The role of radiation therapy in inverted papilloma of the nasal cavity and paranasal sinuses. Int J Radiat Oncol Biol Phys 20:777-780, 1991

9.	Hug EB, Wang CC, Montgomery WW, et al: Management of inverted papilloma of the nasal cavity and paranasal sinuses: importance of radiation therapy. Int J Radiat Oncol Biol Phys 26:67-72, 1993

10.	Mak ACA, van Andel JG, van Woerkom-Eijkenboom WMA: Radiation therapy of carcinoma of the nasal vestibule. Eur J Cancer 16:81-85, 1980

11.	McCollough WM, Mendenhall NP, Parsons JT, et al: Radiotherapy alone for squamous cell carcinoma of the nasal vestibule: management of the primary site and regional lymphatics. Int J Radiat Oncol Biol Phys 26:73-79, 1993

12.	McNeese MD, Chobe R, Weber RS, Hogstrom KR: Carcinoma of the nasal vestibule: Treatment with radiotherapy. Cancer Bull 41:84-87, 1989

13.	Mendenhall NP, Parsons JT, Cassisi NJ, et al: Carcinoma of the nasal vestibule treated with radiation therapy. Laryngoscope 97:626-632, 1987

14.	Parsons JT, Mendenhall WM, Mancuso AA, et al: Malignant tumors of the nasal cavity and ethmoid and sphenoid sinuses. Int J Radiat Oncol Biol Phys 14:11-22, 1988

15.	Trimas SJ, Stringer SP: The use of nasal endoscopes in the diagnosis of nasal and paranasal sinus masses. Am J Rhinol 8:1-5, 1994

16.	Wong CS, Cummings BJ, Elhakim T, et al: External irradiation for squamous cell carcinoma of the nasal vestibule. Int J Radiat Oncol Biol Phys 12:1943-1946, 1986

Principles and Practice of Clinical Physics and Dosimetry
Michael L.F. Lim, CMD, ACT
Advanced Medical Publishing, Inc., USA

—— *CHAPTER 19* ——

Cancer of the Salivary Glands

I. INTRODUCTION

There are three pairs of salivary glands that drain the saliva into the mouth. The salivary glands are the parotid gland, the submandibular gland and the sublingual gland. The parotid gland is the largest and lies between the external auditory meatus, the mastoid process and the mandible. The submandibular gland lies under the mandibular and the sublingual gland under the mucous membrane of the floor of mouth.

Cancer incidence of the salivary gland in male and female are about equal. Nutritional deficit and radiation exposure are among the known causes of cancer of the salivary gland.

Presentations are swelling, tenderness, trismus and swollen lymph nodes.

Radiographic studies, CT, physical examination and biopsy are the diagnostic procedures used for cancer of the salivary gland.

The common glands involved are the parotid and the submandibular glands. In the early stage, surgery followed by radiation therapy is the treatment of choice. In later stage, radiation therapy is the treatment of choice due to the difficulties of removing all the tumor without sacrifice of the facial, lingual or hypoglossal nerve.

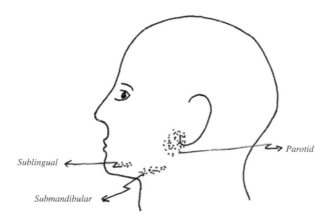

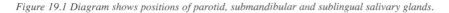

Figure 19.1 Diagram shows positions of parotid, submandibular and sublingual salivary glands.

II. LOCALIZATION

The patient lies on his unaffected side with his head resting on a head rest. The shoulder is pulled inferiorly to allow for room for treatment set up. A plastic immobilization shell is fabricated for the patient in this position. Anterior and lateral films are taken. Field centers are drawn on the shell for referencing. Radio-opaque markers are taped on the field centers on the shell. The radio-opaque markers would show up on CT for centering at the time of planning. The patient is CT. After exporting the CT images to the planning computer, the radiation oncologist delineates the GTV and the organs at risk. Results from the physical examination, biopsy and radiographic studies are used to localize the tumor. Margins are created to form the CTV/PTV

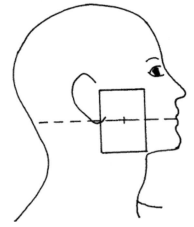

Figure 19.2 Set-up for treating cancer of the parotid salivary gland.

III. TREATMENT PLANNING

Coverage of the target volume is achieved with a pair of 30° wedged fields as shown in Figure 19.3. After plan approval by the radiation oncologist, the plan isocenter with reference to the original center is documented on the plan. This plan isocenter is set up at simulation for plan check. The plan fields are simulated as per plan and films are taken for documentation. The new field centers are marked on the shell for treatment set up.

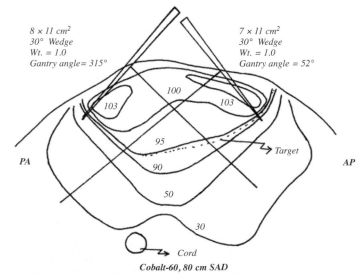

Figure 19.3 Dose distribution of wedged pair in the treatment of parotid salivary gland tumor.

IV. PUBLICATIONS OF INTERESTS

1. Elkon D, Colman M, Hendrickson FR: Radiation therapy in the treatment of malignant salivary gland tumours. Cancer 41:502,1978.

2. Matsuba HM, Thawley SE, Devineni VR, et al: High grade malignancies of the parotid gland: Effective use of planned combined surgery and irradiation. Laryngoscope 95:1059,1985.

3. Moss WT: The salivary glands. In Cox JD, ed: Moss Radiation Oncology: Rationale, Technique, Results, ed 7, pp 121-131. St. Louis, MO, Mosby-Year Book, 1994

4. Rafla S: Malignant parotid tumours: Natural history and treatment. Cancer 40:136,1977.

5. Smith SA: Radiation-induced salivary gland tumours. Arch Otolaryngol 102:561,1976.

6. Soni SC, Kahn FR, Paul JM, et al: Electron beam treatment of malignant tumours of salivary glands. J Radiol Electrol 58:677,1977.

7. Spitz MR: Risk factors for salivary gland cancer- a review. Cancer Bull 37(3):153,1985.

8. Tapley NdV:Irradiation treatment of malignant tumours of the salivary glands. Ear,nose, throat J 56:39,1977

9. Wang CC, Goodman M: Photon irradiation of unresectable carcinomas of the salivary glands. Int J Radiat Oncol Biol Phys 21:569-576, 1991

Principles and Practice of Clinical Physics and Dosimetry
Michael L.F. Lim, CMD, ACT
Advanced Medical Publishing, Inc., USA

— *CHAPTER 20* —

Cancer of the Tongue

I. INTRODUCTION

The tongue is located in the floor of the mouth. Its base is connected to the hyoid bone, epiglottis and pharynx. Anterior two-third of the tongue lies in the mouth and posterior one-third lies in the oropharynx. The mucous membrane of the under surface of the tongue is smooth while the dorsum of the tongue is covered with papillae.

The tongue is made up of extrinsic and intrinsic muscles, nerves and blood vessels. The extrinsic muscles are attached to bone and the intrinsic muscles lie in the tongue. About one third of cancer of the tongue arise in the posterior third and afflict males more than females. The possible leading causes of tongue cancer are alcohol and tobacco.

The common presentations are ulceration, pain, difficult in swallowing and in more advanced cases, a mass in the neck.

Diagnosis is by visual inspection, palpation and laryngoscopy.

Radiotherapy is the treatment of choice for the obvious reason of preservation of the tongue and its function. Radiotherapy may be administered in one of three ways or a combination of the three ways. The choice depends of the size, location and possible spread of the tumor. Generally, the small anterior tumors are treated by either the intra-oral technique or by implant of radium needles. The larger posterior tumors are treated by opposed laterally fields with an anterior field to cover the cervical and clavicular nodes. Tumor on one side of the tongue may be treated with a pair of wedged fields.

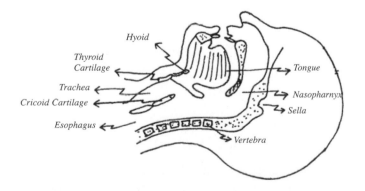

Figure 20.1 Diagram shows the tongue and surrounding structures.

II. LOCALIZATION

The patient lies in a supine position for simulation and treatment. An immobilization shell is fabricated for the head and neck. The patient is simulated to localize the treatment volume. Localization of small oral tongue cancer is by visual inspection and palpation. Localization of large cancer at base of tongue is by imaging techniques. The target volume is dependent on the possible spread pattern of the tumor.

For small anterior tongue tumors, a pair of wedged fields are sufficient. For large tumors and tumors at the posterior tongue, the treatment fields are large opposed lateral fields with an anterior supraclav field to treat the potential spread of the disease. In this set-up, the anterior supraclav field is simulated first. The collimator of the lateral fields are angled to match the divergence of the anterior supraclav field.

With this set-up and angle, the inferior edge of the lateral field is just at the superior edge of the anterior field. To prevent over or under dosage at this junction, the junction is moved once or twice during the course of the treatment. This is achieved by increasing the inferior border of the lateral fields by 1cm and decreasing the superior border of the anterior field by 1 cm.

III. TREATMENT PLANNING

There are three radiation treatment modalities. They are: 1) external beam radiotherapy, 2) intra-oral radiotherapy; and 3) interstitial implant of Iridium-192 needles.

IV. EXTERNAL BEAM RADIOTHERAPY

A. Wedged pair

If the tumor is situated on one side of the tongue and is on the anterior third of the tongue, a pair of wedge fields usually covers the target volume well. A plan is generated using a pair of wedged fields as shown in Figure 20.2.

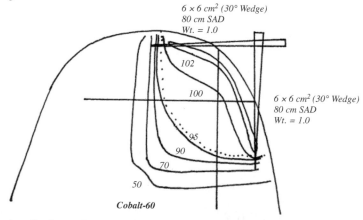

Figure 20.2 Wedged pair dose distribution for cancer of the tongue.

B. Opposed lateral with single anterior supraclav field

With large posterior tumors and potential spread to the cervical and clavicular nodes, large opposed lateral fields with an anterior supraclav field are used. The lateral fields treat the tumor bed while the anterior supraclav field treats the cervical and clavicular nodes.

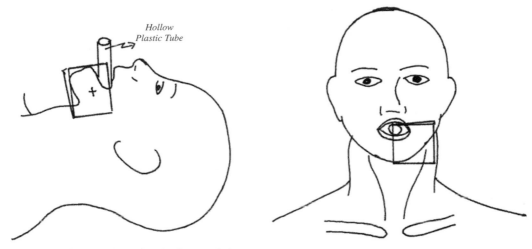

Figure 20.3 Field set-up showing wedged pair technique.

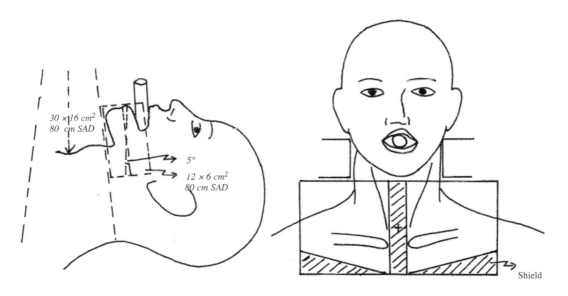

Figure 20.4 Field set-up showing lateral opposed fields and an anterior field.

V. INTRA-ORAL RADIOTHERAPY

For small localized tumor on the anterior third of the tongue, intra-oral radiotherapy may be used. A suitable size cone from a 200kV (DXR) treatment unit is placed on the tongue to cover the tumor adequately giving a total applied dose of 6000 cGy in 30 fractions in 6 weeks.

Intra-oral radiotherapy may also be used as a boost to the large lateral fields. In this situation, the opposed lateral fields deliver a tumor dose of 4000 cGy in 20 fractions in 4 weeks to mid-depth and the intra-oral field delivers an applied dose of 2000 cGy in 20 fractions in 2 weeks.

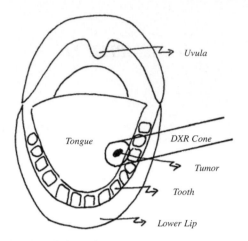

Figure 20.5 Intra-oral treatment set-up using a DXR applicator or electron applicator.

VI. PUBLICATIONS OF INTERESTS

1. Dally V: The place of radiotherapy in the treatment of tumours of the base of the tongue. Am J Roentgenol 93:20,1965.

2. Frazell E, Lucas J Jr: Cancer of the tongue. Cancer 15:218, 1967.

3. Mak AC, Morrison WH, Garden AS, et al: Base of tongue carcinoma: Treatment results using concomitant boost radiotherapy. Int J Radiat Oncol Biol Phys 33:289, 1995

4. Novack A: Treatment of carcinoma of the base of the tongue and the larynx. Laryngoscope 89:1332, 1975.

5. Parsons JT, Million RR, Cassisi NJ: Carcinoma of the base of the tongue: Results of radical irradiation with surgery reserved for irradiation failure. Laryngoscope 92:689, 1982

6. Riley RW, LeeWE, Goffinet D, et al: Squamous cell carcinoma of the base of the tongue. Otholaryngol Head Neck Surg 91:143, 1983.

7. Rollo J, Rosenbom C, Thawley S, et al: Squamous carcinoma of the base of the tongue. Cancer 47:333,1981.

8. Scanlon PW, Soule EH, Devine KD, et al: Cancer of the base of the tongue. Radiology 1054:26,1969.

— CHAPTER 21 —

Cancer of the Pituitary Gland

I. INTRODUCTION

The pituitary gland sits in the sella turcica and is attached to the base of the brain by a thin stalk. It is made up of two lobes, the anterior lobe and the posterior lobe. Superior to the pituitary is the optic chiasm and inferior to the pituitary is the sphenoid sinus.

The two most common pituitary tumors are the chromophobe tumor and the eosinophilic tumor. The chromophobe tumors are usually benign. They are non functioning tumors and cause problems by pressure on surrounding structures such as the optic chiasma causing visual defects and on the eosinophic cells of the pituitary causing hypopituitarism which in turn affect organs like the thyroid, gonads and adrenals. Due to the pressure, headache is a common complaint.

The eosinophilic tumors are small benign tumors. With the growth of the tumors, increase growth hormone is produced causing acromegaly. It also presses on the optic chiasma and causes visual defects.

The common presentations are acromegaly, headache, visual defect, fatigue, obesity, hypertension and a hosts of other endocrine related manifestations.

Diagnostic procedures are endocrinological tests, radiographic studies, CT and visual tests.

Treatment of choice is surgery and/or radiation therapy depending on the size and extent of the disease. Radiation therapy may be given externally or by implantation of radioactive sources such as ^{90}Y or ^{198}Au.

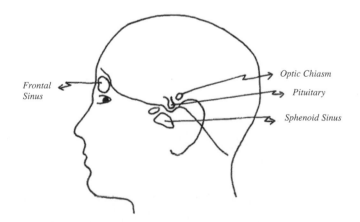

Figure 21.1 Diagram shows the position of the pituitary in the skull.

II. LOCALIZATION

The patient is simulated and anterior and lateral films are taken. Field centers are drawn on the shell for referencing. Radio-opaque markers are taped on the field centers on the shell. The radio-opaque markers would show up on CT for centering at the time of planning. The patient is CT. After exporting the CT images to the planning computer, the radiation oncologist delineates the GTV and the organs at risk. Margins are created to form the CTV/PTV. The entire sella turcica plus margin all round must be included in the target volume.

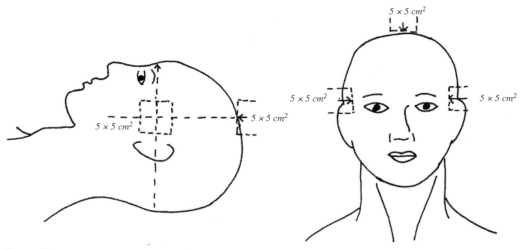

Figure 21.2 Field set-up for treatment of the pituitary tumor.

III. TREATMENT PLANNING

The intersection of the AP and lateral CT marks on the central CT slice are localized and centered for referencing. Coverage of the target volume is achieved a pair of lateral opposed fields and a vortex field *(or an anterior superior oblique field)*. After plan approval by the radiation oncologist, the plan isocenter with reference to the original center is documented on the plan. This plan isocenter is set up at simulation for plan check. The plan fields are simulated as per plan and films are taken for documentation. The new field centers are marked on the shell for treatment set-up.

The three field plan is shown in Figure 21.3.

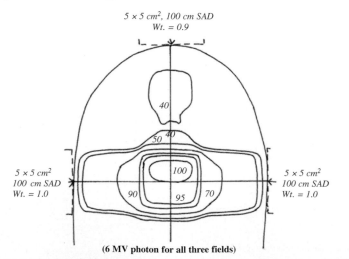

Figure 21.3 Dose distribution for three-field plan in the treatment of carcinoma of the pituitary. (6 MV photons)

IV. PUBLICATIONS OF INTERESTS

1.   Eastman RC, Gordon P, Roth J: Conventional supervoltage irradiation is an effective treatment for acromegaly. J Clin Endocrinol Metab 48:931,1979.

2.   Edmonds MW, Simpton WJK, Meakin JW: External irradiation of the hypophysis for Cushing's disease. Calif Med Assoc J 107:860,1972.

3.   Heuschele R, Lampe I: Pituitary irradiation for Cushing's syndrome. Radiol Clin Biol 36:27,1967.

4.   Levin S: Manifestations and treatment of acromegaly. Calif Med 116:57,1972.

5.   Pistenmaa DA, Goffinet DR, Bagshaw ME, et al: Treatment of acromegaly with megavoltage radiation therapy. Int J Radiat Oncol Biol Phys 1:885,1976.

6.   Pistenmaa DA, Goffinet DR, Bagshaw MA, et al: Treatment of chromophobe adenomas with megavoltage irradiation. Cancer 35:1574, 1975.

7.   Rush SC, Newall J: Pituitary adenoma: The efficacy of radiotherapy as the sole treatment. Int J Radiat Oncol Biol Phys 17:165, 1989

8.   Schoenthaler R, Albright NW, Wara WM, et al: Reirradiation of pituitary adenoma. Int J Radiat Oncol Biol Phys 24:307, 1992

9.   Sheline GE: The role of conventional radiation therapy in the treatment of functional pituitary tumours. In Linfoot JA(ed): Recent advances in the diagnosis and treatment of pituitary tumours, pp 289-313. New York, Raven Press,1979.

10.   Sheline GE: Treatment of nonfuntioning chromophobe adenomas of the pituitary. AJR 120:553, 1974.

11.   Thoren M, Rahn T, Guo WY, et al: Stereotactic radiosurgery with cobalt-60 gamma unit in the treatment of growth hormone-producing pituitary tumors. Neurosurgery 29:663, 1991

12.   Tsang RW, Brierley JD, Panzarella T, et al: Radiation therapy for pituitary adenoma: Treatment outcome and prognostic factors. Int J Radiat Oncol Biol Phys 30:557, 1994

13.   Zierhut D, Flentje M, Adolph J, et al: External radiotherapy of pituitary adenomas. Int J Radiat Oncol Biol Phys 33:307, 1995

—— *CHAPTER 22* ——

Cancer of the Thyroid

I. INTRODUCTION

The thyroid gland sits at the upper part of the trachea and is made up of two lobes joined at the lower part by the isthmus that lies over the second and third tracheal ring. Each lobe is pear shaped and measures about 3.5 cm long by 2 cm wide by 1.5 cm thick. The thyroid gland wraps around the trachea.

Thyroid tumors are of the differentiated and the undifferentiated type. The differentiated type consists of: a) the papillary adenocarcinoma; b) the follicular carcinoma; c) the medullary carcinoma; and d) anaplastic carcinoma.

The leading cause of thyroid cancer is radiation to the thyroid. Radiation from exposure to the atomic bomb, nuclear testing, childhood tonsillar irradiation and thymus irradiation are the common causes. Irradiation to the thyroid in mantle technique for Hodgkin's disease has also been reported to cause thyroid cancer. Long standing nontoxic goiters have been known to lead to thyroid cancer.

Presentations are solitary nodule in neck, enlarged lymph node in neck and hoarseness. Diagnosis is by radioisotopic scanning of the thyroid using ^{123}I or ^{Tc}99m, needle biopsy and ultra sound.

Treatment of choice is by surgery followed by administration of ^{131}I and/or external beam irradiation. At surgery, as much of the diseased thyroid is removed. If tumors are not all removed as shown by a ^{131}I uptake scan, a therapeutic dose of ^{131}I is given orally. The therapeutic dose is in the range of 100-200 mCi depending on the size of the tumor. External beam irradiation is necessary if there is gross disease in the tumor bed and involvement of nodal areas.

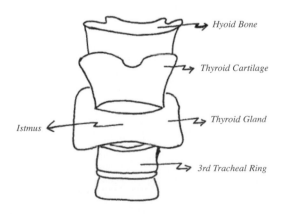

Figure 22.1 Anterior view of the thyroid and surrounding structures.

II. LOCALIZED TUMOR

A) Localization

An immobilization shell is fabricated for the patient in the supine position. The patient is simulated and anterior and lateral films are taken. Field centers are drawn on the shell for referencing. Radio-opaque markers are taped on the field centers on the shell. The radio-opaque markers would show up on CT for centering at the time of planning. CT planning is done to accurately locate the depth of the spinal cord and to delineate the target volume for treatment planning. After exporting the CT images to the planning computer, the radiation oncologist delineates the GTV and the organs at risk. Margins are created to form the CTV/PTV.

B) Treatment Planning

The intersection of the AP and lateral CT marks on the central CT slice are localized and centered for referencing. Coverage of the target volume, without excessive dose to the spinal cord may be achieved with photon arc rotation or with a direct electron field as shown in Figures 22.2 and 22.3. For the photon arc rotation, the isocenter is located at the anterior cord and field is brought in past the central axis in order to shield the cord. *(This may be also be achieved with a symmetric field by placing a central block in the field.)* After plan approval by the radiation oncologist, the plan isocenter with reference to the original center is documented on the plan. This plan isocenter is set up at simulation for plan check. The plan fields are simulated as per plan and films are taken for documentation. The new field centers are marked on the shell for treatment set-up.

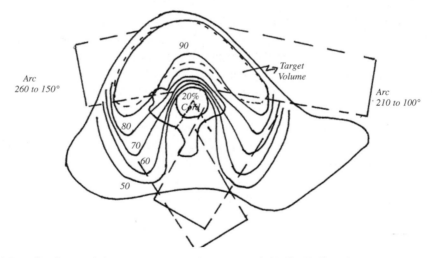

Figure 22.2 Dose distribution of photon arc rotation with asymmetric field. (6 MV photons)

III. LARGE TUMOR WITH NODAL INVOLVEMENT

A) Localization

An immobilization shell is fabricated for the patient in the supine treatment position. The chin is extended by resting the neck on a clear hollow plastic neck rest. *(This allows a posterior neck field to be employed without much attenuation through the neck rest.)*

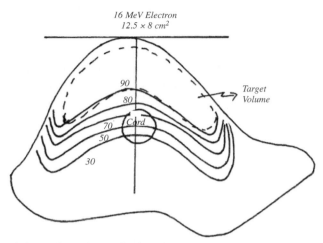

Figure 22.3 Dose distribution of electron beam therapy for thyroid cancer.

The target volume is localized at simulation. Localization of the tumor is from operative reports and imaging studies. Depending on the tumor size and spread, the field may include the neck nodes, thyroid bed, supraclavicular nodes and mediastinal nodes.

The patient is simulated from the anterior and a film is taken. The anterior field typically covers the thyroid bed, cervical nodes, the clavicular nodes and the superior mediastinum. The field center and borders are marked on the shell. A solder wire is taped along the sagittal midline of the patient on the anterior and posterior surface. A lateral film is taken ensuring the anterior surface solder wire and spinal cord are visible on the film. The target volume and spinal cord are delineated on the lateral film. The outline of the wire on the lateral simulator film forms the sagittal contour for treatment planning. Desired areas to be shielded such as the lungs and normal tissue are drawn on the anterior film by the radiation oncologist.

B) Treatment Planning

For external beam planning, the lateral sagittal contour, the target volume and the spinal cord position from the lateral film are digitized into the planning computer using the correct de-magnification factor. In this example, coverage of the target volume is with an anterior field 18 × 18 cm^2 at 100 cm SSD, an inferior posterior field 12 cm long × 8 cm wide *(45° wedge)* at 100 cm SSD and a superior posterior field 6.5 cm long × 10 cm wide at 100 cm SSD. The weightings are 1.0, 0.3 and 0.1 on the 6 MV photon unit. The plan is shown in Figure 22.4.

After the radiation oncologist has approved the plan, the patient is simulated again to localize and verify the two posterior fields. The large field anterior center is set-up to 100 cm SSD. The couch is moved superiorly by 4.2 cm to the exit of the inferior posterior field. This center is marked on the shell. The gantry is rotated 180° to the posterior and SSD is set at 100 cm. A field size of 12 cm × 8 cm wide at 100 cm SSD is set. A film is taken. The gantry is rotated back to the anterior at 0 degree and set to the anterior center at 100 cm SSD. The couch is moved inferiorly by 6cm to the exit of the superior posterior field. This center is marked on the shell. The gantry is rotated 180 degree to the posterior and SSD is set at 100 cm. A field size of 6.5 cm × 10 cm *(wide)* at 100 cm SSD is set. A film is taken.

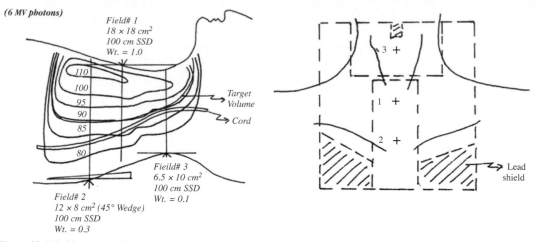

Figure 22.4 Field set-up and dose distribution for carcinoma of the thyroid.

IV. PUBLICATIONS OF INTERESTS

1.   Beierwaltes WH: The treatment of thyroid carcinoma with radioactive iodine. Semin Nucl Med 8:79,1978.

2.   Blahd WH: Treatment of malignant thyroid disease. Semin Nucl Med 9:95,1979.

3.   Blair TJ, Evans RG, Buskirk GJ, et al: Radiotherapeutic management of primary thyoid lymphoma. Int J Radiat Oncol Biol Phys 11:365,1985.

4.   Clark DE: Association of irradiation with cancer of the thyroid in children and adolescents. JAMA 159:1007,1955.

5.   Chung CT, Sagerman RH, Ryoo MC: External irradiation for malignant thyroid tumours. Radiology 136:753,1980.

6.   Edmonds CJ: Treatment of thyroid cancer. Clin Endocrinol Metab 8:223,1979.

7.   Greefield LD: Thyroid cancer:The role of radiotherapy in treatment. Int J Radiat Oncol Biol Phys 2(suppl 2):131,1977.

8.   Hellman DE, Durie BGM, Wollfenden JM, et al: Multidisciplinary management of carcinoma of the thyroid. Arizona Med 37:19, 1980.

9.   Levendag PC, dePorre PMS, van Putten WL: Anaplastic carcinoma of the thyroid gland treated by radiation therapy. Int J Radiat Oncol Biol Phys 26:125, 1993.

10. Linberg RD: Rxternal irradiation in thyroid cancers. In Fletcher GH(ed): Textbook of Radiotherapy, 3rd ed, pp 384-388, Philadelphia, Lea & Febiger, 1980.

11. McDay JB, Danoff BF: External beam radiotherapy in the management of locally invasive carcinoma of the thyroid. Int J Radiat Oncol Biol Phys 4(suppl 2):226, 1978.

12. Parker LN, Belsky JL, Yamamoto T, et al: Thyroid carcinoma after exposure to atomic radiation: A continuing survey of a fixed population, Hiroshima & Nagasaki, 1958-1977.Ann Intern Med 80:600,1974.

13. Simpson WJK: Radiotherapy in thyroid cancer. Can Med Assoc J 113:115,1975.

14. Simpson W, Sutcliffe S, Gospodarowicz M: The thyroid. In Moss W, Cox J, eds: Radiation Oncology: Rationale, Technique, Results, p 262. St. Louis, CV Mosby, 1989.

15. Thambi V, Pedapatti PJ, Murthy A, et al: A radiotherapy technique for thyroid cancer. Int J Radiat Oncol Biol Phys 6:239,1980.

16. Tubiana M: External radiotherapy and radioiodine in the treatment of thyroid cancer. World J Surg 5:75,1981.

17. Tubiana M, Haddad E, Schlumberger M, et al: External radiotherapy in thyroid cancers. Cancer 55:2062, 1985.

Principles and Practice of Clinical Physics and Dosimetry
Michael L.F. Lim, CMD, ACT
Advanced Medical Publishing, Inc., USA

—— *CHAPTER 23* ——

Cancer of the Breast

I. INTRODUCTION

The breasts are hemispherical in shape and are made up of glandular tissues embedded in connective tissue. They lie over the pectoral muscles. Adipose tissues lie between the skin and the glandular tissues and the size of the breasts depend on the adipose tissues.

Lymphatic pathways are mainly to the axillary glands and periphery of breast lymphatics radiate superiorly to infraclavicular nodes, medially to internal mammary nodes and inferiorly to extraperitoneal lymphatics and then to mediastinal nodes.

Breast cancer is the most common cancer in females. It is more common in women with a family history of breast cancer, women with no children or had first child after age 30. It is also more common in countries where the fat intake is high.

The most common site of breast cancer is the upper outer quadrant followed by the central area. Presentation is usually a palpable lump in the breast in the early stage and palpable node in the axilla in the later stage. Spread is by direct infiltration to the surrounding breast tissues and to the axillary, supraclavicular and internal mammary lymph nodes by the lymphatic system. Diagnosis is by physical examination of the breast and surrounding lymph nodes, biopsy and mammography.

Treatment choices for breast cancer are, surgery, radiation therapy, chemotherapy and hormonal therapy. A combination of the above are usually selected depending on several factors such as size of tumor, histology and stage.

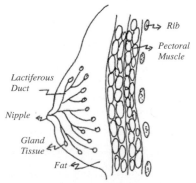

Figure 23.1 Sagittal view of the breast.

II. TREATING ONLY THE BREAST OR CHEST WALL

A) Localization

The patient lies in a supine treatment position with the arm on the treated side stretched out and up to hold on to a handle above the shoulder and with the head turned to the opposite side.

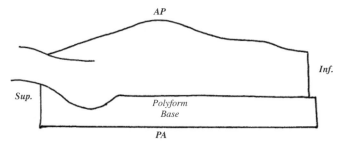

Figure 23.2 Lateral view of patient in treatment position in polyform base.

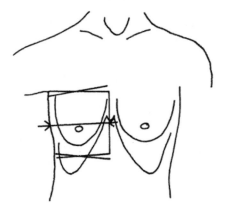

Figure 23.3 Tangential fields.

The radiation oncologist delineates the field borders. A short lead wire is taped on the lateral border. The lateral border is set up to 100 cm SSD using the wall and ceiling lazers. The gantry is angled to match the central axis with the medial border. The SSD reading is taken. The medial border is set to a new SSD of 100 minus 1/2 the separation. The field width is opened to cover the breast/chest wall with a 2 cm margin. The distance x, the drop depth y and the lateral distance z are calculated as shown in the example below. Angle ϕ is set at 50° for adequate coverage of the margins.

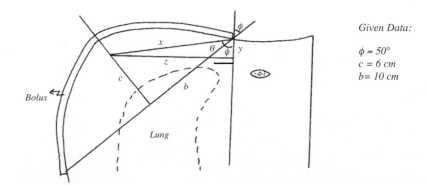

Given Data:

$\phi = 50°$
$c = 6$ cm
$b = 10$ cm

Figure 23.4 Geometric representation for SAD breast set-up for simulation.

Using the top triangle in Figure 23.4 with sides x, y, and z, one could obtain the side y as follow:

$\cos(\theta + \phi) = y/x$, *therefore,* $\rightarrow$ $y = x \cos(\theta + \phi)$, *where* $\phi = 50°$. *In order to calculate y, one has to calculate angle θ and side x as follow:*

1) *angle θ could be calculated from the triangle with sides b, c and x as follow;*

$$tan(\theta) = c/b \rightarrow \theta = tan^{-1}(c/b) = tan^{-1}(6/10) = 31°$$

2) *knowing angle θ, using* triangle in *Figure 23.4* with sides b, c, and x again, one could calculate the side x as follow;

therefore,
$$sin\theta = c/x \rightarrow x = c/sin\theta \rightarrow x = 6 \, cm/sin(31°) = 11.65 \, cm$$

$$y = x \cos(\theta + \phi) = 11.65 \times \cos(31°+50°) = 1.82 \, cm$$

Therefore, the set-up SSD is 98.2 cm. and z could be calculated from the triangle in *Figure 23.4 with sides x, y and z as follow;*

$$tan(\theta + \phi) = z/y \rightarrow z = y \times tan(\theta + \phi) = 1.82 \times tan(31 +50°) = 11.49 \, cm$$

The isocenter is moved 1.82 cm depth vertically on the medial border and 11.49 cm laterally. In order to match the divergence of the field to the base of the treatment volume, the gantry is angled a further *tan⁻¹(1/2 field width)*. The field is visualized under fluoroscope to determine the treatment volume and lung coverage. It is usually acceptable if the lung coverage is less than 3 cm thick as visualized on the simulator monitor. A film is taken for documentation. The gantry is angled to the lateral side and the same process is repeated.

A cross sectional contour is obtained for treatment planning.

B) Treatment Planning

Good dose distribution is achieved with a pair of parallel opposed tangential fields with lung correction as shown in Figure 23.5.

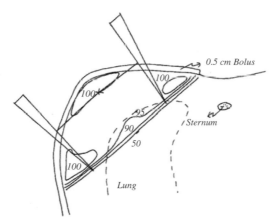

Figure 23.5 Dose distribution for a pair of parallel-opposed tangential fields on 6 MV Linear Accelerator.

III. TREATING THE BREAST *(OR CHEST WALL)*, THE SUPRACLAVICULAR NODES AND THE AXILLARY NODES

A) Localization

The patient lies in the same treatment position as described earlier. An AP field is set to cover the supraclav and axilla at 100 cm SAD. The floor is angled 90° and the gantry is angled inferiorly to match the inferior s/c field border with the superior border of the tangential fields. The angle is set to *Tan⁻¹ [(1/2 field length/width)/(100)]*. An AP film is taken. SSD reading and separation are taken for the axilla and supraclav point for irregular field calculation. A posterior field is simulated for the axilla boost.

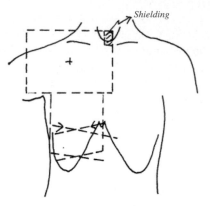

Figure 23.6 Anterior supraclav/axilla field and tangential chest wall fields.

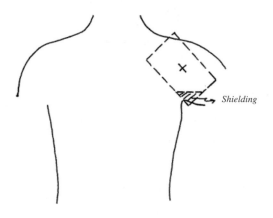

Figure 23.7 Posterior axilla field.

The breast/chest wall tangential fields are simulated as described in section I above. In order to match the divergence of the tangential fields to the inferior border of the AP supraclav field, the tangential fields are angled $\theta°$ by angling the floor. Where $\theta°$ is obtained as follow:

$$\theta° = Tan^{-1} [(1/2\ length)/(100)]$$

B) Treatment Planning

Coverage of the chest wall target volume is with a pair of wedged tangential fields as shown in Figure 23.5.

IV. TREATING THE BREAST *(OR CHEST WALL)*, THE INTERNAL MAMMARY CHAIN NODES, THE SUPRACLAVICULAR NODES AND THE AXILLARY NODES

A) Localization

The patient lies in the same treatment position as described under Section **I** above. An AP inverted L field is simulated to cover the axilla, supraclavicular fossa and the internal mammary chain nodes in the parasternum as shown in Figure 23.8. SSD and separations are taken for the axilla, supraclavicular fossa and parasternum points for irregular field calculation. The dose is prescribed to 3cm depth at the parasternal point and the resulting dose to the anterior axilla and supraclavicular fossa are calculated. The posterior axilla is given an additional boost to bring the dose at mid axilla to the desired dose. The inferior corner of the PA field is shielded to prevent overlap of this field into the chest wall field on the anterior. An AP inverted L field is necessary to treat the internal mammary nodes in the parasternum. If the tangential fields are used to cover these nodes, too much lung volume will be in the fields as shown in Figure 23.14

A cross sectional contour of the chest wall is taken through the tangential chest wall/breast volume for treatment planning.

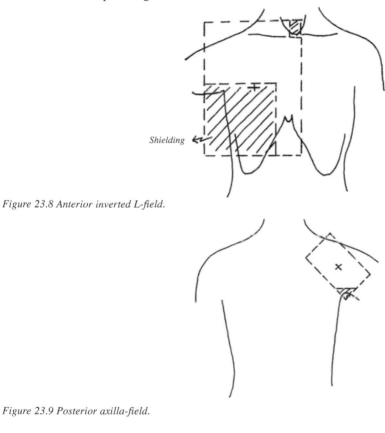

Shielding

Figure 23.8 Anterior inverted L-field.

Figure 23.9 Posterior axilla-field.

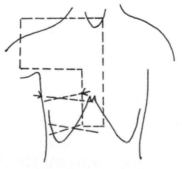

Figure 23.10 Chest wall tangential field showing fields angled to match the border of the axilla field.

B) Treatment Planning

Good coverage of the chest wall and para-sternum is achieved with opposed tangential fields to the chest wall and a direct AP field to the para-sternum giving 4500 cGy to the 95% isodose line for the tangential fields and 4500 cGy to the parasternum at 3 cm depth.

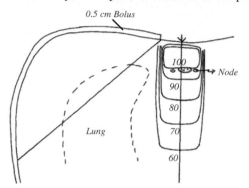

Figure 23.11 Dose distribution for parasternal field. (6 MV photons)

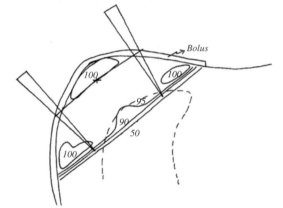

Figure 23.12 Dose distribution for tangential fields. (6 MV photons)

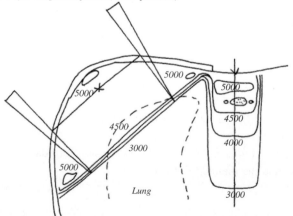

Figure 23.13 Sum dose distribution (in cGy) for tangential fields and parasternal field. (6 MV photons)

V. ELECTRON FIELD THERAPY FOR UNILATERAL CHEST WALL

In patients where the chest wall is too shallow for tangential photon fields, electron fields cover the chest wall rather well without excessive dose to the lung. The selection of the electron energy depends on the thickness of the chest wall.

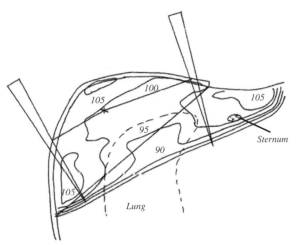

Figure 23.14 Dose distribution for tangential fields to include the internal mammary nodes. (6 MV photons)

Arc electron therapy or fixed static electron therapy provides acceptable dose distribution to encompass the chest wall. Described here are two examples of using static electron fields to treat chest wall.

In order to avoid over or under dose to the junction of the electron fields, the junction should be staggered during the course of the total treatment. This may be achieved by changing the field widths. A treatment unit with variable collimator does this well.

A) Localization

The patient lies in a supine position as described earlier. The radiation oncologist delineates the superior, inferior, medial and lateral border. The delineated area is simulated for record and for referencing for CT planning.

CT images of the patient are obtained and transferred to the treatment planning computer. The radiation oncologist delineates the target volume on each CT slice.

B) Treatment Planning

For the thick chest wall, good dose distribution is achieved with two 10 McV electron fields as shown in Figure 23.15. The junction between the two fields are staggered by opening one side of the field width from 5 cm to 6 cm.

For field 1 set-up, the field center is set to the midline to a SSD of 87.5 cm *(100-depth12.5 cm)*. The gantry is angled 12° and the field center is marked on the skin. For daily treatment, the distance is set to read 100 cm SSD and the planned field size is set.

For field 2, the field center is set to the midline to a SSD of 86.5 cm *(100-depth 13.5 cm)*. The gantry is angled 65° and the field center is marked on the skin. For daily treatment, the distance is set to read 100 cm SSD and the planned field size is set.

As mentioned earlier, one side of the field width is increased by 1cm to stagger the junction half way through treatment.

For the thinner chest wall, the same principle applies as above. The thinner section of the chest wall is bolused up to improve coverage of the target volume and to reduce excessive dose to the underlying lung as shown in Figure 23.16.

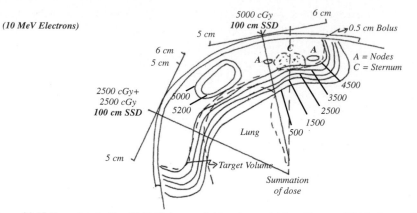

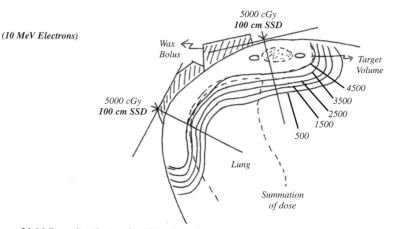

Figure 23.15 Dose distribution 10 MeV electron fields using variable collimator. (Thick chest wall)

Figure 23.16 Dose distribution for 10 MeV electron fields using variable collimator. (Thin chest wall)

VI. ELECTRON FIELD THERAPY FOR BILATERAL CHEST WALL

The same procedure, as described above, applies for the bilateral chest wall. Dose distribution is shown in Figure 23.17.

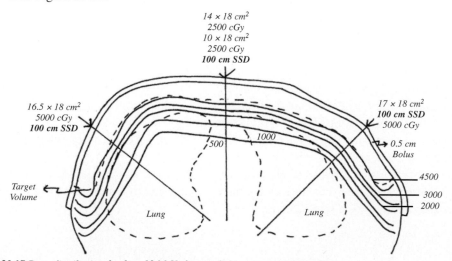

Figure 23.17 Dose distribution for four 10 MeV electron fields using variable collimator.

Electron arc therapy is a more practical way to treat chest wall. This has been described in the chapter on Electron Beam Therapy.

VII. PUBLICATIONS OF INTERESTS

1.   Chu AM, Wood WC, Doncette JA: Inflamatory breast carcinoma treated by radical radiotherapy. Cancer 45:2730,1980.

2.   Danoff BF: the role of radiotherapy in the management of locally advanced non metastatic breast cancer. In Levitt S: Syllabus. Categories course in breast cancer. RSNA Preceedings, 1984.

3.   Deutsch M, Parsons J, Mittal B: Local-regional recurrent breast cancer treatment with radiotherapy (abstract). Int J Radiat Oncol Biol Phys 11(1):101,1985.

4.   Eilber FR, Milne CA, White EC, et al: "Early" carcinoma of the breast: Evaluation of regional therapy and feactures influencing prognosis. South Med J 75:9,1982.

5.   Farrow JH: Current concepts in the detection and treatment of the earliest of the early breast cancers. Cancer 25:468,1970.

6.   Fisher B, Bauer M, Wickerham L, et al: Relation of number of positive axillary nodes to the prognosis of patients with primary breast cancer. An NSABP update. Cancer 52:1551,1983.

7.   Fisher B, Montague E, Redmond C, et al: Findings from NSABP Protocol No.5-04: Comparison of radical mastectomy with alternative treatments for primary breast cancer. Cancer 46:1,1980.

8.   Fraass BA, Robertson PL, Lichter AS: Dose to the contralateral breast due to primary breast irradiation. Int J Radiat Oncol Biol Phys 11:485,1985.

9.   Griscom NT, Wang CC: Radiation therapy of inoperable breast carcinoma. Radiology 79:18,1962.

10.   Harris JR, Hellman S: Primary radiation for early breast cancer. Cancer 51(12): 2547,1983.

11.   Michael L.F.Lim, D.V.Cormack, Treatment of the Chest Wall", Medical Dosimetry, 1988, Vol.13, No.4, page 191-193

12.   Montague ED: Conservation surgery and radiation therapy in the treatment of operable breast cancer. Cancer 53:700,1984.

13.   Prosnitz LR, Goldenberg IS, Packard RA, et al: Radiation therapy as initial treatment for early stage cancer of the breast without mastectomy. Cancer 39:917,1977.

14.   Syed AMN, Puthawala A, Fleming P, et al: Combination of external and intestitial irradiation in the primary management of breast carcinoma. Cancer 46:1360,1980.

— *CHAPTER 24* —

Cancer of the Esophagus

I. INTRODUCTION

The esophagus is a muscular tube measuring about 25 to 28 cm long. It extends from the pharynx to the stomach. The superior border is at the level of C6-C7 vertebrae and the inferior border is at the level of T11-T12 vertebrae. It lies just posterior to the trachea and anterior to the vertebral bodies.

The esophagus is divided into the cervical part and the thoracic part but in tumour classification and in planning treatment, it is divided into the upper, middle and lower third. Poorly differentiated squamous cell carcinoma makes up more than 90% of the cases and occurs mainly in the middle and lower third. The remaining 10% or less are adenocarcinoma which are mostly in the lower third of the esophagus.

The disease occurs mainly in the elderly and is more common in men than in women. The incidence in highest in the Orient particularly in Japan. High incidence have also been reported in the Scandinavian countries.

The common presentations are dysphasia, weight loss, malaise and persistent cough. Diagnosis is by barium swallow under fluoroscope, esophagoscopy with biopsy and CT.

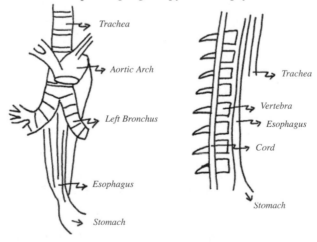

Figure 24.1 Esophagus and surrounding structures (Anterior and lateral view.)

Treatment of choice depends on the stage, location and size of the tumor. Surgery and radiation therapy are chosen for radical treatment. For palliation, radiation therapy is the choice.

II. LOCALIZATION

The tumor is localized from the diagnostic studies. The target volume is localized at simulation with the patient in the supine treatment position. The arms are stretched above the head to keep them out of the posterior oblique fields. Barium is given by mouth and the esophagus obstruction is localized on the fluoroscope when the patient swallows. At least 5 cm margin on both sides of the tumor superiorly and inferiorly are added to ensure adequate coverage. An AP and lateral simulator films are taken and the field marks are drawn on the patient. In this example, the collimator is angled 10° to follow the slope of the esophagus.

Planning CT is done and the images are transferred to the treatment planning computer. The radiation oncologist delineates the target volume on each slice.

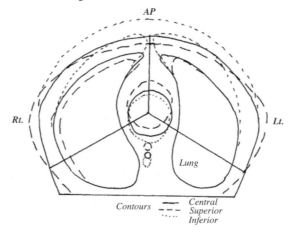

Figure 24.2 Contours and target volumes of the central, superior and inferior slices.

III. TREATMENT PLANNING

Good coverage of the target volume is generally attained with a three field technique; anterior field, right posterior oblique field and left posterior oblique field as shown in Figure 24.3. Lung inhomogeneity is corrected for the posterior oblique fields using Batho-Young correction method. Due to the slope of the chest, the anterior field may require a wedge with the thick end in the superior direction and the thin end in the inferior direction.

Because the treatment plane is non-vertical and the gantry angles for the oblique fields are not horizontal, a new gantry angle, floor angle and collimator angle must be calculated in order to cover the target volume. Coordinate transformation is used to calculate the angles.

1) Anterior field
No change in planned angle.

2) Left posterior oblique
Collimator angle from lateral film $\phi = 10°$, Gantry angle from plan $\theta = 120°$. New gantry angle δ obtained as follow: $\rightarrow$ Cos δ = Cos $(\phi) \times$ Cos$(\theta) \rightarrow \delta$ = Cos^{-1}[Cos$(10°) \times$ Cos$(120°)]$ = 119°
New floor angle: $\rightarrow$ tan γ = sin(ϕ)/tan(θ) = sin$(10°)$/tan$(120°)$ = 0.0887 $\rightarrow \gamma$ = tan^{-1}(0.0887)= 5.7°
New collimator angle: $\rightarrow$ tan α = tan(ϕ)/sin$(\theta) \rightarrow \alpha$ =tan^{-1}{tan$(10°)$/sin$(120°)$} = 11.5°

3) Right posterior oblique
All the angles are the reversed of the left posterior oblique field.

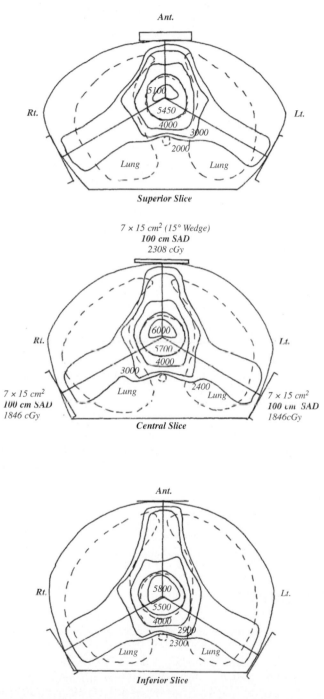

Figure 24.3 Dose distribution for central, superior and inferior planes using three field technique using 10 MV photon beam with lung inhomogeneity correction.

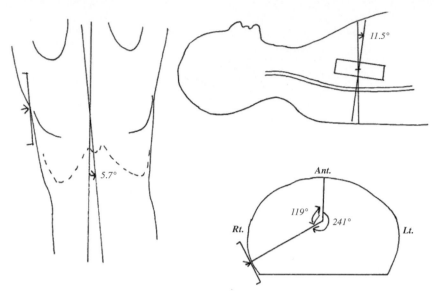

Figure 24.4 Calculated angles for floor, collimator and gantry for left posterior oblique field.

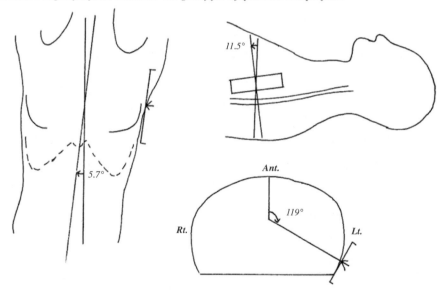

Figure 24.5 Calculated angles for floor, collimator and gantry for right posterior oblique field.

The patient is simulated again after planning to verify and record the planned fields.

IV. INTRACAVITARY THERAPY

The primary site may be supplemented with an additional boost dose of 2000 cGy using ^{192}Ir intracavitary therapy. The isodose distribution is as shown in Figure 24.6. A nasogastric tube is first inserted into the esophagus. A train of dummy pellets are then inserted into the nasogastric tube. An X-Ray film is taken to localize the pellets in relation to the tumor site.

Treatment planning is done to determine the dwell time and positions of the ^{192}Ir source to provide the desired dose distribution. The patient is then hooked up to the remote after loading brachytherapy unit for treatment. The dwell times and positions of the ^{192}Ir source are programmed and the treatment is started remotely.

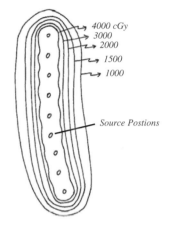

Figure 24.6 ^{192}Ir dose distribution for esophageal intracavitary therapy.

V. PUBLICATIONS OF INTERESTS

1.   Gooduer JT: Surgical and radiation treatment of cancer of the thoracic esophagus. Am J Roentgenol 105:523,1969.

2.   Hancock SL, Glatstein E: Radiation therapy of esophageal cancer. Semin Oncol 11:144,1984.

3.   Newaishy GA, Read GA, Duncan W, et al: Results of radical radiotherapy of squamous cell carcinoma of the esophagus. Clin Radiol 33:347,1982.

4.   Newaishy GA, Read GA, Duncan W, et al: Results of radical radiotherapy of squamous cell carcinoma of the oesophagus. Clin Radiol 33:347, 1982.

5.   Rosenberg JC, Lichter AS, Leichman LP: Cancer of the esophagus. In DeVita VT, Hellman S, Rosenberg SA, eds: Cancer: Principles and Practice of Oncology, ed 3, p 725. Philadelphia, JB Lippincott, 1989.

6.   Schaer J, Katon RM, Ivancev K, et al: Treatment of malignant esophageal obstruction with silicone-coated metallic self-expanding stents. Gastrointest Endosc 38:7, 1992.

7.   Seydel HG, Wichman L, Byhhardt R, et al: Preoperative radiation and chemotherapy for localized squamous cell carcinoma of the esophagus: An RTOG study. Int J Radiat Oncol Biol Phys 14:33, 1988.

8.   Smoron G, O"Brien C, Sullivan C: Tumour localization and treatment technique for cancer of the esophagus. Radiology 111:735,1974.

9.   Tate T, Brace JA, Morgan H, Skeggs DBL: Conformation therapy: A method of improving the tumour treatment volume ratio. Clin Radiol 37:267, 1986.

10. Thompson WM: Esophageal cancer. Int J Radiat Oncol Biol Phys 9:1533, 1983.

11. Younghusband JD, Aluwihare APR: Carcinoma of the esophagus: Factors influencing survival. Br J Surg 57:422,1970.

PRINCIPLES AND PRACTICE OF CLINICAL PHYSICS AND DOSIMETRY
Michael L.F. Lim, CMD, ACT
Advanced Medical Publishing, Inc., USA

— CHAPTER 25 —

Hodgkin's Disease

I. INTRODUCTION

Hodgkin's disease is a special form of malignant lymphoma involving the lymph glands. The disease is divided into four classifications. They are: a) lymphocyte-predominant, b) mixed cellularity, (c) lymphocyte-depleted; and d) nodular sclerosis. Nodular sclerosis nodes are larger than the other three classes and often remains localized in the upper thorax.

Spread of the disease is by direct infiltration and by circulatory system to the spleen, bone marrow, liver and bone.

The disease is divided into four stages. Stage I is involvement of a single lymph node region. Stage II is involvement of two or more lymph node regions on the same side of the diaphragm. Stage III is involvement of lymph node regions on both sides of the diaphragm and/or spleen. Stage IV is involvement outside the lymph nodes. The above stages may include A for asymptomatic and B for symptoms such as fever, night sweats and weight loss.

The disease is more common in males than in females with 50% of the cases occurring in the 20-40 age group. Children under 15 have only about 10% of the cases. There have been reports of higher risk of getting Hodgkin's disease after infectious mono-nucleosis. Also, radiation induced Hodgkin's disease has been reported. The presentations are swollen lymph glands *(usually in the cervical region)*, fever, night sweats and weight loss of more than 10% body weight. Diagnosis is by biopsy of the enlarged lymph node and confirmation of staging is by CT and laparotomy studies.

Treatment choice is radiation therapy for early stages and combination of radiation therapy and chemotherapy for later stages and for the B substage. For children, total tumor dose of 2000-2500c Gy in 13-16 fractions is sufficient while adults need total tumor dose of about 4500 cGy in 25 fractions.

Possible complications from radiation therapy are, solid tumor induction, growth limitation of bones and muscles, thyroid dysfunction, bone marrow suppression, radiation pneumonitis, pericarditis and infection. Prognosis is very good with 5 year survival in the 75-95% region.

II. MANTLE FIELD

A) Localization

A contoured polyform base is fabricated for the patient in the supine treatment position. Hands are placed on the hips and chin is extended. The mantle field is simulated by setting a field size large enough to cover from the chin to a level just below the diaphragm and laterally to include both axillae. A typical field size is about 40 × 40 cm^2 at 100 cm SSD. Small lead pellets are placed on selected calculation points on the patient as shown in the list below. After fluoroscopy, an AP film is taken. Shielding is drawn on the films. Field marks are drawn on the patient's skin and SSD readings and separations are taken for the selected calculation points. A PA film is also taken.

B) Treatment Planning

An irregular field calculation is put through the planning computer. Dose to the calculation points are added and are listed below. MU setting is calculated for each of the fields. In some patients, the lower mediasternum dose may be lower than desired. This may be taken to the desired dose with an additional boost to the region or a compensator may be fabricated to even the dose to the selected points.

Table 25.1 Calculated doses to selected points.

Point	Dose(cGy)
Center	4500
Rt.Neck	5160
Lt.Neck	5095
Rt.s/c	5084
Lt s/c	5090
Rt. Axilla	4974
Lt. Axilla	4930
Lower mediasternum	4454

III. INVERTED Y FIELD

A) Localization

The inverted Y field is simulated to cover the paraaortic lymph nodes, the pelvic nodes and the inguinal nodes. A gap is calculated to match the mantle and inverted Y field at mid depth between the fields.

To further safe guard the cord from radiation overdose, a small shielding may be included in the inverted Y field at the superior border at midline. Small lead pellets are placed on selected calculation points on the patient as shown in the list below. After fluoroscopy, an AP film is taken. Field marks are drawn on the patient's skin and SSD readings and separations are taken for the selected calculation points. Shielding is drawn on the films. A PA film is also taken.

B) Treatment Planning

After the mantle field, the patient has a month's rest before returning for the inverted Y field. An irregular field calculation is put through the planning computer. Dose to the calculation points are added and are listed below. MU setting is calculated for each of the fields

Table 25.2 Calculated doses to selected points.

Point	Dose(cGy)
Center	4500
Para-aortic	4372
Rt.inguinal	4434
Lt.inguinal	4500

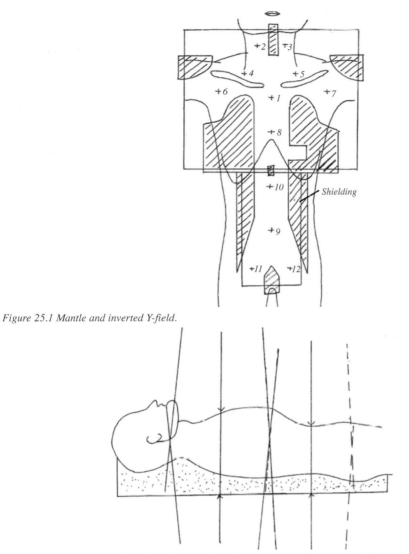

Figure 25.1 Mantle and inverted Y-field.

Figure 25.2 Lateral view of mantle and inverted Y-field showing polyform contoured base and gap between fields.

IV. PUBLICATIONS OF INTERESTS

1. Carmel RJ, Kaplan HS: Mantle irradiation in Hodgkin's disease: An analysis of technique, tumour eradication and complications. Cancer 37:2813,1976.

2. Hancock SL, Tucker MA, Hoppe RT: Breast cancer after treatment of Hodgkin's disease. J Natl Cancer Inst 85:25-31, 1993.

3. Hellman SH, Mauch P, Goodman RL, et al: The place of radiation therapy in the treatment of Hodgkin's disease. Cancer 42:971,1978.

4. Hoppe R: Radiation therapy in the management of Hodgkin's disease. Semin Oncol 17:704-715, 1990.

5. Hoppe RT: Treatment planning in the radiation therapy of Hodgkin's disease. Front Radiat Ther Oncol 21:270-287, 1987.

6. Hughes DB, Smith AR, Hoppe R, et al: Treatment planning for Hodgkin's disease: A Patterns of Care study. Int J Radiat Oncol Biol Phys 33:519-524, 1995.

7. Johnson RE, Faw FL, Glenn DW, et al: Clinical and technical aspects of total nodal irradiation for Hodgkin's disease. In Fletcher GH(ed): Textbook of Radiotherapy. Philadelphia, Lea & Febiger, 1973.

8. Kinsella TJ, Fraass BA, Glatstein E: Late effects of radiation therapy in the treatment of Hodgkin's dis-

ease. Cancer Treat Rep 66:991,1982.

9.   Krikorian JG, Portlock CS, Mauch PM: Hodgkin's disease presenting below the diaphragm: A review. J Clin Oncol 4:1551-1562, 1986.

10. Lutz WR, Larsen RD: Technique to match mantle and paraaortic fields. Int J Radiat Oncol Biol Phys 9:1753-1756, 1983.

11. Marks JE, Haus AG, Sutton HG, et al: The value of frequent treatment verification films in reducing localization error in the irradiation of complex fields. Cancer 37:2755,1976.

12. Mueller N, Evans A, Harris NL, et al: Hodgkin's disease and Epstein-Barr virus: Altered antibody pattern before diagnosis. N Engl J Med 320:689, 1989.

13. Page V, Gardner A, Karzmark C: Physical and dosimetric aspects of radiotherapy of malignant lymphomas. I. The mantle technique. Radiology 96:609,1970.

14. Palos B, Kaplan HS, Karzmark C: The use of thin lung shields to deliver limited whole lung irradiation during mantle field treatment of Hodgkin's disease. Radiology 96:441,1971.

Principles and Practice of Clinical Physics and Dosimetry
Michael L.F. Lim, CMD, ACT
Advanced Medical Publishing, Inc., USA

—— *CHAPTER 26* ——

Cancer of the Lung

I. INTRODUCTION

The two lungs in the chest cavity are separated by the mediastinum. They are cone shaped with a base and an apex projecting upwards behind the clavicle. The base is concave and rest upon the diaphragm. There are two lobes in the left lung and three lobes in the right lung. The lobes are separated by the fissues. The bronchi enter the lungs at the hila.

There are four major histologic cell types of lung carcinoma. They are: i) squamous cell (or epidermoid carcinoma), ii) small cell (or oat cell carcinoma), iii) adenocarcinoma; and iv) large cell *(or large cell anaplastic carcinoma)*. The most common is squamous cell carcinoma.

Lung cancer is the leading cause of death from cancers in males and fast becoming the same for females due to increasing number of female smokers. Lung cancer is commonly seen in the 55-65 age group and at time of diagnosis, most of the patients have metastasis in the neighboring nodes and even distant sites such as brain, liver, bones and kidneys. Due to the spread, age of the patients, difficulties in removing all the tumor and the radioresistance of the tumor, the death rate is very high.

The leading cause of lung cancer is tobacco smoking. With increase smoking, the risk is increases. Pollutants such as asbestos, coal tar fumes, nickel, etc have also been associated with lung cancer.

The usual presentations are cough, chest pain, blood stained sputum and dyspnea.

Diagnosis is by chest X-Ray, bronchoscopy, cytological studies and CT.

Due to the frequent spread to the supraclavicular and/or mediastinal lymph nodes, treatment fields usually cover the supraclav and/or mediastinum. To be effective at all in controlling the disease, the tumor dose is usually high, 6000 cGy in 30 fractions or 6960 cGy in 58 fractions in 6 weeks twice a day. Palliative dose is usually around 4500cGy in 23 fractions in 5 weeks.

For the radical treatment, parallel opposed AP-PA fields alone are not acceptable due to excessive dose to the normal lung and to the cord. Some centers treat AP-PA parallel opposed fields to about 4000 cGy and then oblique fields are employed to go off cord to ensure cord dose is less than 4500 cGy. With this technique, the cord may be acceptable but the total dose to normal lung tissues may be high enough to cause pneumonitis. Due to these problems, it is wise to plan a radical course of treatment very carefully right from the start. CT planning helps a great deal in tumor localization and planning by employing beam directing and beams eye view for shielding in order to spare maximum normal tissue.

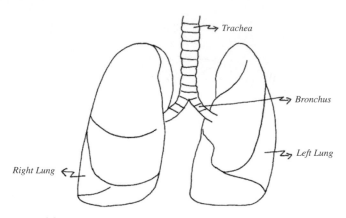

Figure 26.1 Anterior view of the lungs and trachea.

II. LOCALIZATION

The patient is simulated in the supine position with arms above the head. An AP and lateral field are simulated to adequately cover the maximum tumor margin as documented on diagnostic CT, chest X-Ray and other diagnostic tests. AP and lateral simulator films are taken. Field centers are drawn on the patient's skin for referencing. In addition to these marks, lateral horizontal lines are also marked on the sides of the patient to ensure patient is not rotated on repeated setup for planning and treatment. Radio-opaque markers are taped on the field centers. The radio-opaque markers would show up on CT for centering at the time of planning. The patient is CT. After exporting the CT images to the planning computer, the radiation oncologist delineates the GTV and the organs at risk. Margins are created to form the CTV/PTV

III. TREATMENT PLANNING

The intersection of the AP and lateral CT marks on the central CT slice are localized and centered for referencing. Planning is done to achieve good coverage of the target volume without going over the tolerance dose to the lungs and the cord. The example shown here is a three field arrangement using a left anterior oblique, a right anterior oblique and a right posterior oblique field to reduce the dose to the cord and the lungs. Correction is made for lung inhomogeneity. Shielding is constructed using beams eye view. After plan approval by the radiation oncologist, the plan isocenter with reference to the original center is documented on the plan. This plan isocenter is set up at simulation for plan check. The plan fields are simulated as per plan and films are taken for documentation. The new field centers are marked on the shell for treatment set-up.

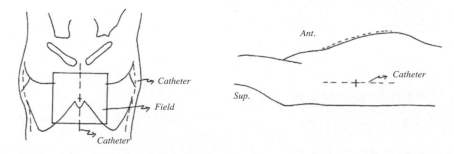

Figure 26.2 Anterior and lateral view of patient in treatment position for CT scan.

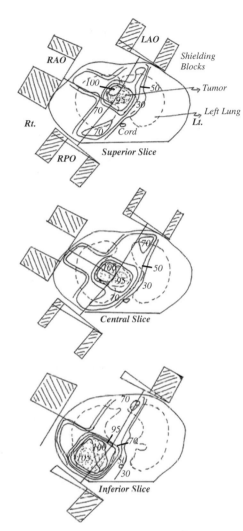

Figure 26.3 Dose distribution of three-field plan for superior, central and inferior slice on the 10 MV photon.

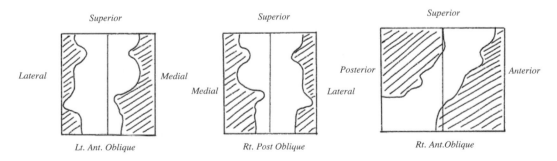

Figure 26.4 Beams eye view for Left anterior oblique, right posterior oblique and right anterior oblique fields.

IV. PUBLICATIONS OF INTERESTS

1. Bangma PJ: Post-operative radiotherapy. In Deeley TJ (ed): Modern radiotherapy. Carcinoma of the bronchus, p 163, New York, Appleton-Century-Crofts, 1972.

2. Bleehan NM, Bumn PA, Cox JD: et al: Role of radiation therapy in small cell anaplastic carcinoma of the lung. Cancer treatment rep 67:11, 1983.

3. Choi NC: Curative radiation therapy for unresectable non small cell carcinoma of the lung: Indications, techniques, results. In Choi NC, Grillo HC (eds): Thoracic Oncology, p 163, New York, Raven Press, 1983.

4. Cohen MH: Signs and symptoms of bronchogenic carcinoma. In Strauss MJ (ed): Lung cancer clinical diagnosis and treatment, p 85. New York, Grune and Stratton, 1977.

5. Emami B, Melo A, Carter BL, et al: Value of computed tomography in radiotherapy of lung cancer. AJR 131:63, 1978.

6. Emami B: Three-dimensional conformal radiation therapy in bronchogenic carcinoma. Semin Radiat Oncol: 92-97, 1996.

7. Graham M, Matthews J, Harms W, et al: 3-D radiation treatment planning study for patients with carcinoma of the lung. Int J Radiat Oncol Biol Phys 29:1105-1117, 1994.

8. Perez CA, Purdy J, Razek A: Radiation therapy of cancer of the lung and esophagus. In Levitt SH, Tapley ND (eds): Technological basis of radiation therapy: Practical clinical applications, p138. Philadelphia, Lea and Febiger, 1984.

9. Prasad S, Pilepich MV, Perez CA: Contribution of CT to quantitive radiation therapy planning. AJR 136:123,1981.

10. Seydel HG, Kutcher GJ, Steiner RM, et al: Computed tomography in planning radiation therapy for bronchogenic carcinoma. Int J Radiat Oncol Biol Phys 6:601,1980.

—— *CHAPTER 27* ——

Cancer of the Gall Bladder

I. INTRODUCTION

The gall bladder is a conical bag situated in a fossa on the under surface of the right lobe of the liver. It is divided into the fundus, body and neck. It is joined at the neck to the hepatic duct by the cystic duct. Most tumors of the gall bladder are adenocarcinoma with a small number being squamous cell carcinoma. It is a rare but fatal disease. Females are affected four times more than females. The average age for the disease is 70 years old and is more common in patients with gall stones. The patient usually complains of abdominal pain and weight loss is common. The patient is jaundice and nausea and vomiting may be present. Diagnosis is by X-Ray of the gall bladder, CT and lobotomy tests. Surgery is the treatment of choice. Radiotherapy is given for palliation and if operation is not possible.

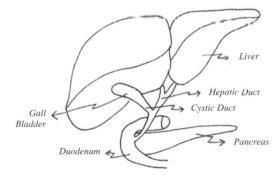

Figure 27.1 Gall bladder and surrounding organs.

II. LOCALIZATION

Due to the proximity of sensitive organs near by, CT planning should be done to accurately localize the gall bladder for planning. The patient lies in a supine position with arms above the head for simulation. An AP and lateral fields are set to cover the target volume and simulator films is taken. Field centers are drawn on the patient's skin for referencing. Radio-opaque markers are taped on the field centers on the skin at CT. The radio-opaque markers would show up on CT for centering at the time of planning. The patient is CT. After exporting the CT images to the planning computer, the radiation oncologist delineates the GTV and the organs at risk. Margins are created to form the CTV/PTV

III. TREATMENT PLANNING

The intersection of the AP and lateral CT marks on the central CT slice are localized and centered for referencing. Planning CT is done to localize the gall bladder and surrounding organs such as the kidneys, intestines, stomach and spinal cord. Coverage of the target volume is achieved with three fields on 10 MV photons as shown in Figure 27.2. After plan approval by the radiation oncologist, the plan isocenter with reference to the original center is documented on the plan. This plan isocenter is set up at simulation for plan check. The plan fields are simulated as per plan and films are taken for documentation. The new field centers are marked on the shell for treatment set up.

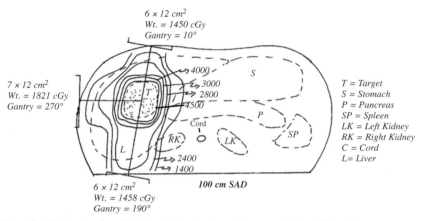

Figure 27.2 Dose distribution for three field plan in the treatment of cancer of the gall bladder.

IV. PUBLICATIONS OF INTERESTS

1.   Fletcher MS, Dawson JL, Wheeler PQ, et al: Traetment of high bile duct carcinoma by internal radiotherapy with Iridium-192 wire. Lancet 2:172,1981.

2.   Goebel RH: Techniques for localized radiation of the biliary tree. ASTR Preceedings. Int J Radiat Oncol Biol Phys 5:80,1979.

3.   Green N, Mikkelsen WP, Kernen JA: Cancer of the common hepatic bile ducts: Palliative radiotherapy. Radiology 109:687,1975.

4.   Hanna SS, Rider WD: Carcinoma of the gallbladder or extra-hepatic bile ducts: The role of radiotherapy. Can Med Assoc J 118:59,1978.

5.   Herskovic A, Heaston D, Engler MJ, et al: Irradiation of biliary carcinomas. Radiology 139:219,1981.

6.   Ikeda H, Kiroda C, Uchida H: Intraluminal irradiation with Iridium-192 wires for extrahepatic bile duct carcinoma.

7.   Johnson DW, Safai C, Goffinet DR: Malignant obstructive jaundice: Treatment with external beam and intracavitary radiotherapy. Int J Radiat Oncol Biol Phys 11:411,1985.

8.   Mahe M, Romestaing P, Talon, et al: Radiation therapy in extrahepatic bile duct carcinoma. Radiother Oncol 21:121, 1991.

9.   Pilipich MV, Lambert PM: Radiotherapy for carcinoma of the extrahepatic biliary system. Radiology 127:767, 1978.

10.   Smoron GL: Radiation therapy of carcinoma of the gallbladder and biliary tract. Cancer 40:1422, 1977.

11.   Sworon GL: Radiation therapy of carcinoma of gallbladder and biliary tract. Cancer 40:1422,1977.

12.   Veeze-Kuypers B, Meerwaldt JH, Lameris JS, et al: The role of radiotherapy in the treatment of bile duct carcinoma. Int J Radiat Oncol Biol Phys 18:63, 1990.

Principles and Practice of Clinical Physics and Dosimetry
Michael L.F. Lim, CMD, ACT
Advanced Medical Publishing, Inc., USA

—— *CHAPTER 28* ——

Cancer of the Liver

I. INTRODUCTION

The liver is situated in the right and left hypochondriac and epigastric region. The superior surface is convex to fit into the concave surface of the diaphragm. The inferior surface is concave and is in contact with the stomach, pylorus, duodenum, colon and the right kidney. The liver is divided into the right and left lobes which are separated from each other by the fissure for ligamentum teres and ligamentum renosum.

Most liver cancers are the adenocarcinoma type. Cancer of the liver is rare but fatal. It is more common in the Orientals and affects males about eight times more than females. The average age at onset of disease is 65 years old. The possible causes are cirrhosis of the liver, intestinal parasitism, alfatoxin from moldy peanuts and hepatitis B virus.

The presentations are, abdominal fullness, dull pain in the upper abdomen, weight loss, tiredness and mild jaundice. Diagnostic tests are radioisotope scan, needle biopsy, CT of the liver and laparotomy.

Surgery is the treatment of choice for resectable localized tumors. Otherwise radiation therapy is given. The whole liver is treated to 1600 cGy in 8 fractions followed by a two week rest and then another course of radiation therapy to the whole liver giving 1000 cGy in 5 fractions. Immediately following the second course, a boost of 600 cGy in 3 fractions is given to the localized nodule. Chemotherapy is given in conjunction with the radiation therapy.

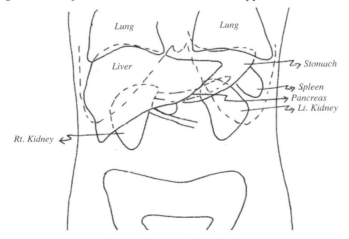

Figure 28.1 Liver and surrounding organs.

II. LOCALIZATION

Due to the proximity of sensitive organs near by, CT planning should be done to accurately localize the liver for planning. The patient positioning for simulation and CT planning are as described for the gall bladder in the previous chapter.

III. TREATMENT PLANNING

A) First and second course whole liver treatment

The slices are planned to ensure good coverage of the whole liver but minimize the dose to the surrounding organs. This is achieved with a pair of parallel opposed oblique fields on the 15 MV unit. The beam parameters are as shown on the plan. Kidney blocking is constructed from beam's eye view. This beam's eye view is transferred to the plan check simulator films for verification of shielding.

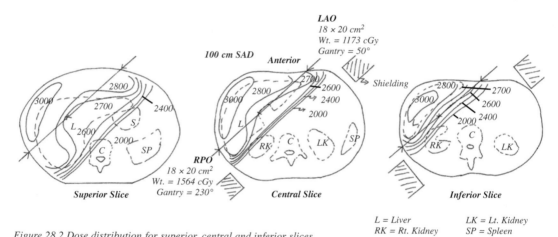

Figure 28.2 Dose distribution for superior, central and inferior slices.

L = Liver	LK = Lt. Kidney
RK = Rt. Kidney	SP = Spleen
C = Cord	S = Stomach

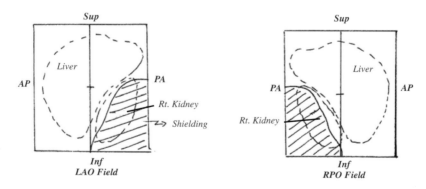

Figure 28.3 Beam's eye view for shielding.

B) Third Course Boost

The slices to be included in the boost are selected by the radiation oncologist. Target volume for each slice is delineated. In this example, good coverage of the target volume is achieved with a pair of oblique wedged fields on the 15 MV photon unit as shown in Figure 28.4

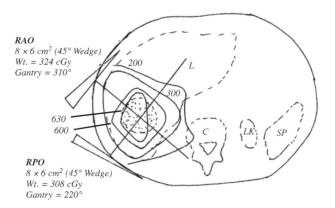

RAO
$8 \times 6\ cm^2$ *(45° Wedge)*
Wt. = 324 cGy
Gantry = 310°

RPO
$8 \times 6\ cm^2$ *(45° Wedge)*
Wt. = 308 cGy
Gantry = 220°

Figure 28.4 Dose distribution for boost.

IV. PUBLICATIONS OF INTERESTS

1.   Issa P: Cancerous hemangioma of the liver: The role of radiotherapy. Br J Radiol 41:26,1968.

2.   Michael L.F.Lim, CT Treatment Planning of the Liver", (Medical Dosimetry, AAMD)1988, Vol.13, No.3, page 119-126

3.   Park WC, Phillips R: The role of radiation therapy in the management of hemangiomas of the liver. JAMA 212:1496,1970.

Principles and Practice of Clinical Physics and Dosimetry
Michael L.F. Lim, CMD, ACT
Advanced Medical Publishing, Inc., USA

—— *CHAPTER 29* ——

Cancer of the Kidney

I. INTRODUCTION

The kidneys are the bean shape excretory organs situated in the abdomen. They measure about 10 cm long by 6cm wide by 3.5 cm thick and they extend from the 11th rib to just above the iliac crest. The right kidney is a little lower than the left kidney due to the liver above the right kidney.

Anterior to the right kidney are the liver, duodenum and colon. Posterior to the right kidney are the ribs. Anterior to the left kidney are the stomach, spleen, pancreas and colon. Posterior to the left kidney are the ribs. The kidneys are embedded in adipose tissue and supported by renal fascia. They are divided into three general regions that are the renal cortex, renal medulla and renal pelvis.

Most cancer of the kidney are adenocarcinoma with transitional cell or squamous cell carcinoma for the rest of the cases. There are four staging for carcinoma of the kidney. Stage I is tumor confined to the kidney. Stage II is tumor spread to the perinephric fat. Stage III is tumor spread to regional lymph nodes. Stage IV is tumor spread to adjacent organs or distant metastasis.

The average age is in the 60 and likely causes are chronic irritation and smoking. The male to female ratio is approximately 2:1.

The presentations are haematuria, pain, mass on palpation and fever. Diagnostic tests to confirm cancer of the kidney are IVP, CT, urine tests and ultrasound.

If the tumor is resectable, radical nephrectomy is the treatment of choice. For pain control or to stop bleeding, palliative nephrectomy may be performed. Radiation therapy is employed only if the tumor is unresectable or if the patient refuses surgery giving a dose of 4500 cGy in 25 fractions. Post-operative irradiation may be employed for residual or recurrent tumors. Chemotherapy has been given in some cases.

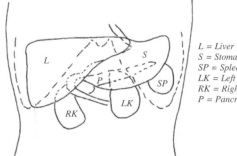

L = Liver
S = Stomach
SP = Spleen
LK = Left Kidney
RK = Right Kidney
P = Pancreas

Figure 29.1 Kidneys and surrounding organs.

II. LOCALIZATION

If the patient has had nephrectomy, surgical clips left behind would help localize the kidney bed. If nephrectomy is not done, IVP or CT would be needed to localize the kidneys. For simulation, the patient lies supine with arms above the head. The affected kidney is localized and a field is set to cover the desired target volume. AP and lateral simulator films are taken. Field marks are drawn on the patient's skin. CT planning is done for treatment planning.

III. TREATMENT PLANNING

The target volume, spinal cord, liver, pancreas and opposite kidney are delineated in the CT by the radiation oncologist. Coverage of the target volume is achieved with three wedged fields as shown in Figure 29.2. Dose to the surrounding sensitive organs must be kept as low as possible. The plan is verified on the simulation at plan check and simulator films are taken for record.

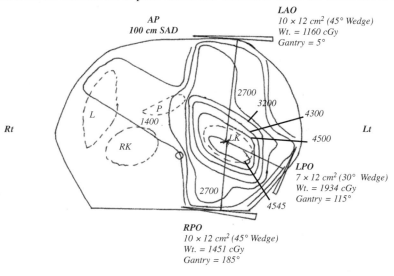

Figure 29.2 Dose distribution for three field plan in the treatment of cancer of the left kidney. (6 MV photons)

IV. PUBLICATIONS OF INTERESTS

1.   Annon J, Karstens J, Durben G, et al: Carcinoma of the renal parenchyma, renal pelvis and ureter:Radiological diagnosis and treatment planning. Cancer Treat Rev 7:29,1980.

2.   Brookland R, Richter M: The postoperative irradiation of the renal pelvis and ureters. J Urol 133:952,1985.

3.   Halperin E, Harisiadis L: The role of radiation therapy in the management of metastatic renal cell carcinoma. Cancer 51:614,1983.

4.   Onufrey V, Mohiuddin M: Radiation therapy in the treatment of metastatic renal cell carcinoma. Int J Radiat Oncol Biol Phys 11:2007, 1985 .

5.   Peeling WB, Mantell BS, Shepheard BG: Post-operative irradiation in the treatment of renal cell carcinoma. Br J Urol 41:23, 1969.

6.   Rubin P, Keller BO, Cox C, et al: Preoperative irradiation in renal cancer: Evaluation of radiation treatment plans. Am J Roentgenol Rad Ther Nucl Med 123:114, 1975.

7.   Schwartz LH, Richaud J, Buffat L, et al: Kidney mobility during respiration. Radiother Oncol 32:84, 1994.

8.   Stein M, Kuten A, Halperin J, et al: The value of postoperative irradiation in renal cell cancer. Radiother Oncol 24:41, 1992.

Principles and Practice of Clinical Physics and Dosimetry
Michael L.F. Lim, CMD, ACT
Advanced Medical Publishing, Inc., USA

—— *CHAPTER 30* ——

Cancer of the Pancreas

I. INTRODUCTION

The pancreas is a hammer shape organ located in the epigastric and left hypochondriac regions of the abdomen. The head of the pancreas fits around the curve of the duodenum and the tail extends to the spleen. The organs around the pancreas are the stomach, liver, spleen, duodenum and kidneys. Due to the proximity of these organs, treatment planning for the pancreas must be very localized and precise to spare the surrounding organs as much as possible.

The pancreas is both an exocrine and endocrine gland. In its exocrine function, pancreatic juices are secreted into the duodenum to help in digestion. In its endocrine function, insulin, glucagon and somatostatin are secreted by the cells of the islets of Langerhans.

Most of the pancreatic tumors are adenocarcinoma with the rest being islet cell tumors. It is a rare tumor but fatal. The common age group is in the 60. There is no known cause although some chemicals, coffee and diabetes have been suggested as causative.

The usual presentations are pain in the epigastric region, weight loss, nausea and jaundice.

Diagnosis is by CT scans, ultrasound, barium meal radiograph and laparotomy.

For localized resectable tumors, surgery is the treatment of choice. Local resection or total pancreatectomy may be performed. For unresectable tumors, radiotherapy is the alternative. It is a radioresistant tumor and high dose of radiation is required to do any good. But surrounding organs are sensitive to radiation. Therefore great care must be taken to localize the tumor well and radiation fields are planned to encompassed just the pancreas as much as possible with minimum dose to other organs. Photon beams of the 10 MV range are commonly used giving a dose of 4500 cGy in 25 fractions. Neutron therapy has been used in some centers and intra-operative electron therapy has also been used due to low dose to surrounding organs. Chemotherapy is also being given in conjunction with radiation therapy.

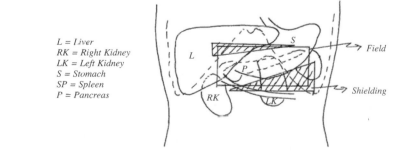

L = Liver
RK = Right Kidney
LK = Left Kidney
S = Stomach
SP = Spleen
P = Pancreas

Figure 30.1 Diagram shows pancreas, surrounding organs and the treatment field.

II. LOCALIZATION

The patient is simulated in the supine position with arms above the head. Using diagnostic results, the pancreas is localized under fluoroscope examination. AP and lateral simulator films are taken. Field marks and lateral lazer lines are marked on the patient's skin to aid in the set up for CT planning and second simulation for plan verification and treatment. The patient is CT and the CT images are transferred to the planning computer where the radiation oncologist would delineate the tumor and surrounding organs at risk.

III. TREATMENT PLANNING

Good coverage of the pancreas is achieved with three wedged fields as shown in Figure 30.2. The left kidney, spleen and some liver are shielded. The plan is simulated for verification and recording.

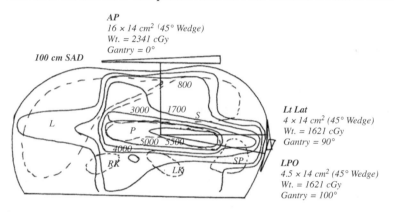

Figure 30.2 Dose distribution for three wedged fields in the treatment of cancer of the pancreas. (10 MV)

IV. PUBLICATIONS OF INTERESTS

1.   Alabdula ASM, Hussey DH, Olson MH, et al: Experience with fast neutron therapy for unresectable carcinoma of the pancreas. Int J Radiat Oncol Biol Phys 7:165,1981.

2.   Bosset JF, Pavey JJ, Gillet M, et al: Conventional external irradiation alone as adjuvant treatment in resectable pancreatic cancer: Results of a prospective study. Short communication. Radiother Oncol 24:191, 1992.

3.   Dobelbower RR: The radiotherapy of pancreatic cancer. Semin Oncol 6:378,1979.

4.   Garton GR, Gunderson LL, Nagorney DM, et al: High-dose preoperative external beam and intraoperative irradiation for locally advanced pancreatic cancer. Int J Radiat Oncol Biol Phys 7:1153, 1993.

5.   Goldson AL, Ashaveri E, Espinoza MC, et al: Single-dose intraoperative electrons for advanced stage pancreatic cancer: Phase I pilot study. Int J Radiat Oncol Biol Phys 7:869, 1981.

6.   Gunderson LL, Martin JK, Earle JB et al: Intraoperative and external beam irradiation +/- resection: Mayo pilot experience. Mayo Clin Proc 59:691,1984.

7.   Haslam JB, Cavanaugh PJ, Stroup SL: Radiation therapy in the treatment of irresectable adenocarcinoma of the pancreas. Cancer 32:1341,1973.

8.   Higgins PD, Sohn JW, Fine RM, et al: Three-dimensional conformal pancreas treatment: comparison of four- to six-field techniques. Int J Radiat Oncol Biol Phys 31:605, 1995.

9.   Roldan GE, Gunderson LL, Nagorney DM, et al: External beam versus intraoperative and external beam irradiation for locally advanced pancreatic cancer. Cancer 61:1110, 1988.

— *CHAPTER 31* —

Cancer of the Stomach

I. INTRODUCTION

The stomach is a muscular bag that serves as container for food in the early stages of digestion. It lies in the epigastric and left hypochondriac regions of the abdomen. The stomach is made up of three distinct regions namely, the fundus, body and pyloric portion. The medial curve of the stomach is the lesser curvature and the lateral curve is the greater curvature. The organs nearby are the liver, kidneys, pancreas, spleen and the duodenum.

Most of the cancers of the stomach are of the adenocarcinoma type (95%) with a small portion of the cancers being squamous cell carcinoma. Cancer of the stomach is relatively rare in North America but is common in Japan, Chile and Iceland. Male to female ratio is about 2:1. Age group is in the 50-60 year old. Some of the causes are in the diet, gastric polyps, pernicious anemia and gastric ulcer.

The presentations are epigastric discomfort, weigh loss, ulcer pain and anemia.

Diagnosis is by endoscopic studies, biopsy, CT and upper GI series..

Treatment of choice is surgery because adenocarcinoma of the stomach is radioresistant and also because the pancreas, liver, spleen, kidneys and small intestines are nearby and will be included in any treatment fields.

Radiotherapy may be given pre or post-operatively or to patients who cannot be operated giving a dose of 4500 cGy in 25 fractions. Chemotherapy may be given in conjunction with the above.

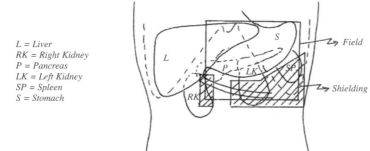

L = Liver
RK = Right Kidney
P = Pancreas
LK = Left Kidney
SP = Spleen
S = Stomach

Figure 31.1 Diagram shows stomach, surrounding organs and the treatment field.

II. LOCALIZATION

The patient is simulated in the supine position with the arms above the head. Barium is given orally during simulation and also when simulator films are taken. The target volume of the stomach is localized under fluoroscope. AP and lateral simulator films are taken with barium in the stomach. Field marks are drawn on the patient. The patient then goes for CT planning. After CT, the images are transferred to the planning computer and the radiation oncologist delineates the target volume and other organs at risk near by such as the spinal cord, liver and kidneys.

III. TREATMENT PLANNING

A plan is generated to deliver a high uniform dose to the stomach but minimum dose to the surrounding organs. A three-field beam arrangement on the 10 MV photon meets the objective as shown in Figure 31.2. The anterior field is weighted more than the posterior and lateral fields. The plan is simulated for verification and· recording.

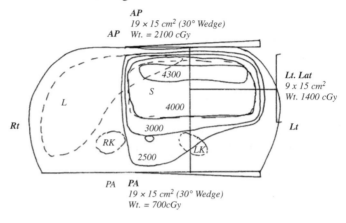

Figure 31.2 Dose distribution for 3-field plan in the treatment of cancer of the stomach. (10 MV photon beam)

IV. PUBLICATIONS OF INTERESTS

1. Abe M, Takahashi M: Intraoperative radiotherapy: The Japanese experience. Int J Radiat Oncol Biol Phys 5:863,1981.

2. Asakawa H, Takeda T: High energy X-Ray therapy of gastric carcinoma. J Jpn Soc Cancer Ther 8:362,1973.

3. Holbrook MA: Radiation therapy. Current concepts in cancer. Gastric cancer: Treatment principles. JAMA 228:1289,1974.

4. Mantell BS: Radiotherapy for dysphagia due to gastric carcinoma. Br J Surg 69:69, 1982.

5. Nordman E: Value of megavolt therapy in gastric carcinoma. Bull Cancer (Paris) 63:217, 1976.

6. Roswit B, Malsky SJ, Reid CB: Radiation tolerance of the gastrointestinal tract. In Vaeth J (ed): Frontiers of radiation therapy oncology, p 160. Baltimore, University Park Press, 1972.

7. Takahashi M, Abe M: Intra-operative radiotherapy for carcinoma of the stomach. Eur J Surg Oncol 12:247, 1986.

8. Tsukiyama I, Akine Y, Kajiura Y, et al: Radiation therapy for advanced gastric cancer. Int J Radiat Oncol Biol Phys 15:123, 1988.

9. Weiland C, Hymmen U: Magavoltage therapy for malignant gastric tumours. Strahlentherapie 40:20,1972.

Principles and Practice of Clinical Physics and Dosimetry
Michael L.F. Lim, CMD, ACT
Advanced Medical Publishing, Inc., USA

—— *CHAPTER 32* ——

Cancer of the Small Intestines

I. INTRODUCTION

Cancer of the small intestines is rare. Treatment of choice is surgery with radiotherapy coming into play only if surgery is not complete or possible. Tumors of the small intestines are radioresistant and the intestinal tract tolerates radiation poorly resulting in diarrhea, nausea and vomiting.

If radiotherapy is given, it is with a pair of parallel opposed fields *(approximately 25 × 35 cm²)* giving a total tumor dose of about 2000 cGy in 20 fractions.

A good dietitian plays an important roll in the management of the patient during treatment to reduce bowel complications and to make sure the patient is eating properly and enough.

Principles and Practice of Clinical Physics and Dosimetry
Michael L.F. Lim, CMD, ACT
Advanced Medical Publishing, Inc., USA

—— *CHAPTER 33* ——

Cancer of the Colon

I. INTRODUCTION

The colon is about 5-6 feet long and is made up of the ascending colon, the tranverse colon ,the descending colon and the sigmoid colon. The sigmoid colon is joined to the rectum. The colon is made up of the mucosa that contains the villi, the muscularis mucosa, the submucosa, circular muscle layer, longitudinal muscle layer and the serosa.

Cancer of the colon is divided into four stages. Stage A is tumor invasion into the submucosa, muscle with no nodal or distant metastasis. Stage B is tumor invasion into the serosa with no nodal or distant metastasis. Stage C is tumor invasion through the serosa and involvement of regional nodes. Stage D is distant metastasis. Cancer of the colon is one of the commonest cancer in the 50-60 year old group. It is commoner in countries where the diet lacks fibre and high fat content. This cause low transit time of the dietary components through the gut. Male to female ratio is about equal. Most cancers of the colon is in the sigmoid colon.

The presentations are anaemia, GI bleeding, abdominal mass, bowel obstruction, abdominal pain, pelvic pain and blood in stool.

Some of the diagnosis that are commonly performed are sigmoidoscopy, rectal ecamination and barium encma.

Surgery is the treatment of choice. But patients who have wide spread disease or who are high risk, radiation therapy is the treatment of choice. In some cases, post-operative radiotherapy is given as a supplement.

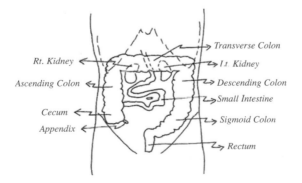

Figure 33.1 Position of colon in relation to organs nearby.

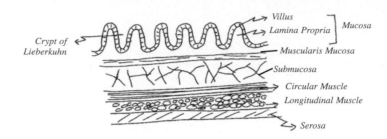

Figure 33.2 Cross section through colon.

II. LOCALIZATION

For simulation, the patient lies in a prone position with arms above the head. A field is set to cover the whole pelvis. A PA simulator film is taken. The lateral target volume is localized and a film is taken. A contour is obtained through the field center.

III. TREATMENT PLANNING

Good coverage of the target volume is achieved with three fields on the 6 MV as shown in Figure 33.4. Wedges are used for the lateral fields to reduce the dose to the posterior target area. Anterior field is avoided to reduce the dose to the intestines. A dose of 4500 cGy in 25 fractions is given.

If necessary, the fields are coned down to give higher dose to the tumor but further reduce the dose to sensitive organs near by such as the intestines. A dose of 540 in 3 fractions is given as a boost.

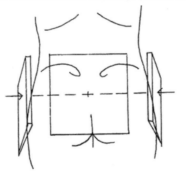

Figure 33.3 Three field set-up to treat cancer of the sigmoid colon.

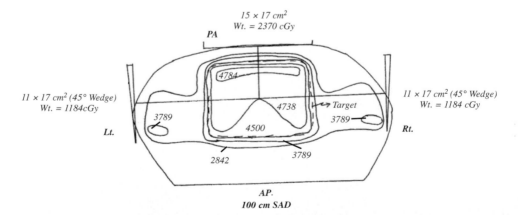

Figure 33.4 Dose distribution for three-field plan on the 6 MV photon unit to treat cancer of the sigmoid colon.

IV. PUBLICATIONS OF INTERESTS

1.	Duttenhaver J, Hoskins RB, Gunderson LL, et al: Adjuvant postoperative radiation therapy in the management of cancer of the colon. Cancer 57:955,1986.

2.	Emani B, Pilepich M, Wilett C, et al: Management of unresectable colorectal carcinoma(preoperative radiotherapy and surgery.) Int J Radiat Oncol Biol Phys 8:1295,1982.

3.	Enker WE: Surgical treatment of large bowel cancer. In Enker WE(ed). Carcinoma of the colon and rectum, p93, Chicago Year Book Medical Publishers, 1978.

4.	Higgins GA Jr, Conn JH, Jordan PH Jr, et al: Preoperative radiotherapy for colorectal cancer. Ann Surg 181:624, 1975.

5.	Jain M, Cook GM, Davis FG, et al: A case-control study of diet and colo-rectal cancer. Int J Cancer 26:757, 1980.

6.	Jensen OM, MacLennan R: Dietary factors and colorectal cancer in Scandinavia. Isr J Med Sci 15:329, 1979.

7.	Jarvinen H, Franssila KO: Familial juvenile polyposis coli: Increased risk of colorectal cancer. Gut 25:792, 1984.

8.	Kopelson G: Adjuvant postoperative radiation therapy for colorectal carcinoma above the peritoneal reflection: I. Sigmoid colon. Cancer 51:1593, 1983.

9.	Liu K, Stamler J, Moss D, et al: Dietary cholesterol, fat, and fibre, and colon-cancer mortality: An analysis of international data. Lancet 2:782, 1979.

10.	Modan B, Barell V, Lubin F, et al: Low-fiber intake as an etiologic factor in cancer of the colon. J Natl Cancer Inst 55:15, 1975 .

11.	Pahhlman L, Glimelius B, Ginman C, et al: Preoperative irradiation of primarily non-resectable adenocarcinoma of the rectum and rectosigmoid. Acta Radiol Oncol 24:35, 1985.

12.	Stevens KR Jr, Allen CV, Fletcher WS: Preoperative radiotherapy for adenocarcinoma of the rectosigmoid. Cancer 37:2866, 1976.

13.	Wang CC, Schulz MD: The role of radiation therapy in the management of carcinoma of the sigmoid, rectosigmoid and rectum. Radiology 79:1,1962.

14.	Welch JP, Donaldson GA: Detection and treatment of recurrent cancer of the colon and rectum. Am J Surg 135:505,1978.

15.	Willett CG, Shellito PC, Tepper JE, et al: Intraoperative electron beam radiation therapy for primary locally advanced rectal and rectosigmoid carcinoma. J Clin Oncol 9:843, 1991.

16.	Withers HR, Cuasay L, Mason KA, et al: Electrive radiation therapy in the curative treatment of cancer of the rectum and rectosigmoid colon. In Stroehlin JR, Romsdahl MM(eds). Gastrointestinal cancer, p351. New York, Raven Press, 1981.

Principles and Practice of Clinical Physics and Dosimetry
Michael L.F. Lim, CMD, ACT
Advanced Medical Publishing, Inc., USA

— CHAPTER 34 —

Cancer of the Rectum

I. INTRODUCTION

The rectum continues from the sigmoid colon to the anus. It measures about 15 cm in length and is divided into the upper, middle and lower third. It is situated in the hollow of the sacrum and coccyx. Histologically, it is very similar to the colon.

Staging, incidence, presentation and diagnosis are similar to the colon.

Surgery is the treatment of choice. Patients who have wide spread disease or who are high risk for surgery, radiation therapy is the choice. Post-operative radiation therapy may be given as a supplement to surgery.

For the early stage, radiation therapy is given using a three-field technique giving a dose of 5000 cGy in 25 fractions.

A two-field technique has been used in some centers giving a dose of 4500 cGy in 25 fractions.

For later stages, a larger four-field box technique is used.

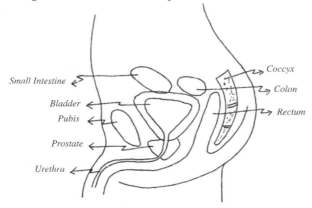

Figure 34.1 Position of rectum and organs nearby (Male).

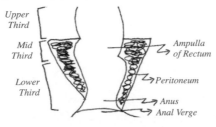

Figure 34.2 Anatomy of the rectum.

II. TWO FIELD TECHNIQUE

A) Localization

For simulation, the patient kneels on a specially constructed platform which is attached to the end of the simulator couch. A lead wire is taped on the patient's back going sagitally from the level of L4 to the scrotum. Barium is put into the rectum. The PA field is set to cover the rectum. A PA simulator film is taken and field marks are drawn on the patient's skin. With the simulator gantry at 90°, the lateral field is set to cover the rectum. A lateral simulator film is taken and field marks are drawn on the patient's skin.

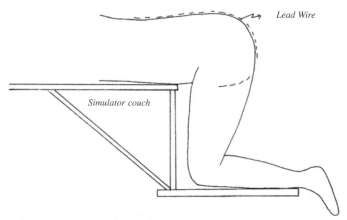

Figure 34.3 Patient in treatment position for simulation.

B) Treatment Planing

The patient's sagittal contour is entered into the planning computer by digitizing the sagittal out-line indicated by the lead wire from the lateral simulator film. The position of the sacrum, coccyx and rectum are also entered. Good coverage of the rectum is with a pair of wedged fields as shown in Figure34.5.

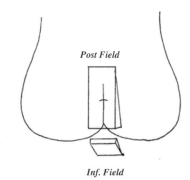

Figure 34.4 Two field set-up to treat cancer of the rectum.

III. THREE FIELD TECHNIQUE

A) Localization

If the tumor is small and is situated in the upper third of the rectum, the anus may be spared by using a posterior and two posterior oblique wedged fields as shown in Figure 34.7. For simulation,

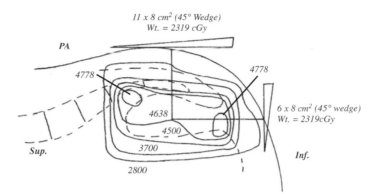

Figure 34.5 Dosimetry for wedged fields in the treatment of cancer of the rectum on 6 MV photon unit.

the patient lies in a prone position with arms above the head. Barium is put into the rectum. Under fluroscopy, the rectum is localized and a PA field size is set to cover the rectum. A PA simulator film is taken and field marks drawn on the patient's skin. With the gantry at the lateral position, the rectum is localized and a lateral field size is set to cover the rectum. A lateral simulator film is taken and field marks drawn on the patient's skin. The patient is scanned (CT) and the images are transferred to the planning computer for target volume delineation by the radiation oncologist.

B) Treatment Planning

Uniform dose distribution around the target volume is achieved with a posterior direct field and two posterior oblique-wedged fields on the 6 MV unit as shown in Figure 34.7. After planning, the patient is taken back to the simulator to simulate the plan for verification and recording. At simulation, barium is put into the rectum to verify field coverage.

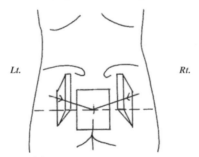

Figure 34.6 Three field set-up to treat cancer of the rectum.

IV. PAPILLON TECHNIQUE (ENDOCAVITARY TECHNIQUE)

This technique is applicable only if the tumor is: i) accessible, ii) small, iii) non-infiltrating; and iv) well differentiated.

V. LOCALIZATION

The patient is set up in a knee-chest position. The tumor mass is visualized with the aid of a rectoscope. After gradual dilation of the anus, the treatment protoscope is inserted. With the aid of the rectoscope, the protoscope is aimed at the tumor mass.

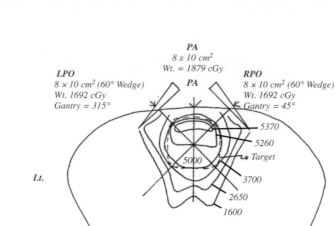

Figure 34.7 Dose distribution for three-field in the treatment of cancer of the rectum on 6 MV photon unit.

VI. TREATMENT PLANNING

Radiation is supplied from a special 50kV SXR unit with short (4 cm) SSD. Surface dose rate is in the region of 2000 cGy/min. Total surface dose is in the region of 10,000 cGy in 3 fractions in 6 weeks treating once every two weeks.

VII. PUBLICATIONS OF INTERESTS

1. Cummings BJ, Rider WD, Harwood AR, et al: External beam radiation therapy for adenocarcinoma of the rectum. Dis Colon Rectum 26:30,1983.

2. Gabriel NB, Dukes C, Bussey HJR: Lymphatic spread in cancer of the rectum. Br J Surg 23:395,1935.

3. Higgins GA, Humphrey EW, Dwight RW, et al: Preoperative radiation and surgery for cancer of the rectum: Veterans Administration Surgical Oncology Group Trial II. Cancer 58:352, 1986.

4. Kligerman MM: Radiotherapy and rectal cancer. Cancer 39(suppl 2):896, 1977.

5. Mohuidden M, derdel J, Marks G, et al: Results of adjuvant therapy in cancer of the rectum. Cancer 55:350,1985.

6. Mohuidden M, Kramer S, Marks G, et al: Combined pre- and postoperative radiation for carcinoma of the rectum. Int J Radiat Oncol Biol Phys 8:133,1982.

7. Papillon J: Rectal and anal cancers: Conservative treatment by irradiation- An alternative to radical surgery. New York, Springer-Verlag, 1982.

8. Papillon J: Intracavitary irradiation of early rectal cancer for cure. Cancer 36:696,1975.

9. Sischy B, Remington JH, Sobel SH: Treatment of rectal carcinomas by means of endocavitary irradiation. Cancer 46:1957,1980.

10. Sischy B, Hinson EJ, Wilkinson DR: Definitive radiation therapy for selected cancers of the rectum. Br J Surg 75:901, 1988.

11. Willett CG, Shellito PC, Tepper JE, et al: Intraoperative electron beam radiation therapy for primary locally advanced rectal and rectosigmoid carcinoma. J Clin Oncol 9:843, 1991.

Principles and Practice of Clinical Physics and Dosimetry
Michael L.F. Lim, CMD, ACT
Advanced Medical Publishing, Inc., USA

—— *CHAPTER 35* ——

Cancer of the Anus

I. INTRODUCTION

Cancer of the anus is treated very much like cancer of the rectum. For small tumor in the anal verge, surgery followed by external beam irradiation giving 3000 cGy in 15 fractions followed by ^{192}Ir implant giving 2000 cGy in 2 to 3 days is the treatment of choice. If the tumor is larger than 4 cm and is in the anal canal, surgery followed by external beam irradiation to the whole pelvis including the perineum giving 4500 cGy is the treatment of choice. External beam irradiation is given using a pair of AP and PA parallel opposed fields.

II. PUBLICATIONS OF INTERESTS

1. Newman G, Calverley DC, Acker BD, et al: The management of carcinoma of the anal canal by external beam radiotherapy: Experience in Vancouver 1971-1988. Radiother Oncol 25:196, 1992.

2. Otim-Oyet D, Ford H, Fisher C, et al: Radical radiotherapy for carcinoma of the anal canal. Clin Oncol 2:84, 1990.

3. Papillon J: Rectal and Anal Cancers: Conservative Treatment by Irradiation. An Alternative to Radical Surgery. Berlin, Springer-Verlag, 1982.

4. Spencer SA, Pareek PN, Brezovich I, et al: Three-port perineal sparing technique. Radiology 180:563, 1991.

5. Svensson C, Goldman S, Friberg B: Radiation treatment of epidermoid cancer of the anus. Int J Radiat Oncol Biol Phys 27:67, 1993 .

6. Wagner JP, Mahe MA, Romestaing P, et al: Radiation therapy in the conservative treatment of carcinoma of the anal canal. Int J Radiat Oncol Biol Phys 29:17, 1994.

—— *CHAPTER 36* ——

Cancer of the Cervix

I. INTRODUCTION

The anatomy of the cervix has been described in association with the anatomy of the uterus. Staging is divided into five stages. Stage 0 is carcinoma in situ. Stage I is tumor confined to the cervix. Stage II is tumor extension beyond cervix but not to the pelvic wall. May involve the upper 2/3 of the vagina. Stage III is tumor extension to the pelvic wall and all of the vagina. Stage IV is tumor extension to the bladder or rectum or beyond the true pelvis.

Cancer of the cervix is the most common gynecological cancer. Age group used to be in the 40-60 year old range but in the last few years, the age group has been getting a lot younger. This is probably due to sexual promiscuity. Early coitus and multipartners predisposes to the development of cancer of the cervix. The incidence is higher in prostitutes but low among nuns. Venereal diseases and herpes virus type II are closely associated with cervical cancer.

The common presentations are post coital bleeding, unexplained vaginal spotting or bleeding, vaginal discharge and pelvic pain.

Diagnosis is by pelvic examination, Schiller test, D&C, cone biopsy and colposcopy.

For stage 0 and I, treatment of choice is surgery especially if the patient is young and desires to have family. Otherwise, brachytherapy and external beam irradiation may be given. For stage II, III and IV, brachytherapy and external beam irradiation are the treatment of choice.

II. LOW DOSE RATE ^{137}Cs TUBE AND COLPOSTAT SOURCES

A) Localization

The intrauterine applicator and colpostats are inserted into the patient's uterus and vagina. This is performed in the operating room *(OR)* with the patient under general anesthetic. Dummy tube sources are inserted into the applicators and a radio opaque rectal marker is inserted into the rectum. An AP film is taken. Radio opaque dye is injected into the bladder catheter and with the rectal marker in place a lateral film is taken. The patient is taken back to the brachytherapy ward after recovery.

B) Treatment Planning

The tube coordinates and source activity *(source strength)* are digitized into the planning computer. The coordinates of the bladder and rectal points are also digitized into the computer. A combination of source activity and source position are planned to achieve the desired dose distribution and dose rate. These are approved by the radiation oncologist before live sources are inserted into the applicator in the order and position as planned. The treatment time is calculated from the prescribed dose over the dose rate.

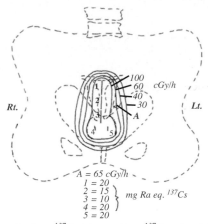

Figure 36.1 Anterior dose distribution for three ^{137}Cs tubes and two ^{137}Cs colpostats.

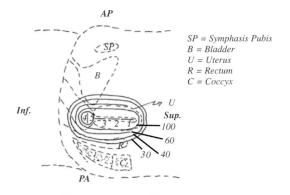

Figure 36.2 Lateral dose distribution for three ^{137}Cs tubes and two ^{137}Cs colpostats.

III. LOW DOSE RATE ^{137}Cs PELLETS

Many centers have replaced the afterloading technique with computerized remote afterloading system such as the 'Selectron'. This system uses 2.5 mm ^{137}Cs pellets which are 20 mCi or 40 mCi each.

A) Localization

The localization procedure is the same as described above. Instead of using dummy tube sources for the planning films, a train of dummy pellets is inserted into each of the applicators.

B) Treatment Planning

Coordinates of the 'active' pellet positions are digitized into the planning computer. A combination of 'active' pellet positions are planned to arrive at the desired dose distribution and dose rate. Dose rates are also calculated for the rectal and bladder points. These are approved by the radiation oncologist before the applicators in the patient are connected to the 'Selectron' and treatment time calculated.

The hoses from the 'Selectron' are connected to the patient's applicators. Each hose is designed to match only the correct applicator. The planned 'active' pellet positions and treatment time are programmed into the 'Selectron' via its keyboard. The displayed 'active' pellet positions and treatment time are checked by a second staff member before loading the sources from the primary safe into the secondary safe. The spaces between 'active' positions are filled with non active pellets. A print out of the programmed 'active' pellet positions and treatment time are checked. All staff members leave the room and the treatment is started from outside the room by pressing the start button.

The pellets are pneumatically transferred from the secondary safe into the patient's applicators. The treatment time counts down. During nursing care and visitation, the treatment may be stopped by pressing the stop button outside the room before entering the room.

In the event of any kind of failure or when the treatment time is completed, he sources automatically return to the secondary safe of the 'Selectron.'

The advantages of this system over the manual afterloading system are: i) no exposure to the radiation oncologist, brachytherapy technologist and the nursing staff, ii) Better nursing care,iii) Treatment is stopped automatically when treatment is finished or when there is any kind of failure; and iv) Greater variation of dose distribution from the many combinations of 'active' source positions. The disadvantages are: i) cost, ii) Need qualified personnel to service the unit, iii) With treatment interruptions, the treatment is prolonged; and iv) Only two patients may be treated at one time if all the three channels are used on each patient.

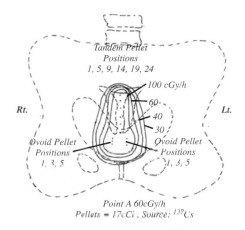

Figure 36.3 Anterior dose distribution for 'Selectron' system with 'active' ^{137}Cs pellets as shown.

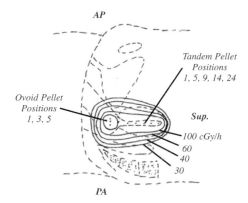

Figure 36.4 Lateral dose distribution for 'Selectron' system with 'active' ^{137}Cs pellets as shown.

IV. HIGH DOSE RATE ^{192}Ir PELLETS

Similar to the technique described above except that the treatment is given in minutes instead of days and a single high activity (10 Ci) source is used to "dwell" at planned positions for a planned time. The treatment is fractionated.

V. EXTERNAL BEAM IRRADIATION

A) Localization

About a week after the second insertion, the patient is brought back to be planned for the external beam radiation treatment. The patient lies in a supine position for simulation. A field is set to cover the whole pelvis. A common field size is 15×15 cm^2 at 100 cm SAD. An AP and a PA simulator film are taken. Field marks are drawn on the patient's skin. A contour is obtained through the field center. A midline shield is drawn on the simulator films. This shielding is about 5 cm across but the width and position may vary depending on the position of the insertions.

B) Treatment Planning

A parallel opposed dose distribution may be generated if required. Due to the midline shielding, normalization, calculation and dose prescription are taken to the center of the unblocked field. An irregular field is put through the treatment planning computer to calculate the MU setting.

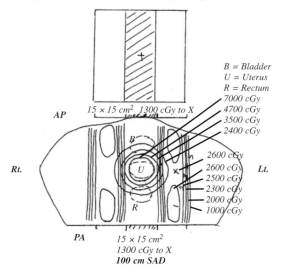

Figure 36.5 Dose distribution for two ^{137}Cs low dose rate insertions and external beam parallel opposed fields with midline shielding.

VI. PUBLICATIONS OF INTERESTS

1.   Ackerman LV, del Regato JA(eds): Cancer: Diagnosis, treatment and prognosis, pp 717-819, St.Louis, CV Mosby,1977.

2.   Adams E, Rawls WE, Melnick JL: The association of herpes virus type 2 infection and cervical cancer. Prev Med 3:122,1974.

3.   Allt WEC: Supervoltage radiation treatment in advanced cancer of the uterine cervix. Can Med Assoc J 100:792,1969.

4.   Castro JR, Issa P, Fletcher GH: Carcinoma of the cervix treated by external irradiation alone. Radiology 95: 163,1970.

5.   Evans SR Jr, Hilaris BS, Barber HRK: External vs intestitial irradiation in unresectable recurrent cancer of the cervix. Cancer 28: 1284, 1971.

6.   Fu KK, Phillips TL: High-dose rate versus low-dose rate intracavitary brachytherapy for carcinoma of the cervix. Int J Radiat Oncol Biol Phys 19:791-796, 1990.

7.   Grigsby PW, Perez CA: Radiotherapy alone for medically inoperable carcinoma of the cervix: Stage IA and carcinoma in situ. Int J Radiat Oncol Biol Phys 21:375-378, 1991.

8.   Jones D, Notley H, Huterk R: Geometry adopted by Manchester radium applicators and Selectron afterloading applicators in intracavitary treatment for carcinom of cervix uteri. Br J Radiol 60:481-485, 1987.

9.   Kapp KS, Stuecklschweiger GF, Kapp DS, et al: Dosimetry of intracavitary placements for uterine and cervical carcinoma: Results of orthogonal film, TLD, and CT-assisted techniques. Radiother Oncol 24:137-146, 1992.

10. Nakano T, Arai T, Morita S, et al: Radiation therapy alone for adenocarcinoma of the uterine cervix. Int J Radiat Oncol Biol Phys 32:1331-1336, 1995.

11. Perez CA, Breaux S, Madoc-Jones H, et al: Radiation therapy alone in the treatment of carcinoma of the uterine cervix: I. Analysis of tumour recurrence. Cancer 51: 1393, 1983.

12. Perez CA, Kuske R, Glasgow GP: Review of brachytherapy techniques for gynecologic tumours. Endocuriether Hypertherm Oncol 1:153,1985.

13. Podczaski E, Stryker JA, Kaminski P, et al: Extended field radiotherapy for carcinoma of the cervix. Cancer 66:251-258, 1990.

14. Potish RA, Gerbi BJ: Role of point A in the era of computerized dosimetry. Radiology 158:827-831, 1986

15. Potish RA, Gerbi BJ: Cervical cancer intracavitary dose specification and prescription. Radiology 165:555-560, 1987

16. Pourquier H, Dubois JB, Deland R: Cancer of the uterine cervix. Dosimetric guidelines for prevention of late rectal and rectosigmoid complications as a result of radiotherapeutic treatment. Int J Radiat Oncol Biol Phys 8:1887,1982.

17. Syed AMN, Feder BH: Techniques of after loading intestitial implants. Radiol Clin North Am 46:458, 1977.

Principles and Practice of Clinical Physics and Dosimetry
Michael L.F. Lim, CMD, ACT
Advanced Medical Publishing, Inc., USA

— *CHAPTER 37* —

Cancer of the Uterus

I. INTRODUCTION

The uterus is a pear shape body situated in the pelvis. It measures about 7 cm long by 4.5 cm wide by 4 cm thick. Anterior to the uterus is the bladder and posterior is the rectum. Superiorly lies the intestines and inferiorly lies the cervix and vagina. The uterus is divided into the fundus, body and neck *(or cervix.)* The uterine artery crosses over the ureter at 2 cm superior and 2 cm lateral from the cervical os. This point has been used for dose prescription for brachytherapy insertion.

Cancer of the uterus are generally adenocarcinoma arising in the body of the uterus. Staging is divided into five stages. Stage 0 is carcinoma in situ. Stage I is tumor confined to the corpus uteri. Stage II is tumor invasion of the corpus uteri and cervix. Stage III is tumor extension outside the uterus but not outside the true pelvis. Stage IV is tumor extension outside the true pelvis.

The incidence of carcinoma of the uterus is commoner in menopausal and post menopausal women and among Jewish women. It has been observed to be commoner in obese and diabetic women and in women who has a history of irregular menstruation.

The common presentations are abnormal vagina bleeding in menopausal and post menopausal women, presence of uterine polyps and low back pain.

To diagnose the disease, a complete menstrual history must be obtained. Endoscope examination and D & C are also required.

Surgery is the treatment of choice. Total hysterectomy and bilateral salpingo-oophorectomy are performed. Post-operative radiotherapy is given to the pelvis to reduce the chance of recurrence from seeding. A four field box technique may be used to deliver a total tumor dose of 4000 cGy in 20 fractions. If surgery is not possible, radiation therapy is the choice. A combination of brachytherapy and external beam radiation is commonly used. Brachytherapy is given in two insertions and the external radiation is given with a pair of AP and PA parallel opposed fields with central shield of about 5 cm wide.

Chemotherapy and hormonal therapy may also be given.

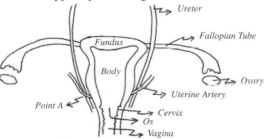

Figure 37.1 Diagram shows uterus and surrounding organs and vessels.

II. LOW DOSE RATE ^{137}Cs TUBE SOURCES

A) Localization

The intrauterine applicator is inserted into the patient's uterus. This is performed in the operating room (OR) with the patient under general anesthetic. Dummy tube sources are inserted into the applicator and a radio opaque rectal marker is inserted into the rectum. An AP film is taken. Radio opaque dye is injected into the bladder catheter and with the rectal marker in place, a lateral film is taken. The patient is taken back to the brachytherapy ward after recovery.

B) Treatment Planning

The tube coordinates and source activity (source strength) are digitized into the planning computer. The coordinates of the bladder and rectal points are also digitized into the computer. A combination of source activity and source position are planned to achieve the desired dose distribution and dose rate. These are approved by the radiation oncologist before live sources are inserted into the applicator in the order and position as planned. The treatment time is calculated from the prescribed dose over the dose rate.

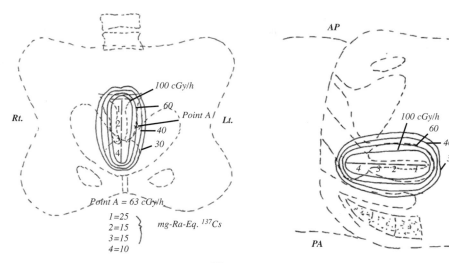

Figure 37.2 Anterior dose distribution for four ^{137}Cs tube sources.

Figure 37.3 Lateral dose distribution for four ^{137}Cs tube sources.

III. EXTERNAL BEAM IRRADIATION

A) Localization

About a week after the second insertion, the patient is brought back to be planned for the external beam radiation treatment. The patient lies in a supine position for simulation. A field is set to cover the whole pelvis. A common field size is 15×15 cm^2 at 100 cm SAD. An AP and a PA simulator films are taken. Field marks are drawn on the patient's skin. A contour is obtained through the field center. A midline shield is drawn on the simulator films. This shielding is about 5 cm across but the width and position may vary depending on the position of the insertions.

B) Treatment Planning

A parallel opposed dose distribution may be generated if required. Due to the midline shielding, normalization, calculation and dose prescription are taken to the center of the unblocked field. An irregular field is put through the treatment planning computer to calculate the MU setting.

IV. PUBLICATIONS OF INTERESTS

1.   Badib AO, Vontgama C, Kurohara SS, et al: Radiotherapy in the treatment of sarcomas of the corpus uteri. Cancer 24:724,1969.

2.   Brady LW, Lewis GC, Antoniades J, et al: Evolution of therapeutic techniques. Gynecol Oncol 2:253,1974.

3.   Gagnon JD, Moss WT, Gabourel LS, et al: External irradiation in the managemenet of stage II endometrial carcinoma.Cancer 44:1247,1979.

4.   Hasumi K, Matsuzawa M, Chen HF, et al: Computed tomography in the evaluation and treatment of endometrial carcinoma. Cancer 50:904,1982.

5.   Nori D, Hilaris BS, Batata MA, et al: Remote afterloading in cancer management: II. Clinical applications of remote afterloading. In Hilaris BS, Batata MA, eds: Brachytherapy Oncology: 1983, pp 101-118. New York, Memorial Sloan-Kettering Cancer Center, 1983.

6.   Perez CA, Kuske R, Glasgow GP: Review of brachytherapy for gynecologic tumours. Endocurietherapy/Hypertherm Oncol 1:153,1985.

7.   Simon N, Silverstone SM: Intracavitary radiotherapy of endometrial cancer by afterloading. Gynecol Oncol 1:13, 1972.

8.   Ziel HK, Finkle WD: Increased risk of endometrial carcinoma among users of conjugated estrogens. N Engl J Med 293:1167,1975.

Principles and Practice of Clinical Physics and Dosimetry
Michael L.F. Lim, CMD, ACT
Advanced Medical Publishing, Inc., USA

— CHAPTER 38 —

Cancer of the Vagina

I. INTRODUCTION

The vagina is a dilatable canal measuring about 7 cm at the anterior wall and 9cm at the posterior wall. It extends from the vulva to the uterus where it widens to form the fornices.

There are four staging for cancer of the vagina. Stage I is tumor limited to the vaginal wall. Stage II is tumor extension to the cervix or vulva but not to the lateral pelvic walls, bladder or rectum. Stage III is tumor extension to the pelvic walls. Stage IV is tumor extension to the bladder, rectum or beyond the true pelvis.

It is a very uncommon gynecological cancer and accounts for less than 2% of all cancers. Age group with the disease is in the 55-65 year old. Most tumors are squamous cell carcinoma.

The presentations are visible and palpable lesions, vaginal discharge or bleeding, pain and groin masses.

Only very early and small tumors are treated by surgery. The most common treatment for stage I and II is by brachytherapy using ^{137}Cs loaded vaginal applicator placed in the vagina. For stages III and IV, external beam irradiation to the whole pelvis is the treatment of choice using a four field box technique treating to a total dose of 4000-5000 cGy in 20-25 fractions.

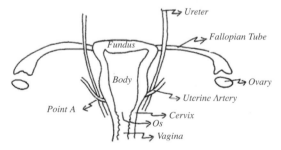

Figure 38.1 Diagram shows position of vagina in relation to surrounding organs.

II. BRACHYTHERAPY

A) Localization

The appropriate vaginal applicator is inserted into the vagina in the OR. Dummy pellets are placed inside the lumen of the vaginal applicator and a radio-opaque rectal marker is placed in the rectum. An AP film is taken. Radio-opaque dye is injected into the bladder catheter and a lateral film is taken. The patient is taken back to the brachytherapy ward after recovery.

B) Treatment Planning

The coordinates of standard 'active' pellet positions for the applicator size, rectal and bladder points are digitized into the planning computer. The desired dose distribution uniform along the surface of the applicator as shown in Figure 38.2. Dose to the bladder and rectum are also calculated to ensure they are within the acceptable range. The treatment time is calculated and the *"Selectron"* is set up and programmed as described in cancer of the cervix.

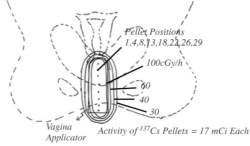

Figure 38. Dose distribution for a 3 × 8 cm² vaginal applicator using 8 of ^{137}Cs pellets at 17 mCi each.

PUBLICATIONS OF INTERESTS

1.   Chau PM: Radiotherapeutic management of malignant tumours of the vagina. Am J Roentgenol Radium Ther Nucl Med 89:502,1963.

2.   Daw E: Primary carcinoma of the vagina. J Obstet Gynaecol Br Common W 78:853,1971.

3.   Hintz GL, Kagan AR, Chan P, et a;" Radiation tolerance of the vaginal mucosa. Int J Radiat Oncol Biol Phys 6:711, 1980.

4.   Kucera H, Vavra N: Radiation management of primary carcinoma of the vagina: Clinical and histopathological variables associated with survival. Gynecol Oncol 40:12-16, 1991.

5.   Lee RA, Symmonds RE: Recurrent carcinoma in situ of the vagina in patients previously treated for in situ carcinoma of the cervix. Obstet Gynecol 48:61,1976.

6.   Lee WR, Marcus RB, Sombeck MD, et al: Radiotherapy alone for carcinoma of the vagina: The importance of overall treatment time. Int J Radiat Oncol Biol Phys 29:983 988, 1994.

7.   Leung S, Sexton M: Radical radiation therapy for carcinoma of the vagina: Impact of treatment modalities on outcome. Peter MacCallum Cancer Institute experience 1970-1990. Int J Radiat Oncol Biol Phys 25:413-418, 1993.

8.   MacNaught R, Symmonds RP, Hole D, et al: Improved control of primary vaginal tumors by combined external beam and interstitial radiotherapy. Clin Radiol 37:29-32, 1986.

9.   Perez CA, Arneson AN, Dehner LP, et al: Radiation therapy in carcinoma of the vagina. Obstet Gynecol 44:862,1974.

10. Perez CA, Korba A, Sharma S: Dosimetric considerations in irradiation of carcinoma of the vagina. Int J Radiat Oncol Biol Phys 2:639-649, 1977.

11. Prempree T, Viravathana T, Slawson RG, et al: Radiation management of primary carcinoma of the vagina. Cancer 40:109,1977.

12. Reddy S, Lee MS, Graham JE, et al: Radiation therapy in primary carcinoma of the vagina. Gynecol Oncol 26:19-24, 1987.

13. Sharma SC, Gerbi B, Madoc-Jones H: Dose rates for brachytherapy applicators using 137Cs sources. Int J Radiat Oncol Biol Phys 5: 1893, 1979.

14. Shimm DS, Ropar M: Radiation therapy of carcinoma of the vagina. Acta Obstet Gynecol Scand 65:449-452, 1986.

15. Spirtos NM, Doshi BP, Kapp DS, et al: Radiation therapy for primary squamous cell carcinoma of the vagina: Stanford University experience. Gynecol Oncol 35:20-26, 1989.

16. Stock RG, Mychalczak B, Armstrong JG, et al: The importance of brachytherapy technique in the management of primary carcinoma of the vagina. Int J Radiat Oncol Biol Phys 24:747-753, 1992.

Principles and Practice of Clinical Physics and Dosimetry
Michael L.F. Lim, CMD, ACT
Advanced Medical Publishing, Inc., USA

—— *CHAPTER 39* ——

Cancer of the Ovaries

I. INTRODUCTION

The ovaries are almond shape structures measuring about 4 cm in length by about 3 cm in width. They are located on each side of the uterus below the fallopian tube. The ovaries are attached to the uterus by the ovarian ligament. Anterior to the ovaries is the broad ligament.

There are four staging for cancer of the ovaries. Stage Ia is tumor limited to one ovary with no ascites. Stage Ib is tumor limited to both ovaries with no ascites. Stage Ic is tumor in both ovaries with ascites. Stage IIa is tumor extension to the uterus or tubes. Stage IIb is tumor extension to other pelvic tissues. Stage IIc is similar to IIa and IIb with ascites. Stage III is tumor spread outside the pelvis. Stage IV is distant metastasis.

The commonest age group to get cancer of the ovary is 40-60 year old. Some of the contributing factors are disorder of the endocrine function, use of stilbestrol, contact with asbestos, obesity and use of talc powder.

Most patients present symptoms when the cancer has grown to a considerable size. When this happens, the usual complains are abdominal distention, edema of the lower limbs and intestinal obstruction.

The diagnostic methods to diagnose cancer of the ovary are pelvic examination, ultrasound and CT. Laparotomy and histological examination of the tumor are necessary to establish diagnosis.

Treatment of choice for early disease is surgery where bilateral salpingo-oophorectomy and hysterectomy are performed. When surgery is not possible, external beam irradiation is the treatment of choice with chemotherapy or hormonal therapy as adjunct. External beam irradiation is with a pair of parallel opposed AP and PA fields given in two courses. For the first course, a large field is used to include the whole peritoneal cavity. The boost field covers only the pelvis.

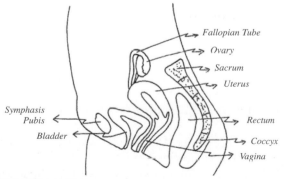

Figure 39.1 Ovaries and surrounding organs.

II. LOCALIZATION

For simulation, the patient lies in a supine position with hands on chest. The large field is localized and AP and PA simulator films are taken. Field marks are drawn on the patient. Calculation points to the left and right kidneys and liver are indicated on the AP film.

The boost field may be simulated at this point.

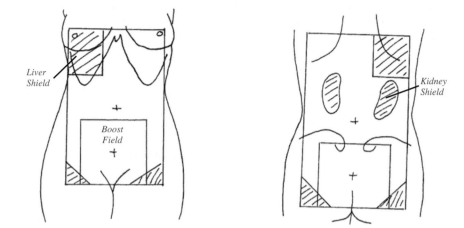

Figure 39.2 Large field (with liver and kidney shielding) and boost field.

III. TREATMENT PLANNING

A) First course (Large field)

The total tumor dose for the large field is 2520 cGy in 14 fractions with kidney shielding at 1800 cGy to the kidneys and liver shielding at 2000 cGy. Point dose calculation is done for the center, liver and kidneys in order to shield them at their appropriate doses.

B) Second course (boost field)

The total tumor dose for the boost field is 2160 cGy in 12 fractions.

IV. PUBLICATIONS OF INTERESTS

1. Aure JC, Hoeg K, Kolstad P: Radioactive colloidal gold in the treatment of ovarian carcinoma. Acta Radiol Ther(Stockh) 10:399,1971.

2. Bakri YN, Given FT, Peeples WJ, et al: Complications from intraperitoneal radioactive phosphorus in ovarian malignancies. Gynecol Oncol 21: 294,1985.

3. Bush RS: Ovarian cancer: Contribution of radiation therapy to patient management. Radiology 153: 17,1984.

4. Delclos L, Smith JP: Ovarian cancer with special regard to types of radiotherapy. Natl Cancer Inst Monogr 42:129,1975.

5. Demko AJ, Bush RS: Radiation therapy of ovarian carcinoma. In Griffiths CT, Fuller AF(eds): Gynecologic Oncology, pp263-298,Boston, Maritinus. Nijhoff,1983.

6. Dembo AJ, Van Dyk J, Japp B, et al: Whole abdominal irradiation by a moving strip technique for patients with ovarian cancer. Int J Radiat Oncol Biol Phys 5:1933,1979.

7. Eltringham JR: Radiation therapy for ovarian carcinoma. Clin Obstet Gynecol 22:967,1979.

8. Hacker NF, Berek JS, Burnison CM, et al: Whole abdominal radiation as salvage therapy for epithelial ovarian cancer. Obstet Gynecol 65:60-66, 1985.

9. Kong JJS, Peters LJ, Wharton JT, et al: Hyperfractionated split course whole abdominal radiotherapy for ovarian carcinoma: Tolerance and toxicity. Int J Radiat Oncol Biol Phys 14:737, 1988.

10. Martinez A, Schray MF, Howes AE, et al: Postoperative radiation therapy for epithelial ovarian cancer: The curative role based on a 24 year experience. J Clin Oncol 3:901-910, 1985.

11. Mychalczak BR, Fuks Z: The current role of radiotherapy in the management of ovarian cancer. Hematol Oncol Clin North Am 6:895-913, 1992 .

12. Perez CA, Walz BJ, Jacobson PL: Radiation therapy in the management of carcinoma of the ovary. Natl Cancer Inst Monogr 42: 119, 1975.

13. Qazi F, McGuire WP: The treatment of ovarian cancer. CA Cancer J Clin 45:88-101, 1995.

14. Reinfuss M, Kojs Z, Skolyszewski J: External beam radiotherapy in the management of ovarian cancer. Radiother Oncol 26:26-32, 1993.

15. Thomas GM, Dembo AJ: Integrating radiation therapy into the management of ovarian cancer. Cancer 71:1710-1718, 1993

16. Thomas L, Pigneux J, Chauvergne J, et al: Evaluation of whole abdominal irradiation in ovarian carcinoma with a four orthogonal field technique. Int J Radiat Oncol Biol Phys 30:1083-1090, 1994.

17. Townsend R, Glassburn JR, Brady LW, et al: Whole abdominal irradiation for carcinoma of the ovary. Cancer Clin Trials 2:351,1979.

18. Toznor A, Polychronopalla A, Hsieh CC, et al: Hair dyes, tranquilizers and perineal talc application as risk factors for ovarian cancer. Int J Cancer 55:408-410, 1993.

19. Vergote IB, Winderen M, DeVos LN, et al: Intraperitoneal radioactive phosphorus therapy in ovarian carcinoma. Cancer 71:2250-2260, 1993.

20. Wharton JT, Delclos L, Gallager S, et al: Radiation hepatitis induced by abdominal irradiation with the cobalt-60 moving strip technique. Am J Roentgel Rad Ther Nucl Med 117:73,1973.

Principles and Practice of Clinical Physics and Dosimetry
Michael L.F. Lim, CMD, ACT
Advanced Medical Publishing, Inc., USA

— CHAPTER 40 —

Cancer of the Penis

I. INTRODUCTION

The penis is the male external genital organ. It is made up of highly erectile tissue. Through it passes the urethra that is the outlet for urine and sperms. The erectile tissue is made up of two cylindrical masses that are the corpus cavernosum penis on the ventral end and the corpus spongiosum penis on the dorsal end. The distal end of the penis is made up of glans penis which is covered by the prepuce *(skin)* in an uncircumcised male. Cancer of the penis is divided into four stages. Stage I is tumor confined to the glan. Stage II is tumor extension onto the shaft of the penis. Stage III is when there is inguinal metastasis. Stage IV is distant metastasis.

Cancer of the penis is a very rare disease in countries where hygiene is good. It is never seen in males who are circumcised at birth. Most of the cancer are of the squamous cell type. An ulcerating and discharging lesion is the usual presentation. In later stages, a mass may be felt at the inguinal region. Biopsy confirms diagnosis. Confirmation of nodal involvement is also by biopsy.

Probably the best treatment is surgery but the psychological trauma is not acceptable. Fortunately, radiation therapy is a good alternative. Operable nodes are removed surgically. Inoperable nodes are treated by radiation. The small tumors are treated with superficial X-Rays (100 kV) taking care to shield surrounding tissues. Deeper and more advanced tumors are treated on the ^{60}Co unit with a pair of parallel opposed fields through a wax block which holds the penis up and acts as build up and provide dose uniformity.

Cylindrical mold using Radium or Caesium sources may be used but do not provide as good a dose distribution as the parallel opposed ^{60}Co unit treatment. The dose on the surface is higher than at the center of the penis by as much as 30-50%.

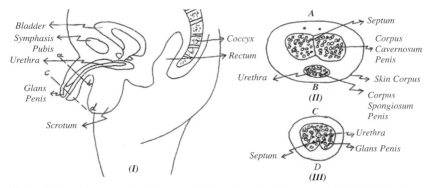

Figure 40.1 (I) Penis and surrounding structures. (II) Cross section of the penis at level a-b. (III) Cross section of the penis at level c-d.

II. EXTERNAL BEAM IRRADIATION

A) Localization

Localization is by visual inspection to ensure penis is inside the mold for the parallel opposed ^{60}Co treatment or for brachytherapy.

B) Treatment Planning

i. Superficial X-Ray

This is the treatment of choice for very small superficial tumors. The applicator is directed at the lesion and lead sheets are placed on the scrotum to shield the testis. Total surface dose is in the region of 5000 cGy in 20 fractions.

ii. Cobalt-60

For larger and deeper lesions, the ^{60}Co beams are necessary to achieve a good depth dose. A wax block is fabricated to immobilize the penis in the same treatment position. The wax block also acts as a build up to prevent skin sparing and provide dose uniformity. Treatment is with a pair of parallel opposed beams using a field size of about 4.5 cm wide by 7 cm long at 80 cm SAD. A plan may be generated if desired. Scrotal shielding should be used to reduce dose to the testis.

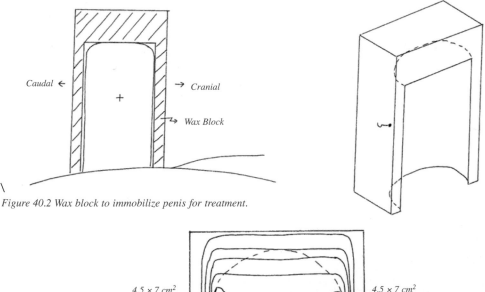

Figure 40.2 Wax block to immobilize penis for treatment.

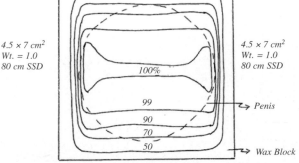

Figure 40.3 Dose distribution for parallel opposed fields on Cobalt-60 unit.

III. BRACHYTHERAPY

A) Localization

As described under external beam irradiation.

B) Treatment Planning

Eight radium needles, at 4 mg each, are placed around the circumference of the wax mold. With this arrangement, homogenous dose distribution is achieved around the penis. The 50 cGy/h isodose line covers the target volume(top half of the penis) in the sagittal and cross sectional planes. The treatment time is calculated from the total tumor dose over the chosen dose rate. In this example, the total tumor dose is 5000 cGy and the dose rate is 50 cGy/h. The treatment time is 100 hours. At 10 hours a day, the patient is treated over 10 days. Due to the length of treatment time per day and due to the possibility of dysuria from radiation urethritis, the patient is catheterized during treatment.

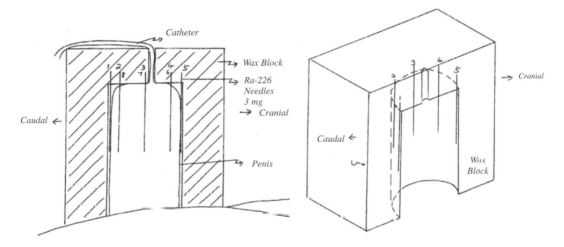

Figure 40.4 Wax mold with Radium needles.

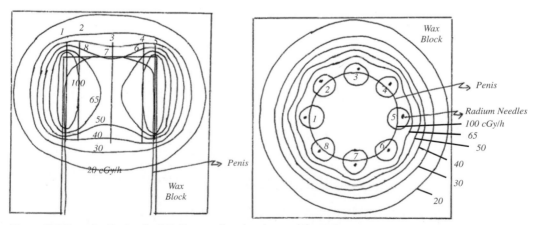

Figure 40.5 Dose distribution for 8 Radium needles placed around the penis.

IV. PUBLICATIONS OF INTERESTS

1.   Almgand LE, Edsmyr F: Radiotherapy in treatment of patients with carcinoma of the penis. Scand J Urol Nephrol 7:1,1973.

2.   Cabanas RM: An approach for the treatment of penile carcinoma. Cancer 39:456,1977.

3.   Duncan W, Jackson SM: the treatment of early cancer of the penis with magavoltage X-Rays. Clin Radiol 23:246,1972.

4.   Haile K, Delclos L: The place of radiation therapy in the treatment of carcinoma of the distil end of the penis. Cancer 45:1980,1980.

5.   Kelley CD, Arthur K, Rogoff E, et al: Radiation therapy of penile cancer. Urology 4:571-573, 1974.

6.   Knudsen OA, Brennhovd IO: Radiotherapy in the treatment of the primary tumour in penile cancer. Acta Chir Scand 113:69-71, 1967.

7.   Mazeron JJ, Langlois D, Lobo PA, et al: Interstitial radiation therapy for carcinoma of the penis using iridium 192 wires: The Henri Mondor experience (1970-1979). Int J Radiat Oncol Biol Phys 10:1891-1895, 1984.

8.   Murrell DS, Williams JL: Radiotherapy in the treatment of carcinoma of the penis. Br J Urol 37:211-222, 1965.

9.   Newaishy GA, Deeley TJ: Radiotherapy in the treatment of carcinoma of the penis. Br J Radiol 41:519-521, 1968.

10.   Rozan R, Albuisson E, Giraud B, et al: Interstitial brachytherapy for penile carcinoma: A multicentric survey (259 patients). Radiother Oncol 36:83-93, 1995.

11.   Sagerman RH, Yu WS, Chung CT, Puranik A: External-beam irradiation of carcinoma of the penis. Radiology 152:183-185, 1984.

— *CHAPTER 41* —

Cancer of the Prostate

I. INTRODUCTION

The prostate is a muscular and glandular organ situated at the neck of the bladder. It is chestnut in shape and size and measures about 3.5 cm across by 3 cm long. Superior to it is the bladder, anterior is the pubis, posterior is the rectum and inferior is the urethra. On each side of the prostate attached to the superior and posterior surface are the seminal vesicles.

The staging for carcinoma of the prostate is divided into four stages. Stage A is occult tumor. Stage B is tumor confined within the prostate capsule. Stage C is tumor extension outside the capsule and surrounding structures and pelvic nodes may be involved. Stage D is distant metastasis from tumor of the prostate.

It is the most common cancer in men over 50 years old. The tumors are mostly adenocarcinoma with some sarcoma. The cause may be hormonal related.

Some of the common presentations are difficulty in starting stream, dribbling and even bladder retention. Some may have urinary bleeding. On rectal examination, an enlarge lump may be felt anterior to the rectum.

Diagnosis is by rectal examination, CT scan, laboratory tests, bone scan and needle biopsy.

Surgery is the treatment of choice for early prostate cancer although there are controversies regarding the pros and cons of surgery verses radiation therapy related to impotence and incontinence. For later stages, radiation therapy is the choice. Interstitial brachytherapy with I-125 seeds is sometimes used and hormonal therapy may be given in conjunction with radiation therapy.

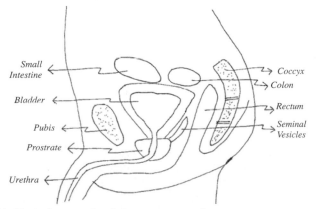

Figure 41.1 Position of bladder and prostate in relation to organs nearby.

II. LOCALIZATION

The patient is encouraged to keep a full bladder before simulation. A full bladder helps to push much of the small bowels and bladder out of the radiation field. The patient lies in a supine position with hands on chest. Urethrogram may be done to more accurately localize the apex of the prostate in planning. AP and lateral fields are simulated and field centers are marked on the patient's skin on the AP and the lateral. The AP field is approximately 15×15 cm^2 and covers the whole pelvis. The lateral field is approximately 11×15 cm^2 covering the pubic symphysis anteriorly and mid sacrum level posteriorly. Radio-opaque markers are taped on the field centers on the skin. The radio-opaque markers would show up on CT for centering at the time of planning. The patient is CT and the images are transferred to the planning computer. The prostate, rectum, bladder, seminal vesicles and heads of femur are delineated. Margins are added for the PTV.

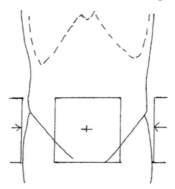

Figure 41.2 Localization of large fields to treat cancer of the prostate using four field technique.

III. TREATMENT PLANNING

A. Early T1 tumor

The intersection of the AP and lateral CT marks on the central CT slice are localized and centered for referencing. A four field plan is generated using the field sizes as simulated. For the AP and PA fields, the corners are shielded to reduce dose to the bowels. For the lateral fields, the superior anterior corners are shielded to reduce dose to the bowels. Dose distribution is shown in Figure 41.3. Total dose is 4500 cGy in 25 fractions to 100% at isocenter.

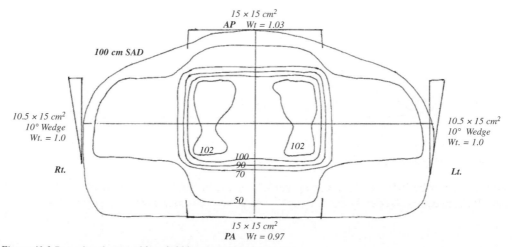

Figure 41.3 Dose distribution of four field box using 18 MV photons.

B. Mid T2 tumor

For T2 tumor, a dose of 4500 cGy is inadequate. An additional dose of 2160 cGy in 12 fractions is needed. To reduce the dose to the heads of femur, six fields are used. A margin of 1 cm is added to the CTV (prostate) to form the PTV. To reduce the dose to the rectum posteriorly, the margin is 0.5 cm posteriorly from CTV. If the seminal vesicles are involved, they are included in the CTV. The six fields are as shown in Figure 41.4. As much of the bladder and rectum are shielded.

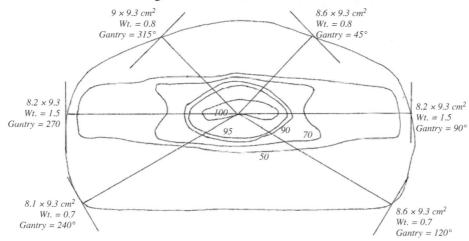

Figure 41.4 Field arrangement and dose distribution of six field boost 1 using 18 MV photons.

C. Late T3 tumor

For T3 tumors a further dose of 720 cGy in 4 fractions is given. The PTV margin is 0.7 cm around the CTV and 0.5 cm margin posteriorly and the seminal vesicles are included in the CTV. The six fields are as shown in Figure 41.5. As much of the bladder and rectum are shielded.

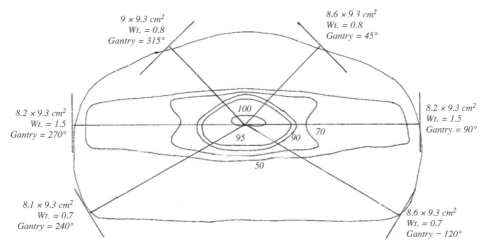

Figure 41.5 Field arrangement and dose distribution of six field boost 2 using 18 MV photons. The field sizes are kept the same but the MLCs are adjusted tighter around the rectum and bladder.

The plans described above are summed and DVHs are generated to document the dose to the prostate, PTV, rectum, bladder, seminal vesicles and heads of femur as shown in Figure 41.6

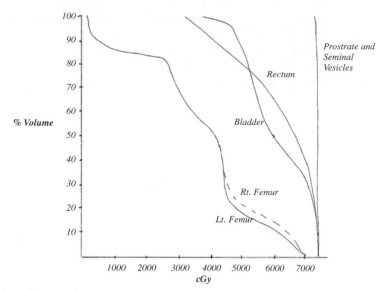

Figure 41.6 Sum plan DVH for prostate + seminal vesicles, rectum, bladder, and heads of femur. The sum plans are four field box, 6 field boost 1 and 6 field boost 2. Total dose = 4500 cGy + 2160 cGy + 720 cGy

D. Intensity Modualated Radiation Therapy (IMRT)

IMRT have increasingly been used as boost to the prostate. An example of a prostate plan using IMRT on 18 MV photons is given below. As shown in the diagram, the coverage of the boost PTV (prostate + seminal vesicles + margin) is good and the dose to the rectum, bladder and heads of femur.

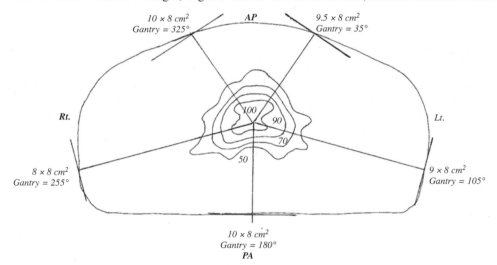

Figure 41.7 Dose distribution for 5 field IMRT on 18 MV photons.

IV. PUBLICATIONS OF INTERESTS

1.   Batata MA, Hilaris BS, Chu FCH, et al: Radiation therapy in adenocarcinoma of the prostate with pelvic lymph node involvement on lymphadenectomy. Int J Radiat Oncol Biol Phys 6:149,1980.

2.   Blennerhassett JB, Vickery AL: Carcinoma of the prostate gland: An anatomical study of tumour location. Cancer 19:980,1966.

3.   Charyulu KKN: Transperineal intestitial implantation of prostate cancer: A new method. Int J Radiat Oncol Biol Phys 6:1261,1980.

4. Crook JM, Raymond Y, Salhani D, et al: Prostate motion during standard radiotherapy as assessed by fiducial markers. Radiother Oncol 37:35-42, 1995.

5. Dewit L, Ang KK, Vander Schueren E: Acute side effects and late complications after radiotherapy of localized carcinoma of the prostate. Cancer Treat Rev 10:79,1983.

6. Diaz A, Roach M III, Marquez C, et al: Indications for and the significance of seminal vesicle irradiation during 3D conformal radiotherapy for localized prostate cancer. Int J Radiat Oncol Biol Phys 30:323-329, 1994.

7. Flocks RH, Culp D, Porta R: Lymphatic spread from prostatic cancer. J Urol 81:194,1959.

8. Forman JD, Mesina CF, He T, et al: Evaluation of changes in the location and shape of the prostate and rectum during a seven week course of conformal radiotherapy. Int J Radiat Oncol Biol Phys 27(suppl 1):222, 1993.

9. Gibbons RP, Mason JT, Correa RJ, et al: Carcinoma of the prostate: Local control with external beam radiation therapy. J Urol 121:310,1979.

10. Goffinet DR, Martinez A, Freiha F, et al: Iodine-125 prostate implants for recurrent carcinomas after external beam irradiation: Preliminary results. Cancer 45:2717,1980.

11. Gore RM, Moss AA: Value of computed tomography in intestitial 125I brachytherapy of prostate carcinoma. Radiology 146:453,1983. Guinan P, Bush I, Ray V, et al: The accuracy of the rectal examination in the diagnosis of prostate carcinoma. N Engl J Med 303:499,1980.

12. Hanks GE: Optimizing the radiation treatment and outcome of prostate cancer. Int J Radiat Oncol Biol Phys 11:1235,1985.

13. Hussey DH, Chan R, delclos L, et al: Radiotherapy for carcinoma of the prostate. Cancer Bull 30:131,1978.

14. Lee WR, Hanks GE, Hanlon AL, et al: Lateral rectal shielding reduces late rectal morbidity following high dose three-dimensional conformal radiation therapy for clinically localized prostate cancer: Further evidence for a significant dose effect. Int J Radiat Oncol Biol Phys 35:251-257, 1996.

15. Ling CC, Burman C, Chui CS, et al: Conformal radiation treatment of prostate cancer using inversely-planned intensity-modulated photon beams produced with dynamic multileaf collimation. Int J Radiat Oncol Biol Phys 35:721-730, 1996.

16. Low NN, Vijayakumar S, Rosenberg I, et al: Beam's eye view based prostate treatment planning: Is it useful? Int J Radiat Biol Phys 19:759-768, 1990.

17. Melian E, Kutcher G, Leibel S, et al: Variation in prostate position: Quantitation and implication for three-dimensional conformal radiation therapy. Int J Radiat Oncol Biol Phys 27(suppl 1):137, 1993.

18. Neal AJ, Oldham M, Dearnaley DP: Comparison of treatment techniques for conformal radiotherapy of the prostate using dose-volume histograms and normal tissue complication probabilities. Radiother Oncol 37:29-34, 1995.

19. Oldham M, Neal A, Webb S: A comparison of conventional "forward planning" with inverse planning for 3D conformal radiotherapy of the prostate. Radiother Oncol 35:248-262, 1995.

20. Perez CA, Pilepich MV, Zivnuska F: tumour control in definitive irradiation of localized carcinoma of the prostate. Int J Radiat Oncol Biol Phys 12:523,1986.

21. Perez CA, Lee HK, Georgiou A, et al: Technical and tumor-related factors affecting outcome of definitive irradiation for localized carcinoma of the prostate. Int J Radiat Oncol Biol Phys 26:565-581, 1993.

22. Perez CA, Purdy JA, Harms W, et al: Three-dimensional treatment planning and conformal radiation therapy: Preliminary evaluation. Radiother Oncol 36:32-43, 1995.

23. Pickett B, Roach M III, Verhey L, et al: The value of nonuniform margins for six-field conformal irradiation of localized prostate cancer. Int J Radiat Oncol Biol Phys 32:211-218, 1995.

24. Pilepich MV, Prasad SC, Perez CA: Computed tomography in definitive radiotherapy of prostatic carcinoma. Part 2: Definition of target volume. Int J Radiat Oncol Biol Phys 8: 235,1982.

25. Roach M III, Faillace-Akazawa P, Malfatti C, et al: Prostate volumes defined by magnetic resonance imaging and computerized tomographic scans for three-dimensional conformal radiotherapy. Int J Radiat Oncol Biol Phys 35:1011-1018, 1996.

26. Roach M III, Pickett B, Weil M, et al: The "critical volume tolerance method" for estimating the limits of dose escalation during three-dimensional conformal radiotherapy for prostate cancer. Int J Radiat Oncol Biol Phys 35:1019-1025, 1996.

27.   Roeske JC, Forman JD, Mesina CF, et al: Evaluation of changes in the size and location of the prostate, seminal vesicles, bladder, and rectum during a course of external beam radiation therapy. Int J Radiat Oncol Biol Phys 33:1321-1329, 1995.

28.   Rudat V, Schraube P, Oetzel D, et al: Combined error of patient positioning variability and prostate motion uncertainty in 3D conformal radiotherapy of localized prostate cancer. Int J Radiat Oncol Biol Phys 35:1027-1034, 1996.

29.   Schild SE, Casale HE, Bellefontaine LP: Movements of the prostate due to rectal and bladder distension: Implications for radiotherapy. Med Dosim 18:13-15, 1993.

30.   Song, PY, Washington M, Vaida F, et al: A comparison of four patient immobilization devices in the treatment of prostate cancer patients with three dimensional conformal radiotherapy. Int J Radiat Oncol Biol Phys 34:213-219, 1996.

31.   Ten Haken RK, Forman JD, Heimburger K, et al: Treatment planning issues related to prostate movement in response to differential filling of the rectum and bladder. Int J Radiat Oncol Biol Phys 20:1317-1324, 1991.

32.   van Herk M, Bruce A, Kroes APG, et al: Quantification of organ motion during conformal radiotherapy of the prostate by three dimensional image registration. Int J Radiat Oncol Biol Phys 33:1311-1320, 1995.

—— *CHAPTER 42* ——

Cancer of the Testis

I. INTRODUCTION

The testis are two glandular male sex organs which are suspended in the scrotum by the spermatic cords. Each testis measures about 4×3×3 cm³. Each testis is made up of two main parts. They are the body and the epididymis. The body is divided into septa and each septum contains the semiferous tublues. The epididymis is made up of a long and convoluted duct that receives the efferent ductules. These are shown in Figure 42.1

Cancer of the testis is divided into four stages. Stage I is tumor confined to the testis and spermatic cord. Stage II is tumor spread beyond the testis but limited to regional lymphatics below the diaphragm. Stage IIa is retroperitoneal metastasis measuring about 2 cm. Stage IIb is retroperitoneal metastasis measuring less than 5cm. Stage IIc is retroperitoneal metastasis measuring greater than 5cm.Stage III is metastasis beyond the diaphragm. Stage IIIa is metastasis beyond the diaphragm but confined to mediastinum or supraclavicular lymphatics. Stage IIIb is metastasis outside lymph nodes. About 97% of the cancer of the testis are from germinal origin with the remaining 3% or so from non-germinal origin. Of the cancer of the testis from germinal origin, most are seminoma. The next group is the so called mixed tumors which are the teratoma, embroynal carcinoma and choriocarcinoma.

Seminomas are very radiosensitive and generally a total tumor dose of 2500 cGy in 20 fractions is enough. The mixed tumors are very radioresistant and a total tumor dose of 4000 cGy in 30 fractions is necessary. Cancer of the testis is very rare, accounting for about 1% of all cancers in males. Age group is 30-40 years old. The left and right testis are equally affected.

The most frequent presentation is an enlarging painless mass in the scrotum.

Diagnosis is by palpation, transillumination, IVP, surgical exploration, HCG and AFP (Human chorionic gonadotropin and Alpha fetoprotein.)

Treatment is a combination of surgery, post-operative radiation therapy and chemotherapy. During surgery, inguinal exploration and high cord ligation and orchietomy are performed. Post-operative radiation therapy is given with a pair of parallel opposed AP and PA fields. The field coverage is dependent of the stage of the disease.

II. STAGE I AND IIA

A) Localization

The patient lies supine for simulation with arms by the side. The radiation field covers the inguinal, iliac and paraaortic nodes from AP and PA. For unilateral tumor, only the nodes on the affected side are covered. For bilateral tumors, the nodes on both sides are covered. AP and PA simulator films are taken and field marks are drawn on the patient. Shielding is drawn on the films and calculation points are indicated on the films.

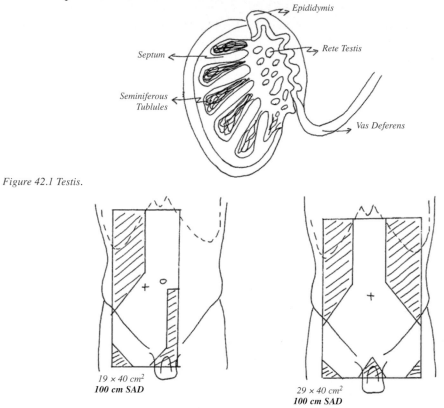

Figure 42.1 Testis.

19 × 40 cm²
100 cm SAD

29 × 40 cm²
100 cm SAD

Figure 42.2 Portals for unilateral and bilateral testicular tumors for stage I and IIA.

B) Treatment Planning

Irregular field calculation is put through the planning computer to calculate MU and the dose to points of interest.

Unilateral lesion

Point	Dose(cGy)
Center	2500
Para-aortics	2436
Lt.groin	2673

Bilateral lesion

Point	Dose(cGy)
Center	2500
Para-aortics	2360
Rt.groin	2582
Lt.groin	2567

III. STAGE IIB AND IIC

A) Localization

The patient lies supine for simulation with arms by the side. The radiation field covers the whole abdomen and pelvis. AP and PA simulator films are taken and field marks drawn on the patient. Shielding is drawn on the films and calculation points are indicated on the films.

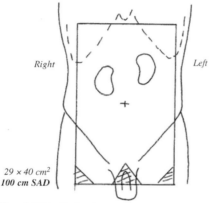

Figure 42.3 Portals for stage IIB and IIC testicular tumors.

B) Treatment Planning

Irregular field calculation is put through the planning computer to generate the block factor to be used for MU setting calculation and to calculate the dose to the calculation points. Kidney shielding is necessary to keep the dose under 1800 cGy.

Point	Dose(cGy)
Center	2000
Rt.groin	2144
Lt.groin	2144
Rt.kidney	1763
Lt.kidney	1747

IV. STAGE III AND IIIA

A) Localization

i) Lower field

The patient lies supine for simulation with arms by the side. The AP and PA field cover the inguinal, iliac and paraaortic nodes. For unilateral tumor, only the nodes on the affected side are covered. For bilateral tumor, the nodes on both sides are covered. AP and PA simulator films are taken and field marks are drawn on the patient. Shielding is drawn on the films and calculation points are indicated on the AP film. A gap between the lower and upper field is calculated.

ii) Upper field

The AP field covers the mediastinal nodes and the left supraclavicular fossa. The PA field covers only the mediastinal nodes. AP and PA simulator films are taken and field marks are drawn on the patient. Shielding is drawn on the films and calculation points are indicated on the films.

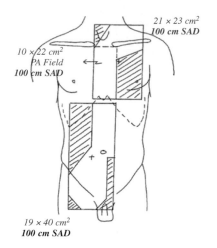

Figure 42.4 Portals for stage III and IIIA unilateral testicular tumors.

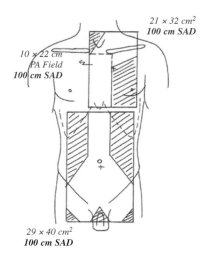

Figure 42.5 Portals for stage III and IIIA bilateral testicular tumors.

B) Treatment Planning

Irregular field calculation is put through the planning computer to generate the block factor to be used for MU setting calculation and to calculate the dose to the calculation points.

Upper field

Point	Dose(cGy)
Mediastinal	2500
Lt.s/c	2500

V. PUBLICATIONS OF INTERESTS

1.   Earle JD, Bagshaw MA, Kaplan HS: Supervoltage radiation therapy of the testicular tumours. Am J Roentgenol 117:653,1973.

2.   Maier JG, Mittemeyer BT: Carcinoma of the testis. Cancer 39:981,1977.

3.   Peckham MJ, McElwain TJ: Radiotherapy of testicular tumors. Proc R Soc Med 67:300, 1974.

4.   Smalley SR, Evans RG, Richardson RL, et al: Radiotherapy as initial treatment for bulky stage II testicular seminomas. J Clin Oncol 3:1333, 1985.

5.   Thomas GM, Rider WD, Dembo AJ, et al: Seminoma of the testis: Results of treatment and patterns of failure after radiation therapy. Int J Radiat Oncol Biol Phys 8:165,1982.

6.   Ytredal DO, Bradfield JS: Seminoma of the testicle: Prophylactic mediastinal irradiation verses periaortic and pelvic irradiation alone. Cancer 3: 628,1972.

7.   Zagars GK, Babaian J: The role of radiation in stage II testicular seminoma. Int J Radiat Oncol Biol Phys 13:163, 1987.

Principles and Practice of Clinical Physics and Dosimetry
Michael L.F. Lim, CMD, ACT
Advanced Medical Publishing, Inc., USA

—— *CHAPTER 43* ——

Cancer of the Bladder

I. INTRODUCTION

The bladder is a muscular sac that serves as a reservoir for urine. It lies in the pelvis behind the pubis. In the male, it is anterior to the rectum and superiorly it is in contact with the colon and small intestines. Inferiorly, is the prostate gland and the urethra.

In the female, it is anterior to the uterus and vagina and superiorly it is in contact with the small intestines. Inferiorly, is the urethra.

Staging for cancer of the bladder is divided into five stages. Stage I is carcinoma in situ. Stage II is tumor confined to the submucosa. Stage III is tumor invasion into the muscle. Stage IV is tumor penetration through the bladder serosa. Stage V is widespread metastasis from tumor of the bladder.

Cancer of the bladder is the most common cancer of the urinary tract. Over 80% of the tumors are situated on the lateral and posterior walls of the bladder. It is found commonly in the 50 to 70 year age group and male to female ratio is approximately 2:1.

Associated causes of bladder cancer are aniline dye, smoking and chronic bladder infection.

The most common presentations are haematuria and dysuria.

Diagnosis may be obtained from urine tests, IVP, cystoscopy and CT. Surgery is the treatment of choice for early stages. If surgery is not possible, radiation therapy is given in two courses using four field box technique for the first course and cone down for the second course boost using either four field box technique or rotational technique. Interstitial brachytherapy with Tantalum-182 wire or Gold-198 seeds may also be used. Chemotherapy has limited benefit. Five year survival is about 40%.

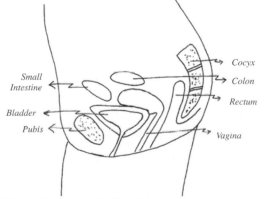

Figure 43.1 Position of bladder and organs nearby (female).

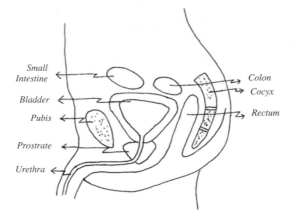

Figure 43.2 Position of bladder and organs nearby (male).

II. LOCALIZATION

The patient is encouraged to empty the bladder before simulation. The patient lies in a supine position with hands on the chest. Cystogram is performed and localization of the bladder is achieved under fluoroscopy. Both courses of treatment may be planned together. For the first course, a large field measuring 15×15 cm^2 is set for the AP and PA and 8×15 cm^2 for the laterals. For the second course, the field is reduced to a 9×9 cm^2 for the AP and PA and 8×9 cm^2 for the laterals. Anterior and lateral simulator films are taken and field marks are drawn on the patient. Lateral lazer lines are drawn on the sides of the patient to aid in daily reproducibility of treatment set up. A contour through the field center is obtained for planning.

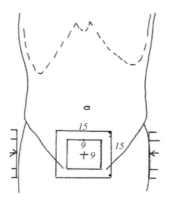

Figure 43.3 Localization for large and boost fields to treat cancer of the bladder using four-field box technique.

III. TREATMENT PLANNING

After delineation of the target volume and rectum, a plan is generated to give a uniform dose to cover the bladder but spare the rectum as much as possible. A composite plan is generated for the two courses of treatment as shown in Figure 43.4 using four field box.

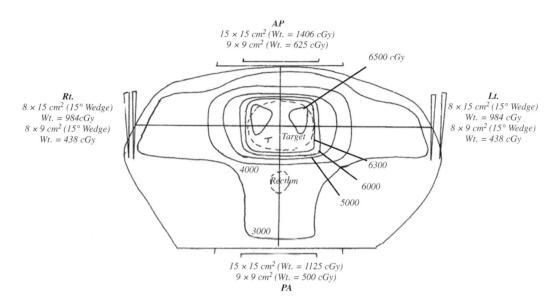

Figure 43.4 Dose distribution for four field box technique using a composite of large and boost fields on 10 MV photons.

IV. PUBLICATIONS OF INTERESTS

1. Batto H, Pervin JL, Auvert J et al: Treatment of malignant bladder tumours by iridium-192 wiring. Urology 16:467,1980.

2. Emami B, Pilepich MV: Anatomic considerations in radiotherapeutic management of bladder cancer. Am J Clin Oncol 6:593,1983.

3. Finney R: The treatment of carcinoma of the bladder by external irradiation. A clinical trial II. Clin Radiol 22:225,1971.

4. Gospodarowicz MK, Hawkins NV, Rawlings GA, et al: Radical radiotherapy for muscle invasive transitional cell carcinoma of the bladder: Failure analysis. J Urol 142:1448-1453, 1989.

5. Hope-Stone HF, Blandy JP, Oliver RTD, et al: Radical radiotherapy and salvage cystectomy in the treatment of invasive carcinoma of the bladder. In Oliver RTD, Hendry WF, Bloom HJG, eds: Bladder Cancer: Principles of Combination Therapy, pp 127-138. London, Butterworth, 1981 .

6. Jahnson S, Pedersen J, Westman G: Bladder carcinoma: A 20-year review of radical irradiation therapy. Radiother Oncol 22:111 117, 1991.

7. Matsumoto K, Kakizoe T, Mikuiya S, et al: Clinical evaluation of intraoperative radiotherapy for carcinoma of the urinary bladder. Cancer 47:504,1981.

8. Morgan RW, Jain MG: Bladder cancer: Smoking, beverages and artificial sweeteners. Can Med Assoc J 3:1067,1974.

9. Quilty PM, Duncan W: Radiotherapy for squamous carcinoma of the urinary bladder. Int J Radiat Oncol Biol Phys 12:861-865, 1986.

10. Radwin HM: Radiotherapy and bladder cancer: A critical review. J Urol 124:43-46, 1980.

11. Sagerman RH, Veenema RJ, Guttmann R, et a;: Preoperative irradiation of carcinoma of bladder. Am J Roentgenol Radium Ther Nucl Med 102:577,1968.

12. Shipley WU: Radiation therapy for patients with bladder carcinoma: Rationale, results, techniques, and possible innovations. In Bonney WW, Prout GR Jr, eds: Bladder Cancer, pp 243-259. American Urological Association Monographs, vol 1. Baltimore, Williams & Wilkins, 1982.

13. Shipley WU: Radiation therapy of bladder carcinoma. ASTRO refresher course, Los Angeles, CA, 1983.

14. Villar A, Munoz J, Aguilo F, et al: External beam irradiation for T1, T2-3 and T4 transitional cell carcinoma of the urinary bladder. Radiother Oncol 9:209-215, 1987.

—— CHAPTER 44 ——

Radiation Reaction

I. INTRODUCTION

Radiation reaction of an organ depends on several factors. These factors may be broken down into two main categories. They are: i) cellular characteristics and ii) physical characteristics of the radiation. The cellular characteristics which govern the sensitivity of a tissue are its differentiation and cell population. The more differentiated the cells, the less radiosensitive the tissue. The physical characteristics of the radiation which govern the reactions of a tissue are: i) LET, ii) dose rate , iii) volume of tissue treated, iv) total dose given; and v) fractionation. Generally, high LET, high dose rate, large volume of tissue treated, large total dose and small fraction size produce higher radiation reaction.

Following are the possible radiation reactions of several organs that may be encountered in radiotherapy. Their reactions are dependent on the factors mentioned above and the doses quoted are average doses assuming the normal fractionated dose of 180-200 cGy per fraction treating five times a week.

II. SKIN

The radiation reactions may be classified under acute or chronic. Some acute reactions may lead to chronic changes. With megavoltage units, due to skin sparing, there is usually very little skin reactions.

a) Acute

Some of the possible acute radiation reactions of the skin are erythema, dry desquamation, moist desquamation and necrosis. Erythema is due to capillary congestion and moist desquamation is due to serum secretion. A few hundred cGy may cause erythema while a few thousand cGy may cause dry and moist desquamation. Where there are skin creases or friction, there is more likelihood of moist desquamation. About 500 cGy may cause epilation in 2-3 weeks. If the dose is not high, hair will grow again but may be of different colour, texture and form. A dose of 3000 cGy or grater may cause dry skin. Dry skin may lead to infection and necrosis.

b) Chronic

Over time and if high doses are given, pigmentation, fibrosis, telangiectasia and malignancy will result.

III. BONE

Matured bones are very radioresistant but growing bones in children are moderately sensitive to radiation. In treating some childhood cancers, care must be taken to include the whole width of the bone such as the vertebra rather than half the vertebrae. This is to prevent scoliosis. Fractionated total dose around 3000 cGy will produce changes in the bones of children.

IV. CNS

The CNS is very radioresistant. Moderate doses will only cause some functional changes and edema but steroid therapy will control the swelling. At high doses, myelitis, necrosis and fibrosis occur. Doses exceeding 5500 cGy to the brain may cause radiation necrosis. Doses greater than 5000 cGy to a small volume of the spinal cord or greater than 4500 cGy to a large volume of the spinal cord will cause radiation myelitis. These are late changes and are due to vascular damage in the first instance.

V. EYE

A dose of around 1500 cGy to the eye lashes will cause epilation and the lachrymal glands may dry up, not unlike drying of the skin. Desquamation and inflammation around the nasolacrimal duct and sac will lead to blockage and thereby cause a watery eye. A few thousand cGy to the cornea will cause inflammation. Doses exceeding 4000 cGy may cause keratitis and doses exceeding 6000 cGy will cause ulceration. The lens is sensitive to radiation. A single dose of 200 cGy will cause partial opacity while 400 cGy or more causes cataract. A dose of around 2500-3000 cGy to the retina may cause constriction of the retinal veins which lead to decrease visual acuity. Higher doses in the region of 6000 cGy to the retina will cause retinal hemorrhage and detachment. A dose of 4000 cGy or more to the iris will cause iridocyclitis which leads to glaucoma. If severe damage is done to the globe, it will have to be enucleated.

VI. EAR

A total dose of 4000-6000 cGy in 4-6 weeks may cause edema and may block the Eustachian tube. Partial loss of hearing will result. Infection if not treated will damage the drum causing permanent hearing loss.

VII. THYROID

A radiation of around 4000 cGy to the thyroid from treatment to nearby structures decreases thyroid function. Higher protracted doses will lead to carcinogenesis.

VIII. LARYNX

Doses exceeding 6000 cGy will cause temporary loss of voice due to inflammation. Late cartilage necrosis with infection can occur after similar doses.

IX. BUCCAL MUCOSA

The mucosa is moderately sensitive to radiation and a dose around 3000 cGy will cause inflammation. Doses exceeding 5000 cGy will cause fibrosis.

X. MANDIBLE

Over 6000 cGy will cause osteonecrosis due to damage of small blood vessels, osteocytes and injury to periosteum.

XI. TEETH

In children, a dose of less than 1000 cGy may stop growth of the teeth buds. Greater than 3000 cGy will destroy the buds. After radiation, growing teeth may present with various abnormalities. High doses to adult teeth will cause radiation dental caries, inflammation and bleeding gums.

XII. SALIVARY GLANDS

A total dose of around 3000 cGy to the salivary glands may cause swelling. Saliva production is scanty and thick and will be bothersome. Swallowing is difficult. Due to the reduction in saliva or thick saliva, dental caries will be the result. The taste is altered due to damage of the taste buds and the thick saliva. Much higher doses will cause fibrosis of the salivary gland that gives it the hard feel.

XIII. ESOPHAGUS

The epithelium lining the esophagus is moderately sensitive to radiation. Doses above 4000 cGy will produce dysphagia due to edema. Ulceration and esophageal perforation are rare and very high doses are needed.

XIV. HEART

Doses higher than 6000 cGy to the whole heart will produce some cardiac damage. However, damage is more usual in the pericardium producing acute pericarditis or chronic pericarditis at a fractionated total dose of around 4500 cGy. There is also functional ECG change.

XV. LUNG

After a moderate dose of radiation, the cilia lining the epithelium cease to function. A dry mucosa causes secretions to thicken and accumulate. A non productive cough results. If radiation is continued to over 2500 cGy, acute radiation pneumonitis is the result. The patient coughs up thick white sputum, is dyspnea and develops a fever. Chronic radiation fibrosis if limited may be symptomless. Higher doses will produce pulmonary fibrosis in the long term.

XVI. STOMACH

After a dose of about 1500 cGy, the gastric mucosa starts to thin and radiation gastritis begins in a few days. The thinning of the gastric mucosa is due to sloughing. Both hydrochloric acid and pepsin secretion are decreased. These reactions are only temporary if the dose does not go much higher. Very high doses, over 5000 cGy, will produce necrosis and even perforation in some cases.

XVII. SMALL INTESTINES AND RECTUM

The epithelium of the small intestines is very radiosensitive. After a single dose of less than 1000 cGy to the villi, they show destruction in 3-4 days. In the treatment of carcinoma of the uterus or bladder, a total dose of more than 5000 cGy in 5 weeks to the small intestines will cause the changes mentioned. With higher doses, late changes such as fibrosis, ulceration, stricture and obstruction will follow.

XVIII. LARGE INTESTINES

The large intestines are often in the field, to a lesser or greater extent, in the treatment of carcinoma of the cervix, uterus, bladder and prostate. The early reactions are diarrhea and tenesmus. If radiation is continued, diarrhea will be worse and may be bloody. A few days of rest from treatment will usually remedy the problem. The late reactions are fibrosis and bowel irritations, rectal bleeding or obstruction. These are usually rare with good treatment planning.

XIX. LIVER

The liver is a moderately radiosensitive organ. The larger the area treated the lower the dose needed to cause radiation hepatitis and liver failure. Doses greater than 2500 cGy to the whole liver will produce radiation hepatitis.

XX. KIDNEYS

A dose over 2300 cGy to either whole kidney will cause radiation nephritis with proteinuria and hypertension. If only one kidney is affected it may be removed to prevent hypertension. If only half or a third of a kidney is in the field, the tolerance dose is higher.

XXI. BLADDER

The bladder is not radiosensitive and hence can tolerate high doses of radiation. A total dose of greater than 7000 cGy in 6-7 weeks will cause acute cystitis. Increase bladder irritability causes a slight reduction in bladder capacity that leads to frequency. Not unlike any other organ, much higher doses will cause fibrosis and a contracted bladder.

XXII. TESTIS

Due to the very active regeneration of sperms, the testis are very sensitive to radiation. Very small dose of radiation (200 cGy) will depress sperm production but more importantly, genetic mutations will take place. Therefore great care must be exercised at all time to shield the testis when organs in the vicinity are treated. Dose of around 500 cGy will cause permanent sterility.

XXIII. OVARY

The same principles apply to the ovary as to the testis.

XXIV. BONE MARROW AND CIRCULATING BLOOD CELLS

In children, the bone marrow are mostly situated in the long bones. In adults they are mostly in the vertebrae and pelvic bones. In the treatment of Hodgkin's disease, the blood count will drop due to the large area of bone treated in the mantle and inverted Y field. This is due to damage of the stem cells and other inmatured blood cells such as erythroblasts, myelocytes and megakaryocytes.

A short rest from treatment is usually sufficient to bring about recovery of the blood cells. In circulating blood cells, only the lymphocytes are radiosensitive. The rest of the matured blood cells are radioresistant.

XXV. PUBLICATIONS OF INTERESTS

1.   Andrews JR: The radiobiology of human cancer radiotherapy. Philidelphia, W B Saunders, 1968.

2.   Brown JM, Berry J: Effects of X-irradiation on cell population kinetics in a model tumour and normal tissue system: Implications for treatment of human malignancies. Br J Radiol 42:372,1969.

3.   Emami B, Lyman J, Brown A, et al: Tolerance of normal tissue to therapeutic irradiation. Int J Radiat Oncol Biol Phys 21:109-122, 1991.

4.   Fowler JF: Current aspects of radiobiology as applied to radiotherapy. Clin Radiol 23: 257,1972.

5.   Frija J, Ferme C, Baud L, et al: Radiation-induced lung injuries: A survey by computed tomography and pulmonary function tests in 18 cases of Hodgkin's disease. Eur J Radiol 8:18-23, 1988.

6.   Gilbert CW, Lajitha LG: The importance of cell population kinetics in determining response to irradiation of normal and malignant tissues. In Cellular Radiation Biology. Baltimore, Williams and Wilkins, 1965.

7.   Gogna NK, Morgan G, Downs K, et al: Lung dose rate and interstitial pneumonitis in total body irradiation for bone marrow transplantation. Aust Radiol 36:317-320, 1992.

8.   Goldstein HM, Rogers LF, Fletcher GH, Dodd GD: Radiological manifestations of radiation-induced injury to the normal upper gastrointestinal tract. Radiology 117:135-140, 1975.

9.   Hopewell JW: Mechanisms of action of radiation on skin and underlying tissues. Br J Radiol 19(suppl):39-47, 1986.

10.   Jirtle RL, Anscher MS, Alati T: Radiation sensitivity of the liver. Adv Radiat Biol 14:269-311, 1990.

11.   Lawrence TS, Ten Haken RK, Kessler ML, et al: The use of 3D dose volume analysis to predict radiation hepatitis. Int J Radiat Oncol Biol Phys 23:781-788, 1992.

12.   Leibel SA, Sheline GE: Tolerance of the brain and spinal cord to conventional irradiation. In Gutin PH, Leibel SA, Sheline GE, eds: Radiation Injury to the Nervous System, pp 239-256. New York, Raven, 1991.

13.   Lepke RA, Libshitz HI: Radiation-induced injury of the esophagus. Radiology 148:375-378, 1983.

14.   Mah K, Van Dyk J, Keane TJ, Poon PY: Acute radiation-induced pulmonary damage: A clinical study on the response of fractionated radiation therapy. Int J Radiat Oncol Biol Phys 13:736-743, 1986.

15.   Marcus RB, Million RR: The incidence of myelitis after irradiation of the cervical spinal cord. Int J Radiat Oncol Biol Phys 19:3-8, 1990.

16.   McDonald S, Rubin P, Phillips TL, Marks LB: Injury to the lung from cancer therapy: Clinical syndromes, measurable endpoints, and potential scoring systems. Int J Radiat Oncol Biol Phys 31:1187-1203, 1995.

17.   Morgan GM, Freeman AP, McLean RG, et al: Late cardiac, thyroid, and pulmonary sequelae of mantle radiotherapy for Hodgkin's disease. Int J Radiat Oncol Biol Phys 11:1925-1931, 1985.

18.   Nimierko A, Goitein M: Modeling of normal tissue response to radiation: The critical volume model. Int J Radiat Oncol Biol Phys 25:135-145, 1993.

19.   Orton CG, Cohen L: A unified approach to dose-effect relationships in radiotherapy. I. Modified TDF and linear quadratic equations. Int J Radiat Oncol Biol Phys 14:549-556, 1988.

20.   Rotstein S, Lax I, Svane G: Influence of radiation therapy on lung-tissue in breast cancer patients: CT assessed density changes and associated symptoms. Int J Radiat Oncol Biol Phys 18:173-180, 1990.

21.   Rubin R, Casaret GW: Clinical Radiation Pathology, Vol I, Philidelphia, W B Saunders, 1968.

22.   Rubin P: Radiation toxicology: Quantitative radiation pathology for predicting effects. Cancer 39(suppl):21:729-736, 1977.

23.   Safdari H, Fuentes JM, Dubois JB, et al: Radiation necrosis of the brain: Time of onset and incidence related to total dose and fractionation of radiation. Neuroradiology 27:44-47, 1985.

24. Schultheiss TE: Spinal cord radiation "tolerance": Doctrine vs. data. Int J Radiat Oncol Biol Phys 19:219-221, 1990.

25. Schultheiss TE, Kun LE, Ang KK, Stephens LC: Radiation response of the central nervous system. Int J Radiat Oncol Biol Phys 31:1093-1112, 1995.

26. Stewart JR, Fajardo LF, Gillette SM, Constine LC: Radiation injury to the heart. Int J Radiat Oncol Biol Phys 31:1205-1211, 1995.

27. Travis EL: Primer of Medical Radiobiology. Year Book Medical Publishers, Inc, Chicago, 1979.

—— CHAPTER 45 ——

Total Body Irradiation (TBI)

I. INTRODUCTION

Total body irradiation may be given using either a linear accelerator or a modified ^{60}Co unit. TBI is a treatment choice for patients with non-Hodgkin's lymphoma, hairy cell leukemia, multiple myeloma, metastasis, mycosis fungoides, chronic phase of granulocytic leukemia or acute lympho-cytic leukemia. The total tumor dose and treatment technique varies with each of the diseases and treatment centers. For this chapter, TBI and bone marrow transplantation *(BMT)* will be discussed for acute lymphocytic leukemia. The fractionated dose is 1000 cGy in 5 fractions given once a day.

II. CLINICAL

Bone marrow transplantation and total body irradiation are performed on patients with acute lymphocytic leukemia *(ALL)* only if, (i) goes into remission from high dose chemotherapy, (ii) matching donor marrow could be obtained *(or marrow from self when in remission)*, and (iii) full understanding and consent of the patient. TBI is given to further eradicate the malignant cells and to suppress hose immune reactivity. BMT is performed to replace the host's marrow.

Before BMT is performed, high dose chemotherapy is given to the patient to eradicate the malignant cells and to suppress host immune reactivity enough to prevent rejection of allogenic marrow transplantation. The bone marrow for BMT could come from autologous marrow *(self marrow)* if the patient is in remission, syngeneic marrow *(marrow from identical twins)* or allo-gencic marrow *(marrow from different genetic origin)*.

For autologous marrow transplantation, 500-800 ml of the patient's marrow is harvested from the sternum and iliac crests before TBI. The marrow is screened to remove fat and bone particles and is stored for later infusion into the patient after TBI.

For syngeneic marrow transplantation and allogeneic marrow transplantation, 500-800 ml of the donor's marrow is harvested while the patient is undergoing TBI. The marrow is screened and is infused into the patient after TBI. With allogeneic marrow transplantation, complications such as graft verses host disease*(GVHD)*, interstitial pneumonitis and infections often develop. GVHD is due to donor T lymphocytes reaction against host tissues especially the skin, liver and gut. GVHD can be treated with cyclosporin and methotrexate enough to control its severity but not to prevent it because GVHD also has antileukemic effect.

III. PHYSICS

If a modified ^{60}Co unit is used for TBI, the adjustable secondary collimator assembly is removed to provide a field 2 meters in diameter at 150 cm source to mid patient distance. A specially constructed copper flattening filter is placed in the path of the radiation beam to improve beam uniformity and to remove electron contamination. Without the filter, the dose at the peripheral will be lower than near the central axis due to oblique filtration through the source capsule, lower scatter contribution at the beam edge and oblique incidence in the phantom. The filter provides a uniform flat 80% isodose line encompassing 180 cm in diameter in a phantom. Output calibration is measured for the above set up at 150 cm source mid patient distance and large field TAR is also measured in a large water phantom.

IV. TREATMENT SET-UP

The patient lies supine with arms by side in a specially constructed box measuring 65 cm × 200 cm × 28 cm deep. The head is turned to the left. The mid length and width of the patient is lined up with the central axis of the beam. TLD are placed on the lateral neck, lateral abdomen and lateral pelvis. Bolus bags are then placed on and around the patient to achieve a uniform flat surface. The separation of the patient *(with the bolus)* is taken and a treatment distance of 150 cm source mid patient is set. The same set up is repeated for the posterior field with the patient in a prone position. The patient's head should remain turned to the left in order to treat the left side of the head.

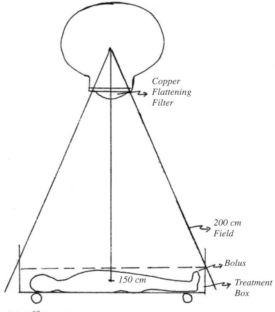

Figure 45.1 Set-up for TBI on the modified ^{60}Co unit.

V. PUBLICATIONS OF INTERESTS

1.   Bekkum van DW, Lowenberg B: Bone marrow transplantation: Biological mechanisms and clinical practice. Dekker, New York,1985.

2.   Breneman JC, Elson HR, Little R, et al: A technique for delivery of total body irradiation for bone marrow transplantation in adults and adolescents. Int J Radiat Oncol Biol Phys 18:1233, 1990.

3.   Briot E, Dutreix A, Bridier A: Dosimetry for total body irradiation. Radiother Oncol 18(suppl 1):16, 1990.

4.   Broerse JJ, Dutreix A: Physical aspects of total body irradiation. Proc meeting at Leiden, J Eur Radiother 3:157-264,1982.

5.   Chaffey JT, Rosenthal DS, Moloney WC, et al: Total body irradiation as treatment for lymphosarcoma. Int J Radiat Oncol Biol Phys 1:399, 1976.

6.   Chou RH, Wong GB, Kramer JH, et al: Toxicities of total body irradiation for pediatric bone marrow transplantation. Int J Radiat Oncol Biol Phys 34:843, 1996.

7.   Deeg HJ, Flournoy N, Sullivan KM, Sheehan K, Buckner CD, Sanders JE, Storb R, Witherspoon RP, Thomas ED: Cataracts after total body irradiation and marrow transplantation: A sparing effect of dose fractionation. Int J Radiat Oncol Biol Phys 10:957-964,1984.

8.   Dominique C, Schwartz LH, Lescrainier J, et al: A modified **60Co teletherapy unit for total body irradiation. Int J Radiat Oncol Biol Phys 33:951, 1995.

9.   Dutreix A, Bridier A: Total body irradiation: Techniques and dosimetry. Pathol Biol 27:373-378,1979.

10.   Galvin JM: Calculation and prescription of dose for total body irradiation. Int J Radiat Oncol Biol Phys 9:1919, 1983.

11.   Galvin JM: Physics considerations for total body irradiation. In Purdy JA, ed: Advances in Radiation Oncology Physics: Dosimetry, Treatment Planning, and Brachytherapy. New York, American Institute of Physicists, 1992.

12.   Grinsky T, Socie G, Ammarguellat H, et al: Consequences of two different doses to the lungs during a single dose of total body irradiation: Results of a randomized study on 85 patients. Int J Radiat Oncol Biol Phys 30:821, 1994.

13.   Hoogenhout J, Brouwer WF, van Gasteren JJ, et al: Clinical and physical aspects of total body irradiation for bone marrow transplantation in Ni Jmegen. Radiother Oncol 18(suppl 1):118, 1990.

14.   Hussein S, el-Khatib E: Total body irradiation with a sweeping **60Cobalt beam. Int J Radiat Oncol Biol Phys 33:493, 1995.

15.   Johnson RE: Treatment of chronic lymphocytic leukemia by total body irradiation alone and combined with chemotherapy. Int J Radiat Oncol Biol Phys 5:159, 1979.

16.   Kim TH, Khan FM, Galvin JM: A report of work party: Comparisson of total body irradiation techniques for bone marrow transplantation. Int J Radiat Oncol Biol Phys 6:779,1980.

17.   Kirby TH, Hanson WF, Cates DA: Verification of total photon irradiation dosimetry techniques. Med Phys 15:364, 1988.

18.   Lam W-C, Order SE, Thomas ED: Uniformity and standardization of single and opposing cobalt 60 sources for total body irradiation. Int J Radiat Oncol Biol Phys 6:245, 1980

19.   Leer JWH, Broers JJ, De Vroome H, et al: Techniques applied for total body irradiation. Radiother Oncol 18(suppl 1):10, 1990.

20.   Miralbell R, Bieri S, Mermillod B, et al: Renal toxicity after allogeneic bone marrow transplantation: The combined effect of total-body irradiation and graft-versus-host disease. J Clin Oncol 14:579, 1996.

21.   Miralbell R, Rouzaud M, Grob E, et al: Can a total body irradiation technique be fast and reproducible? Int J Radiat Oncol Biol Phys 29:1167, 1994.

22.   Molls M, Budach V, Bamberg M: Total body irradiation: The lung as critical organ. Strahlentherapie 162:226, 1986.

23.   Niroomand-Rad A: Physical aspects of total body irradiation of bone marrow transplant patients using 18 MV x rays. Int J Radiat Oncol Biol Phys 20:605, 1991.

24.   Obcemea CH, Rice RK, Mijnheer BJ, et al: Three-dimensional dose distribution of total body irradiation by a dual source total body irradiation. Int J Radiat Oncol Biol Phys 24:789, 1992.

25.   Ray SK, Sontag MR: 3-D photon dose comparison of four different TBI techniques. Med Phys 22:1000, 1995.

26.   Rybka WB, Caplan S, Freeman CR, et al: Experience with single dose and fractionated total body irradiation schedules in bone marrow transplantation. Int J Cell Cloning 4:219, 1986.

27.   Savhn-Tapper G, Nilsson P, Jonsson C, et al: Calculation and measurements of absorbed dose in total body irradiation. Acta Oncol 29:627, 1990.

28.   Scarpati D, Mancini G, Corvo R, et al: Tissue-air ratio in total body irradiation: An in vivo evaluation. Acta Oncol 28:283, 1989.

29.   Sverzellati PE, Zonca G, Stucchi C, et al: Treatment technique and clinical dosimetry in whole-body irradiation. Radiol Med 77:530, 1989.

30.   Syh HW, Chu WK, Kumar PP, et al: Radiation oncology: Estimation of the mean effective organ doses for total body irradiation from Rando phantom measurements. Med Dosim 17:103, 1992.

31.   Van Dyk J: Dosimetry for total body irradiation. Radiother Oncol 9:107-118, Elsevier,1987.

32.   Van Dyk J, Galvin JM, Glasgow GP,   et al: The physical aspects of total and   half body photon   irradiation: A   report of   Task Group   29 Radiation   Therapy Committee,   American Association   of Physicists in Medicine. AAPM Report No. 17, June 1986.

Principles and Practice of Clinical Physics and Dosimetry
Michael L.F. Lim, CMD, ACT
Advanced Medical Publishing, Inc., USA

— *CHAPTER 46* —

Hemi-Body Irradiation

I. INTRODUCTION

Hemi-body irradiation may be given to patients with multiple metastasis using a linear accelerator at an extended treatment distance. Hemi-body irradiation could be for the upper half or lower half body depending on where the multiple metastasis are.

II. TREATMENT SET-UP (UPPER HEMI-BODY)

The patient lies supine with arms by the side in a specially constructed box measuring 65 cm × 200 cm × 28 cm deep. An X-Ray film is placed under the patient. The patient's head is turned to the left. The mid half body length and width of the patient is lined up with the central axis of the beam. A field size is set to cover the upper half body from top of head to umbilicus. The field cross hair projection on the patient is drawn on the patient's skin. Lead pellets are placed on the patient's skin in line with the field cross hair projection. A port film is taken on the treatment unit to show the lungs in order for partial lung shielding blocks to be fabricated. The same is repeated for the posterior field with the patient in a prone position. The patient's head is turned to the right.

The outline of the lungs are drawn on the port film. The port film is laid in the same location in the treatment box. The field cross hair is lined up with the lead pellets shown in the port film. A shielding trolley on wheels is placed over the treatment box. The lung outline from the port film is drawn on the shielding tray on the trolley. Lead is fabricated to cover the outline. The lead thickness is calculated to allow for partial transmission.

The shielding trolley is wheeled into position over the patient lining the field cross hair on the trolley with the field cross hair drawn on the patient. The fabricated lung blocks are placed on the lung outline drawn on the trolley. Bolus bags are then placed on and around the patient to achieve a uniform flat surface. The same set up is repeated for the posterior with the patient in a prone position.

The prescribed tumor dose at mid plane is 600 cGy but the lungs would be limited to 500 cGy through the use of partial transmission lung blocks. The patient is treated using 6 MV photons.

III. CALCULATION

A. Partial transmission through lung blocks

The lung thickness is obtained from either a lateral chest X-Ray or from CT.

Field size (to cover both lungs) = 30 × 30 cm^2

TMR (30 × 30 cm^2 at 9 cm mid lung to lung surface) = 0.852 ◆ *TMR (30 × 30 cm^2 at 12 cm mid lung to skin) = 0.789*

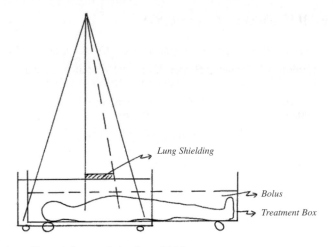

Figure 46.1. Set-up for hemi-body irradiation with partial transmission lung shielding.

Corrected TMR = TMR (12 cm depth) × CF

$$CF = \frac{TMR(9cm)^{0.25-1}}{TMR(12cm)^{1-1}} = \frac{0.852^{0.25-1}}{0.789^{1-1}} = 1.128$$

Therefore, → *Corrected TMR = 0.789 × 1.128 = 0.890*

Dose to mid separation = 300 cGy ♦ *Dose to mid lung = 250 cGy* ♦ *HVL = 1.2486 cm of lead*

Therefore, transmission through lead shielding to deliver 250 cGy to mid lung = 300 × (x)× (0.890/0.789)

Where transmission → *ST = (dose to mid lung/cf)/(dose to mid separation)= (250/1.128)/300 = 0.739*

Transmission → *0.739 = $e^{-\mu x}$, where μ = (0.693/1.2486) = 0.555, x = lead thickness*

Therefore;

$$0.739 = e^{-0.555 \times x} \quad \rightarrow \quad x = \left(\frac{1}{0.555}\right) \times \left(\log\left(\frac{1}{0.739}\right)\right) = 0.545 \ \text{cm of lead}$$

Check:

AP dose to mid depth = 300 cGy

AP dose to mid lung = 300 × 0.739 × (0.890/0.789)= 250 cGy

B. MU calculation

Anterior field

Data: TD = 300 cGy in 1 fraction ♦ *Separation = 26.5 cm & SSD = 194 cm*

Collimator setting = [(100)/(194+13.25)] × (47.7 × 67.4) = 23 × 32.5 cm^2

Output factor(OF) = 1.08 cGy/MU ♦ *PSF_1 (23 × 32.5 cm^2) = 1.045* ♦ *PSF_2 (47.7× 67.4 cm^2) = 1.073*

Field size at mid separation (207.25 cm) = 47.7 × 67.4 cm^2 ♦ *TMR (47.7 × 67.4 cm^2 at 13.25 cm) = 0.805* ♦ *Tray Factor (TF) = 0.970*

$$MU \ setting = \frac{TD}{OF \times IS \times \left(\dfrac{PSF_2}{PSF_1}\right) \times TF \times TMR} = \frac{300}{1.08 \times \left(\dfrac{100}{207.25}\right)^2 \times \dfrac{1.073}{1.045} \times 0.97 \times 0.805} = 1488 \ MU$$

Posterior field

It is same as anterior field.

IV. PUBLICATIONS OF INTERESTS

1. Barrett AJ: Bone marrow transplantation. Cancer Treat Rev 14:203, 1987

2. Cardozo BL, Zoetelief H, van Bekkum DW, et al: Lung damage following bone marrow transplantation. I. The contribution of irradiation. Int J Radiat Oncol Biol Phys 11:907, 1985

3. Curran W, Galvin JM, D'Angio GJ: A simple method for calculation of prescribed dose for total body photon irradiation. Int J Radiat Oncol Biol Phys 17:219, 1989

4. Fitzpatrick PJ, Rider WD: Half body radiotherapy. Int J Radiat Oncol Biol Phys 1:197-207,1976.

5. Fryer C, Fitzpatrick P, Rider W, et al: Radiation pneumonitis: Experience following a large single dose of radiation. Int J Radiat Biol 4:931, 1978

6. Rubin P, Salazar O, Zagars G, et al: Systemic hemibody irradiation for overt and occult metastases. Cancer 55:2210, 1985

7. Salazar OM, Rubin P, Hendrickson FR, et al: Single-dose half-body irradiation for palliation of multiple bone metastases from solid tumors: Final Radiation Therapy Oncology Group report. Cancer 58:29, 1986

8. Tobias JS, Richards JDM, Blackman GM, et al: Hemibody irradiation in multiple myeloma. Radiother Oncol 3:11, 1985

9. Urtasun RC: Hemi-body irradiation technique: A wider use in oncology. Int J Radiat Oncol Biol Phys 9:1585-1586,1983.

10. Van Dyk J, Battisa JJ, Rider WD: Half body radiotherapy: The use of computed tomography to determine the dose to lung. Int J Radiat Oncol Biol Phys 6:463, 1980

11. Van Dyk J, Galvin JM, Glasgow GP, et al: The physical aspects of total and half body photon irradiation: A report of Task Group 29 Radiation Therapy Committee, American Association of Physicists in Medicine. AAPM Report No. 17, June 1986

12. Van Ess J: Single dose half body irradiation for palliation of multiple bone metastases from solid tumours. Cancer: Final Radiation Oncology Group Report 58:29-36,1986.

—— *CHAPTER 47* ——

Brachytherapy

I. INTRODUCTION

Brachytherapy is the treatment of malignant neoplasms with radioactive sources at a very short distance from the neoplasm. These radioactive sources may either be sealed or unsealed. They may be injected, taken by mouth, inserted, implanted or made into a mold worn by the patient. They have the advantage of delivering their radiation very close to the tumor but the dose falls off very rapidly with distance so that the normal tissues receive very low dose.

Brachytherapy may be given using low dose rate sources or high dose rate sources. For low dose rate, treatment is given over days or hours per day. High dose rate treatment is given over minutes in a few fractions.

Examples of brachytherapy are: 1) I-131 in the treatment of thyroid cancer, 2) Cs 137 in the treatment of gynecological cancer, 3) Au-198 seeds in the treatment of prostate cancer; and 4) Ir-192 in the treatment of breast cancer and gynecological cancers. The choice of the radionuclides is dependent on its physical characteristics.

II. PHYSICAL CHARACTERISTICS OF RADIONUCLIDES

The more commonly used radionuclides in brachytherapy and their physical characteristics are provided below in table form.

Table 47.1 Table of physical characteristics of radionuclides used in brachytherapy.

Radio nuclides	Half-life	Exposure rate constant R/cm/mCi/h	Energy (MeV)	Form	Clinical Use
Ra-226	1620y	8.25	0.83	tubes, needles	Gyn
Cs-137	30y	3.28	0.66	tubes, needles	Gyn
Au-198	2.7d	2.38	0.42	seeds	Prostate
Ir-192	74.2d	4.69	0.38	seeds, wires	Breast, Gyn
I-131	8.1d	2.24	0.36	liquid, capsule	Thyroid
I-125	60.3d	1.4	0.03	seeds	Prostate, Eye
P-32	14.3d		1.7	liquid	Bone
Sr-90	29y			plaque	Pterygium

III. HAL-LIFE

It is the time taken to reduce the activity of the radionuclide to half its original activity through decay. For example, a 8000 Curie Cobalt-60 source will decay to 4000 Curie in 5.26 years which is its half life.

The activity of a radionuclide at any time may be calculated using the exponential decay formula.

Example:

A Cobalt-60 source was replaced on the 1st Jan.1984. Its activity was 8000 Curie. Calculate the activity on the 1st July 1986.

Between 1st Jan 1984 and 1st July 1986, there are 30 months. The half-life of Cobalt-60 is 5.26 years. Therefore, the activity on the 1st July 1986. Therefore;

$$A = A_0 e^{-\lambda t} = 8000 \times e^{-\left(\frac{0.693 \times 30}{5.261 \times 12}\right)} = 5755 \ Ci$$

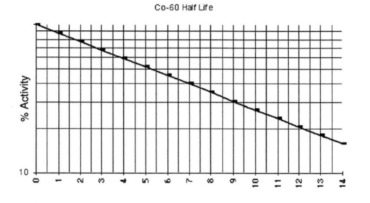

Figure 47.1 Graph of half-life for Cobalt-60.

IV. EXPOSURE RATE CONSTANT

Exposure rate constant is a measure of the intensity of a radionuclide. The unit of measurement is R/cm/mCi/h. This applies if the source is a point source and there is no attenuation of the source by the casing. The measured value is less than the calculated value due to attenuation by the source casing and the source is never a point source. Given the exposure rate constant, the source activity and the distance from source, the exposure rate at some distance may be calculated.

Example:

Calculate the exposure rate in R/min at 80cm from a 8000 Curie source with an exposure rate constant of 12.9 R/cm/mCi/h.

Exposure rate = Exposure rate constant × activity × distance²

$$Exposure \ rate = 12.9 \times 8000 \times 1000 \times \left(\frac{1}{60}\right) \times \left(\frac{1}{80}\right)^2 = 268.8R \ / \ min$$

Note: (i) Since the exposure rate is in mCi, the 8000 Curie is converted to mCi by multiplying by 1000. (ii) Hour is converted to minutes by division of 60.

V. "ALONG AND AWAY" CALCULATION METHOD

As mentioned, if the source is a point source and if there is no attenuation of the source by the source casing, the exposure rate at a distance equals the exposure rate times the activity times the distance square. For linear sources used in brachytherapy, the above does not hold true.

Karen Breitman has calculated "along and away" dose rate*(cGy/hour)* to take into account of the oblique filtration of radiation in the caesium salt and in the casing, and a point in the center of the tube is treated as a point source.

The "along" distance is the distance from the center of a source to a point of interest intersect at right angle. The "away" distance is the distance between the intersection and the point of interest. Referring to Figure 47.2, "along" is from C to I and "away" is from I to A.

Example:

Given below is the source arrangement for three tube sources and two ovoids in the treatment of cancer of the cervix. Calculate the dose rate (cGy/h) at point A. The length of each tube is 2 cm. Point A is 2 cm away from the tube source and 2 cm from the ovoids.

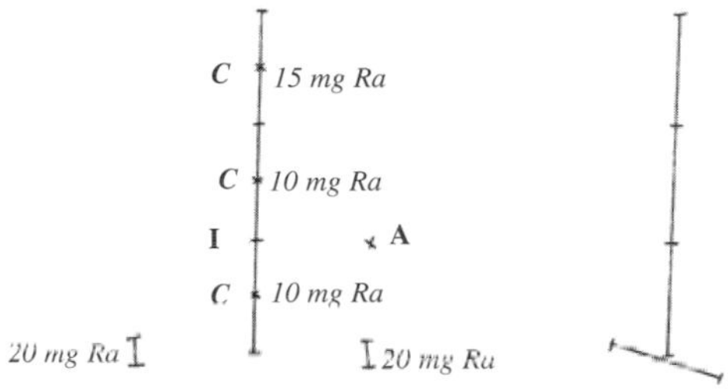

Figure 47.2 Source arrangement in the treatment of cancer of the cervix.

mg Ra Eq.Cs	Along(cm)	Away(cm)	Dose Rate(cGy/h)
15	3	2	0.555 × 15 = 8.3
10	1	2	1.53 × 10 =15.3
10	1	2	1.53×10 = 15.3
20	2	4	0.37× 20 = 7.48
20	2	0	1.58 × 20= 31.6

Therefore dose rate at point A = 77.98 cGy/h.

Table 47.2 "Dose-rate (cGy/hour) for a 137Cs tube of 1 mg-Ra-equivalent, active length: 13.5 mm, total length: 20 mm, filtration: 0.5 mm Pt." From Table I "Dose-rate tables for clinical 137Cs sources sheathed in platinum" by Karen Breitman, BJR 47,657-664,1974.

D(cm)*	Transverse from source center (cm)										
	0	0.5	1	1.5	2	2.5	3	3.5	4	4.5	5
0		21.6	6.91	3.27	1.88	1.21	0.843	0.619	0.472	0.371	0.299
0.5		17.3	6.01	3.01	1.78	1.17	0.821	0.606	0.465	0.366	0.296
1	10.4	7.54	2.06	2.38	1.53	1.05	0.760	0.572	0.444	0.353	0.287
1.5	3.14	2.99	2.43	1.72	1.23	0.896	0.674	0.52	0.411	0.332	0.272
2	1.58	1.5	1.48	1.21	0.947	0.737	0.579	0.462	0.374	0.307	0.255
2.5	0.962	0.905	0.944	0.857	0.724	0.596	0.489	0.402	0.333	0.279	0.235
3	0.648	0.614	0.642	0.619	0.555	0.48	0.408	0.346	0.294	0.25	0.214
3.5	0.467	0..453	0.459	0.46	0.43	0.387	0.34	0.296	0.257	0.223	0.194
4	0.352	0.345	0.343	0.351	0.338	0.314	0.284	0.253	0.224	0.198	0.174

* Distance along source axis

VI. DOSE RECEIVED AT A DISTANCE

Before the era of remote after-loading technique, nursing care was kept to a minimum to reduce radiation exposure to the nurse. It was often educational to calculate the dose received by the nurse while performing nursing duties. An example will be given here.

Example:

A patient has a Fletcher suit insertion for cancer of the cervix with three Cs-137 sources 15,10,10 mg-Radium-equivalent in the uterine tube and one Cs-137 source in each ovoid at 20 mg-Radium equivalent each. If the nurse stands 50 cm from the patient for 5 minutes, what is the dose received by the nurse in mSv? *(Assume the patient absorbs half the radiation.)*

Caluculation:

Exposure rate constant for Cs-137 = 3.28 R/cm² /mCi/h.
Exposure rate constant for Ra-226 = 8.25 R/cm²/mCi/h
Total mg-Radium equivalent = 75 mg
Converting to mCi Cs-137 = (8.25/3.28) × 75 = 188.6 mCi
Exposure rate = exposure rate constant × activity × distance²
Exposure rate = 3.28 × 188.6 × (1/50)² = 0.247 R/h
For 5 mins, the exposure = 0.247 × (5/60)² = 0.021 R
1R = (10 mSv) × (f-factor)
Therefore the nurse receives = (0.021 × 10 × 0.963)/2 = 0.10 mSv.

VII. BRACHYTHERAPY FOR CANCER OF THE CERVIX AND OTHER GYNECOLOGICAL MALIGNANCIES

A. Cancer of the Cervix

Carcinoma of the cervix in the early stage is commonly treated by surgery. For later stages, radiation therapy is often one of the treatment modalities. Radiation therapy is a combination of external beam therapy using a four field box technique and intracavitary therapy using Ra-226 or Cs-137 tubes and ovoids *(Manchester and Fletcher system)* or Cs-137 pellets *(computerized remote after loading system.)*

i. Manchester System

The Manchester system uses a rubber uterine tandem to hold three Ra-226 tubes. The tandem is inserted into the uterus. On each side of the vaginal fornices are placed the ovoids which are separated by a rubber spacer. This system has many disadvantages. The uterine tandem is flexible and as a result, it is sometimes antiverted after insertion causing the dosimetry to deviate from the normal. The sources are inserted before planning is done to determine the best source arrangement. Brachytherapy technologist, operating room nurses, ward nurses and radiation oncologist are all exposed to radiation. Nursing care is kept to a minimum to avoid exposure to radiation.

ii. Fletcher System

The Fletcher after loading system is an improvement over the Manchester system in that the applicators are inserted first in the operating room without the live sources. Orthogonal X-Ray films are taken for planning which determines the source strength and position to achieve a desired plan. The sources are loaded as planned. This system is an improvement over the Manchester system in that the applicators are rigid and placement of the applicators in the desired position is achievable. Planning is done before source insertion resulting in an optimum plan for the insertion. Since the sources are inserted into the applicators in the ward, only the radiation oncologist and the technologist preparing the sources are exposed to some radiation. Radiation exposure here is less than the Manchester system. However, nursing care is still kept to a minimum to avoid exposure to radiation.

iii. Remote After Loading System

The latest system in intracavitary therapy is the computerized remote after loading system. Applicators are inserted in the operating room and a train of dummy sources (stainless steel spheres) are inserted into the applicators. Orthogonal X-Ray films are taken for planning of source positions to achieve the desired plan.

This remote after loading system uses Cs-137 pellets measuring 2.5 mm in diameter. The spaces are 2.5 mm steel pellets to space the Cs-137 pellets to their planned positions. The positions of the Cs-137 pellets and treatment time are programmed according to plan.

The unit then loads the appropriate treatment channels and store the pellets in a secondary safe. The treatment channels are connected to the applicator in the patient. The staff leaves the room and treatment is commenced with a push of the start button. The pellets travel from the secondary safe into the applicators and the planned time counts down. During nursing care and visitation, the treatment may be interrupted by pushing the stop button. The pellets travel from the applicators back to the secondary safe. When treatment is finished, the pellets return to the secondary safe automatically. In case of power failure or machine failure, the pellets return to the secondary safe automatically.

There are numerous advantages with this system. The applicators are rigid and planning is done before source insertion to achieve the best source positions for a desired plan. the use of small pellets provide more versatility to source positioning and different treatment time may be programmed for each treatment channel. Since it is computerized remote after loading, normal nursing care may be provided.

There are some disadvantages compared to the two previous systems. The first is the cost of the unit. The second is treatment is interrupted for nursing care and visitation and therefore treatment is prolonged. Danger of error in the programming of the active pellet positions and treatment time is ever present.

Dose prescription for brachytherapy in the treatment of cancer of the cervix is still largely to point A that is located 2 cm superior to the cervical os and 2 cm lateral to it. Point A is the location where the uterine artery crosses the ureter. Point B is located 3 cm lateral from point A and is of interest because it is where the pelvic nodes are located. Due to the differences in the position and size of tumor in patients, point A should not be the only point of interest in dose prescription. The overall dose distribution should be considered and the tolerance dose of the bladder and rectum should also be borne in mind.

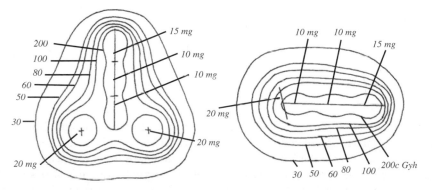

Figure 47.3 Dose distribution of a normal Manchester Radium insertion for cancer of the cervix.

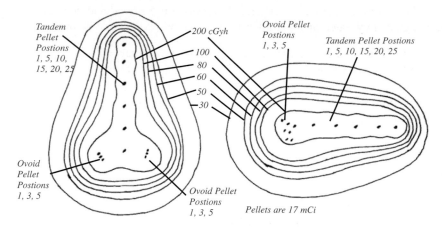

Figure 47.4 Dose distribution of a normal remote afterloading insertion for cancer of the cervix.

B. Cancer of the Vagina

Cancer of the vagina may be treated by brachytherapy. A plastic vagina applicator is inserted into the vagina and held in place during the duration of the treatment. Standard dose distribution for various sizes of vaginal applicator are prepared beforehand. The treatment channel is connected to the applicator and the appropriate plan is used to program the active pellet positions and treatment time.

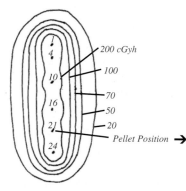

Figure 47.5 Dose distribution of a 2.25 × 7 cm² vaginal applicator.

VIII. MOLD AND IMPLANT

Before the era of computers to generate dose distribution for mold and implant, Paterson and Parker formulated tables and rules of source placements to achieve uniform dose distribution. Even though computers are now used to plan mold and implant brachytherapy, the tables and rules are still widely used.

A. Single Planar Mold

A wax mold is fabricated to fit over the area to be treated. Radium sources are then placed in the wax mold to a pre-determined source distribution. The mold is worn by the patient over the calculated time per day until the desired dose is delivered.

i. Single Ring Mold

Ring mold is used to treat small superficial skin lesion on the head and neck area. The source arrangement is guided by Paterson and Parker rules as shown in the table below.

Table 47.3 Table of distribution rules for surface applicator mold (Paterson and Parker.)
From "The Physics of Radiology" fourth edition by Johns and Cunningham. (Charles C Thomas Publisher)

% of Radium

Diameter/height	less 3	3 to 6	6 to 7.5	7.5 to 10	10
Outer circle	100	95	80	75	70
Inner circle			17	22	27
Center spot		5	3	3	3

Table 47.4 Table of mgh per 1000 cGy at various distances filtered by 0.5 mm Pt. Filtration = 2% per 0.1 mm greater or lesser than 0.5 mm Pt. (Modified from Meredith and Massey by (8.4/8.25)¥(1/0.963) = 1.057.

Treatment Distance

Area	0.5	1	1.5	2	2.5	Area	0.5	1	1.5	2	2.5
0	32	126	283	503	787	42	660	1018	1462	1881	2330
2	102	226	397	628	914	44	681	1047	1501	1930	2384
4	149	294	489	738	1026	46	703	1075	1538	1978	2437
6	187	352	566	827	1127	48	724	1103	1575	2025	2489
8	218	406	633	904	1221	50	746	1132	1601	2072	2540
10	248	458	693	976	1306	52	767	1161	1643	2119	2590
12	276	508	750	1046	1387	54	787	1190	1677	2166	2642
14	304	554	808	1113	1466	56	806	1218	1711	2212	2694
16	333	598	861	1177	1543	58	826	1247	1745	2259	2746
18	362	640	912	1237	1612	60	846	1275	1778	2305	2798
20	390	678	962	1295	1680	62	865	1303	1809	2348	2846
22	415	713	1015	1354	1744	64	884	1331	1840	2391	2893
24	441	747	1065	1411	1810	66	903	1359	1871	2434	2942
26	467	779	1115	1468	1869	68	922	1388	1902	2475	2991
28	493	811	1163	1521	1931	70	941	1417	1932	2516	3040
30	518	841	1207	1572	1988	72	961	1445	1963	2555	3088
32	543	871	1253	1625	2047	74	980	1474	1994	2594	3137
34	567	903	1297	1678	2106	76	999	1052	2024	2633	3185
36	590	929	1341	1732	2165	78	1018	1259	2051	2671	3233
38	614	961	1383	1782	2220	80	1037	1557	2079	2709	3281
40	638	988	1423	1832	2276						

Example:

A flat mold is prepared to treat a circular area 5 cm in diameter and a total dose of 6000 cGy over 8 days. The mold is to be worn for about 10 hours daily. Calculate the total activity of radium required and the source distribution.

Sources Available;

Activity (mg)	Physical length	Active length	Filtration mm Pt
1.5	7.5	5	0.5
2.5	12.5	10	0.5
3	7.5	5	0.5
5	10	10	0.5

Calculation:

$\pi r^2 = 3.142 \times 2.5^2 = 19.6\ cm^2$
mgh per 1000 cGy = 670 mgh (Table 47.4)
Therefore for 6000 cGy = 6 × 670 = 4020 mgh
Total time to be left on = 80 hours
Therefore mg required = 4020/80 = 50.25 mg
Diameter/height = 5/1 = 5

Therefore 95% of source strength to go to the outer circle and 5% to go to the center spot. Therefore 47.7 mg goes to the outer circle and 2.51 mg goes to the center spot. Using the available sources, the outer circle = 16 × 3 mg and the center spot = 1 × 2.5 mg.

Physical length for 3mg source = 0.75 cm
The outer circle circumference = 2πr = 2 × 3.142 × 2.5 = 15.7 cm

Therefore 16 of the 3 mg source gives 16 × 0.75 = 12 cm and will fit evenly on the circumference.

Total Radium (Ra) = 50.5 mg
mgh was 4020, therefore total hour to be left on = 4020/50.5 = 79.6 h
Therefore the mold is to be left on daily for 9.95 h

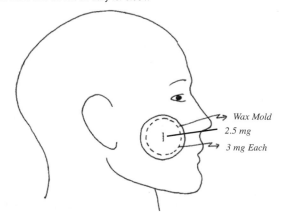

Figure 47.6 Source arrangement on mold.

ii. Double Ring Mold

For larger lesion, a double ring mold is desirable to achieve uniform dose.

Example:

A flat mold is used to treat a circular area 8 cm in diameter at 1.0 cm treatment distance to deliver 6000 cGy over a period of 8 days. The mold is to be worn for about 10 hours daily. Calculate the total activity of the Radium required and their arrangement.

Calculation:

$\pi r^2 = 3.142 \times 4^2 = 50.272\ cm^2$
mgh per 1000 cGy = 1172mg (Table 47.4)
Therefore for 6000 cGy = 6 × 1172 = 7032 mgh
Total time required to be left on = 80 hours
Therefore mg required = 7032/80 = 87.9 mg
Diameter/height = 8/1 = 8

Therefore the outer circle holds 75% of the source and the inner circle holds 22% of the source and the center spot holds 3% of the source.

75% of 87.9 = 65.93 mg, 22% of 87.9 = 19.33 mg, and 3% of 87.9 = 2.64 mg
The outer circle circumference – 2πr = 2 × 3.142 × 4 = 25.1 cm
The inner circle circumference = 2πr = 2 × 3.142 × 2 = 12.6 cm

To achieve an even coverage of the outer circle circumference, 22 × 3 mg are needed. This gives a total circumference of 22 × 0.75 = 16.5 cm. To achieve an even coverage of the inner circle circumference, 8 × 2.5 mg are needed. This gives us a circumference of 8 × 1.25 = 10 cm. The center spot will hold 1 source of 2.5 mg. Total Radium = (1 × 2.5) + (8 × 2.5) + (22 × 3) = 88.5 mg.

The mgh is 7032, therefore total hour to be left on = 7032/88.5 = 79.46 h
Therefore, the mold is to be left on daily for 9.93 h

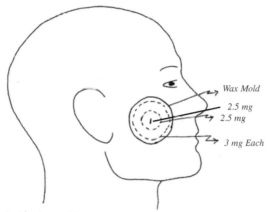

Wax Mold
2.5 mg
2.5 mg
3 mg Each

Figure 47.7 Source arrangement on double ring mold.

iii. Rectangular Mold

For even larger treatment area and depth, a rectangular mold is the choice.

Example:

A chest wall lesion measuring approximately 12 × 6 cm^2 is to be treated to 5000 cGy in 50 hours over 8 days at 1.5 cm. Calculate the total activity of the Radium required and their arrangement.

1) Distribution Rules

Short side < 2 × h *(All radium on periphery.)* Short side > 2 × h *(Add extra Radium parallel to long side and space 2 × h. The extra Radium is 1/2 activity if one bar is used and 2/3 activity if more than one bar is used.), where* h = treatment distance. *From "The Physics of Radiology" fourth edition by Johns and Cunningham. (Charles C Thomas Publisher)*

2) Elongation Correction Factor

From *"The Physics of Radiology"* fourth edition by Johns and Cunningham. *(Charles C Thomas Publisher)*

Ratio of sides of rectangle	1.5:1	2:1	3:1	4:1
Multiply mgh per 1000cGy by	*1.025*	*1.05*	*1.09*	*1.12*

Calculation:

Area = 12 × 6 = 72 cm² & h = 1.5 cm
mgh per 1000 cGy = 1963 mgh (Table 47.4)

Allowing for elongation factor = 1.05 × 1963 = 2061 mgh.
Therefore for 5000 cGy = 5 × 2061 = 10305 mgh.
Over 50 hours, mg-Radium-equivalent required = 10305/50 = 206 mg-Radium-equivalent.

From distance rules, the central bar is 1/2 the activity of the periphery. Total mg-Radium = 206 mg. Therefore, periphery = 137.3 mg and central bar = 68.7 mg. Using 5 mg sources, the periphery needs 28 sources and the central bar needs 12 sources to fit all the sources into the $12 \times 6 \text{ cm}^2$ treatment mold.

Total Radium = 200 mg.
Therefore the mold is to be worn 10305/200 = 51.5 hours over 8 days (or 6.44 hours a day.)

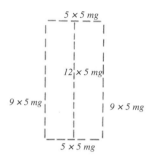

Figure 47.8. Source arrangement for rectangular mold.

B. Single Plane Implant

For deeper tumors, interstitial implant is the treatment choice to deliver the radiation right at the tumor.

1) Distribution Rules

Area	under 25 cm^2	25-100 cm^2	>100cm^2
Peripheral fraction	*2/3*	*1/2*	*1/3*

The parallel needles should not be more than 1 cm apart nor should their active ends be more than 1 cm from the needles at right angles to them which are usually called the 'crossing' needles. The value of the area used to find the approximate mgh per 1000 cGy is that geometric area be less that 10% in the case of one 'uncrossed' end, and less than 20% in the case of both ends 'uncrossed.'

2) Radium Needles in Stock

Mg	Physical length (cm)	Active length (cm)	Filtration (mm Pt)
0.5	*2.5*	*1.5*	*0.6*
1	*4.2*	*3*	*0.6*
1.5	*5.8*	*4.5*	*0.65*
1	*2.5*	*1.5*	*0.6*
2	*4.2*	*3*	*0.6*
3	*5.8*	*4.5*	*0.65*

Filtration correction = 2% per 0.1 mm greater than 0.5 mm Pt.

i. Single Crossed End

Example 1:

An area measuring 5 × 4 cm² is to be treated to 6000 cGy in 160 hours to a treatment distance of 0.5 cm. Calculate the mg-Radium required and their arrangement.

Calculation:

Area to be treated = 5 × 4 cm², Desired dose = 6000 cGy in 160 hours, and the Area = 20 cm² less 10% for one uncrossed end.
Therefore, area = 18 cm² at 0.5 cm treatment distance.
From table 47.4, mgh required per 1000 cGy for 18 cm square at 0.5 cm = 362 mgh.
For 6000 cGy = 6 × 362 = 2172 mgh.
Leaving implant in for 160 hours, mg-Radium required = 2172/160 = 13.6 mg-Radium.
* Area is less than 25 cm square, therefore periphery gets 2/3 and middle gets 1/3 of the 13.6 mg-Radium. Therefore periphery gets 9.1 mg (3 × 3 mg) and the middle gets 4.5 mg (3 × 1.5 mg)*
Corrected for filtration of 3%, the total Radium used = (3 × 3 × 0.97) + (3 × 1.5 × 0.97) = 13.1 mg-Radium.
Therefore total time to leave implant in = 2172/13.1 = 165.8 h

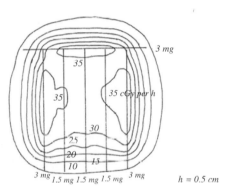

Figure 47.9 Source arrangement and dose distribution for one crossed end implant.

Example 2:

An area measuring 6 x 6 cm² is to be treated to 6000 cGy in 182 hours to a treatment distance off 0.5 cm. Calculate the mg-Radium required and their arrangement.

Calculation:

Area to be treated = 6 × 6 cm²
Desired dose = 6000 cGy in 182 hours.
Area = 36 cm² less 10% for one uncrossed end.
Therefore, area = 32.4 cm² at 0.5 cm treatment distance.
From Table 47.4, mgh required per 1000 cGy for 32.4 cm at 0.5 cm = 548 mgh.
Therefore for 6000 cGy = 6 × 548 =3288 mgh.
Leaving implant in for 182 hours, mg-Radium required = 3288/182 = 18.1 mg.
* Area is greater than 25 cm², therefore periphery gets 1/2 and the middle gets 1/2 of the 18.1 mg-Radium. Therefore the periphery and middle gets 9 mg radium each. Corrected for filtration of 3% for the 3 mg-Radium needles and the 1.5 mg-Radium needles and 2% for the 2 mg needles, total Radium used = (3 × 3 × 0.97) + (2 × 1.5 × 0.97) + (3 × 2 × 0.98) = 17.52 mg.*
* Therefore total time to leave implant in = 3288/17.52 = 187.7 h.*

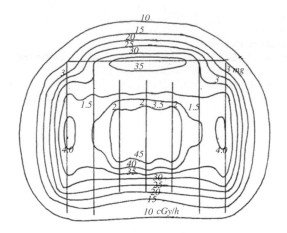

Figure 47.10 Source arrangement and dose distribution for one crossed end implant.

ii. Double Crossed Ends

Example 1:

An area 5 × 4 cm² is to be treated to a total dose of 6000 cGy in 130 hours to a treatment distance of 0.5 cm. Calculate the mg-Radium required and their arrangement. Area to be treated = 5 × 4 cm². Desired dose = 6000 cGy in 130 hours.

Solution:

Area = 20 cm² at 0.5 cm treatment distance.
From table 47.4, mgh required per 1000 cGy = 390 mgh, threfore for 6000 cGy = 6 × 390 = 2340 mgh.
Leaving implant in for 130 hours, mg-Radium required = 2340/130 =18 mg.
    Area is less than 25 cm² , therefore periphery gets 2/3 and the middle gets 1/3 of the 18 mg-Radium. Therefore periphery gets 12 mg and the middle gets 6mg. Corrected for filtration of 2% for the 1 and 2 mg needles and 3% for the 3 mg needles, the total Radium needles = (2 × 2 × 0.98) + (2 × 1 × 0.98) + (4 × 3 × 0.97) = 17.5 mg.
Therefore total time to leave implant in = 2340/17.5 = 133.7 h.

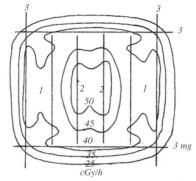

Figure 47.11 Source arrangement and dose distribution for two crossed end implant.

Example 2:

An area 6 × 6 cm² is to be treated to a total dose of 6000 cGy in 130 hours to a treatment distance of 0.5 cm. Calculate the mg-Radium required and their arrangement.

Solution:

Area to be treated = 6 × 6 cm².

Desired dose = 6000 cGy in 130 hours.

Area = 36 cm² at 0.5 cm treatment distance.

From Table 47.4, mgh required per 1000 cGy = 590 mgh. Therefore for 6000 cGy = 6 × 590 = 3540 mgh.

Leaving implant in for 130 hours, mg-Radium required = 3540/130 = 27.2 mg.

Area is greater than 25cm², therefore periphery and middle get 1/2 each of the 27.2 mg-Radium. Therefore each gets 13.6 mg - Radium. Corrected for filtration of 3% for the 3 mg needles, the total Radium used = (9 × 3 × 0.97) = 26.19 mg.

Therefore total time to leave implant in = 3540/26.19 = 135.2 h

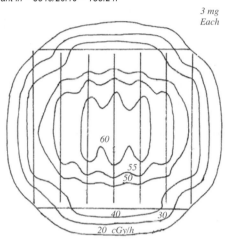

Figure 47.12 Source arrangement and dose distribution for two crossed end implant.

iii. Double Crossed Ends

An area 5 × 4 cm² is to be treated to a total dose of 6000 cGy in 222 hours to a treatment distance of 0.5 cm. Calculate the mg-Radium required and their arrangement. Area to be treated = 5 × 4 cm². Desired dose = 6000 cGy in 222 hours.

Solution:

Area = 20 cm² less 20% for two uncrossed ends.

Therefore area = 16 cm² at 0.5 cm treatment distance.

From table 25.4, mgh required per 1000 cGy = 333 mgh

For 6000 cGy = 6 × 333 =1998 mgh.

Leaving implant in for 222 hours, mg-Radium required = 1998/222 = 9 mg.

Area is less than 25 cm², therefore periphery gets 2/3 and middle gets 1/3 of the 9 mg-Radium. Therefore periphery gets 6mg and middle gets 3mg. Corrected for filtration of 2% for the 1mg and 3% for the 3 mg needles, total Radium used = (2 × 3 × 0.97) + (3 × 1 × 0.98) =8.76 mg-Radium.

Therefore total time to leave implant in = 1998/8.76 = 228.1 h.

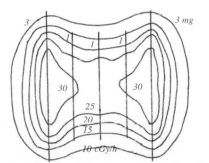

Figure 47.13 Source arrangement and dose distribution for two uncrossed end implant.

C. Two Plane Implant *(Two Ends Crossed)*

One plane implant is good to treat tissues up to 1 cm in thickness. If the thickness is more than 1cm, then single plane implant does not deliver adequate dose to tissues greater than 1cm. In this case, two plane implant should be used.

Example:

A tumor with an area of 5.3 × 5.3 cm² is to be treated to a total dose of 6000 cGy in 80 hours over 8 days to a treatment distance of 1 cm. Calculate the mg-Radium required and their arrangement. Also calculate the dose to 0.5, 1.0, and 1.5 cm depth.

Calculation:

Area to be treated = 5.3 × 5.3 cm²
Desired dose = 6000 cGy in 80 hours.
Area = 28.1 cm² and the treatment distance is 1cm.
From Table 47.4, mgh per 1000 cGy = 813 mgh.
Therefore for 6000 cGy = 6 × 813 = 4878 mgh.
Leaving implant in for 80 hours, mg-Radium required = 4878/80 = 61.0 mg-Radium.
Therefore for two planes, mg-Radium for each plane = 30.5 mg.

Area is greater than 25 cm², therefore periphery and middle each gets 1/2 of the 30. 5 mg-Radium on each plane. Therefore periphery and middle each gets 15.3 mg-Radium for each plane. Corrected for filtration of 3%, the total Radium used = (16 × 3 × 0.97) = 46.56 mg.

Therefore total time to leave implant in = 4878/46.56 = 104.8 h or 13.1 hours a day for 8 days.

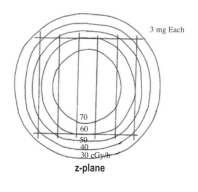

z-plane

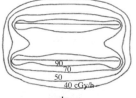

x-plane

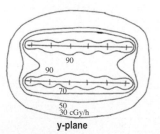

y-plane

Figure 47.14 Source arrangement and dosimetry for two plane implant with two ends crossed.

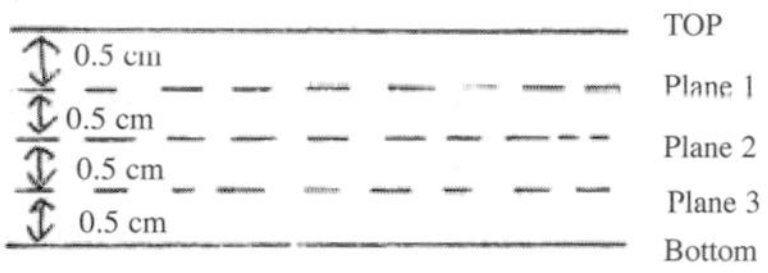

Figure 47.15 Two plane implant with plane of calculation in between.

IX. DOSE CALCULATION TO PLANE 1,2, AND 3

Plane 1

Area = 28.1 cm² and depth from top plane to plane 1 = 0.5 cm
mgh = 494 but mg on top plane = 30.5
Therefore dose to plane 1 = (30.5/494) × 1000 = 61.7 cGy/h
Depth from bottom plane to plane 1 = 1.5 cm
mgh = 1165 but mg on bottom plane = 30.5
Therefore dose to plane 1 = (30.5/1165) × 1000 = 26.2 cGy/h
Therefore total dose to plane 1 from top and bottom plane = 61.7 + 26.2 = 87.9 cGy/h
Therefore for 80 hours = 80 × 87.9 = 7032 cGy.

Note: The 80 hour is used here to obtain the total dose to plane 1 even though the implant is to be left in for 105.2 hours as calculated in the previous section because the actual mg-Radium used is 46.56 mg based on available needles in stock. The dose distribution is adjusted accordingly.

Plane 3

As calculated for plane 1 but in reverse.

Plane 2

Area = 20.1 cm² and depth from top plane to plane 2 = 1.0 cm.
mgh = 813 but mg on top plane = 30.5.
Therefore dose to plane 2 = (30.5/813) × 1000 =37.5 cGy/h

Since the distance from plane 2 to bottom plane is the same as from plane 2 to top plane, the dose is the same as calculated above which is 37.5 cGy/h. Therefore total dose to plane 2 from top and bottom plane = 75 cGy/h.
Therefore for 80 hours = 80 × 75 = 6000 cGy.

D. Cylindrical Volume Implant

For treatment volume larger than 2.5 cm thick, volume implant is necessary to deliver a uniform dose.

Distribution Rules:

Table 47.5 Table of mgh to give 1000 cGy to volume implant filtered by 0.5 mm Pt.
From "The Physics of Radiology" fourth edition by Johns and Cunningham. (Charles C Thomas Publisher)

Volume cm³	5	10	20	30	40	50	60	80	100	140
mgh	106	168	267	350	425	493	556	673	782	979

Belt = 50%, Core = 25% and ends = 12.5% at each end.

For each end uncrossed, volume is reduced by 7.5%. Correction for long cylinder, mgh is increased by;

Length/diameter	1.5	2	2.5	3
Correction	3%	6%	10%	15%

i. One Crossed End

A treatment volume measuring 3 cm inn diameter by 4 cm long is to be treated to 6000 cGy in 168 h with one crossed end. Calculate the mg-Radium required and their arrangement.

Calculation:

Volume of cylinder = Area × height = $\pi r^2 \times L$ = 3.14 × 1.5² × 4 = 28.27 cm³
Corrected for one crossed end, volume = 28.27 × 0.925 = 26.1 cm³
mgh per 1000 cGy (from Table 47.5) = 317.6 mg
Therefore for 6000 cGy = 6 × 317.6 = 1906 mgh.
Since sources are to be left in for 168 h ◆ mg-Radium require = 1906/168 =11.35 mg-Radium.
Therefore belt = 50% of 11.35 = 5.6 mg (6 × 1 mg)
Core = 25% of 11.35 = 2.8 mg (3 × 1 mg)
End = 12.5% of 11.35 = 1.4 mg (2 × 1 mg)
Total = 6+3+2 = 11 mg.
Corrected for 2% filtration, total Radium = (11 × 1 × 0.98) = 10.78 mg.
Therefore total time required to deliver 6000 cGy = 1906/10.78 = 176.8 h.

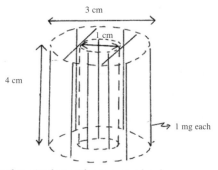

Figure 47.16 Source arrangement for volume implant with one crossed end.

ii. Two Crossed Ends

A treatment volume measuring 3 cm in diameter by 4 cm long is to be treated to 6000 cGy in 168 h with two crossed ends. Calculate the mg-Radium required and their arrangement.

Calculation:

Volume of cylinder = Area × height = $\pi r^2 \times L$ = 3.14 × 1.5² × 4 = 28.27 cm³ ◆ mgh per 1000 cGy = 33 6 mgh
Therefore for 6000 cGy = 6 × 336 = 2016 mg. Since sources are to be left in for 168 h, mg-Radium required = 2016/168 =12.0 mg.
Distribution: Belt = 50% of 12 = 6 mg (6 × 1 mg)
Core = 25% of 12 = 3 mg (3 × 1 mg) ◆ Ends = 12.5% of 12 = 1.5 mg (2 × 1 mg each end) ◆ Total = 6+3+2 = 11 mg-Radium
Correction for 2% filtration, total Radium = (11 × 1 × 0.98) = 10.78 mg
Therefore total time required to deliver 6000 cGy =2016/10.78 = 187 h

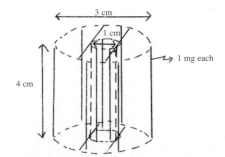

Figure 47.17 Source arrangement for volume implant with two crossed ends.

E. Permanent Implant

For treatment sites such as prostate and bladder, permanent implant may be used instead of partial implant as described in the previous sections. Permanent implants are left in the tissue to decay completely to deliver their full dose. Radionuclide such as Gold-198 seeds is often the choice.

Example:

An area 2 cm circle in diameter is to be treated to 6000 cGy at a depth of 0.5 cm using Au-198 seeds to be left in permanently. Calculate the mCi of Au-198 seeds required.

Exposure rate constant for Au-198 = 2.38 ♦ *Exposure rate constant for Ra-226 = 8.25* ♦ *Half-life for Au-198 = 2.7 days.*

Calculation:

Area of the 2 cm circle = πr^2 = 3.142 × 1 = 3.142 cm^2 ♦ *mgh per 1000 cGy (from Table 47.4) = 128.8 mgh.*
Therefore for 6000 cGy = 6 × 128.8 =773 mgh Radium.
Allowing for full decay, the mCi of Au 198 required,

$$C = \left(M \times \left(\frac{\Gamma_{Radium}}{\Gamma_{Gold}} \right) \right) \times \left(\frac{0.693}{t_{1/2}} \right)$$

where C = mCi of Au-198 ♦ *M = mgh* ♦ *Γ = exposure rate constant* ♦ *$t_{1/2}$ = half-life of Au-198 in hours.*
Therefore,

$$C = \left(773 \times \left(\frac{8.25}{2.38} \right) \right) \times \left(\frac{0.693}{2.7 \times 24} \right) = 28.6 \ mCi$$

X. Sr-90 EYE PLAQUE

Sr-90 is molded into a thin foil and placed inside a cup shape silver eye applicator. The front of the applicator is covered with a very thin layer of silver (0.1 mm) and polythene to provide a smooth surface. The thin layer of silver and polythene also helps to remove the low x- rays. The Sr-90 eye applicator comes in different sizes.

The percentage depth dose and surface dose rate may be obtained by placing TLD discs under the applicator for a set period after which they are read. The surface dose rate of the applicator varies with the activity of the Sr-90. The percentage isodose curves generally follow the shape of the applicator with a slight focusing effect at the center.

The rays from the Sr-90 eye applicator is used to treat pterygium. Pterygium is a layer of tissue that grows over the cornea causing visual defect. The pterygium is surgically removed and the affected eye is treated by placing the Sr-90 eye applicator over the cornea. A single dose of 1500 cGy is given in a single session. Without this treatment, the pterygium has the tendency to regrow after surgical removal.

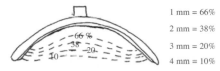

1 mm = 66%
2 mm = 38%
3 mm = 20%
4 mm = 10%

Figure 47.18. Isodose lines for a 18 mm disc Sr-90 eye applicator.

XI. PUBLICATIONS OF INTERESTS

1.   Batley F, Constable WC: The use of the 'Manchester system' for treatment of cancer of the uterine cervix with modern after-loading radium applicators. J Can Assoc Radiol 18:396,1967.

2.   Breitman KE: Dose-rate tables for clinical ^{137}Cs sources sheathed in platinum. Br J Radiol 47:657-664, 1974.

3.   Cunningham DE, Stryker JA, Velkley DE, et al: Intracavitary dosimetry: A comparison of MGHR prescription to doses at points A and B in cervical cancer. Int J Radiat Oncol Biol Phys 7:121-123, 1981.

4.   Fletcher GH: Textbook of Radiotherapy, 2nd ed. Philadelphia, Lea & Febiger, 1973, p620.

5.   Godden TJ: Physical Aspects of Brachytherapy: Medical Physics Handbook 19, pp 41-76. Bristol, Adam Hilger, 1988.

6.   Henschke K, Hilaris BS, Mahan GD: Afterloading intestitial and intracavitary radiation therapy. Am J Roentgenol 90:386,1963.

7.   Hilaris BS(ed): Handbook of Intestitial Brachytherapy. Action, MA, Publishing Science Group,1975.

8.   Horsler AFC, Jones JC, Stacey AJ: Cesium 137 sources for use in intracavitary and intestitial radiotheraph. Br. J Radiol 37:385,1964.

9.   Johns HE, Cunningham JR: The Physics of Radiology, pp 96-100. Springfield, IL, Charles C Thomas, 1983.

10.   Khan FM: The Physics of Radiation Therapy. Baltimore, Williams and Wilkins, 1984, p354-388.

11.   Krishnaswamy V: Dose distribution about Cs-137 sources in tissue. Radiology 105:181,1972.

12.   Krishnaswamy V: Dose tables for ^{125}I seed implants. Radiology 132:727-720, 1979.

13.   Ling CC, Roy JN: Radiobiophysical aspects of brachytherapy. In Williamson JF, Thomadsen BR, Nath R, eds: Brachytherapy Physics: American Association of Physicists in Medicine, 1994 Summer School, pp 39-71. Madison, WI, Medical Physics Publishing, 1995.

14.   Meli JA: Source localization. In Williamson JF, Thomadsen BR, Nath R, eds: Brachytherapy Physics: American Association of Physicists in Medicine, 1994 Summer School, pp 235-253. Madison, WI, Medical Physics Publishing, 1995.

15.   Merredith WJ(ed): Radium dosage. The Manchester System. Edinburgh, Livingstone, Ltd, 1967.

16.   O'Connell D, Joslin CA, Howard N, Ramsey NW, Liversage WE: The treatment of uterine carcinoma using the cathetron. Br J Radiol 40:882,1967.

17.   Paine CH: Modern afterloading methods for intestitial radiotherapy. Clin Radiol 23:263,1972.

18.   Paterson R, Parker HM: A dosage system for gamma-ray therapy. Br J Radiol 7:592, 1934.

19.   Potish RA, Gerbi BJ: Role of point A in the era of computerized dosimetry. Radiology 158:827-831, 1986

20.   Potish RA, Gerbi BJ: Cervical cancer intracavitary dose specification and prescription. Radiology 165:555-560, 1987

21.   Simon N, Silverstone SM: Intracavitary therapy of endometrial cancer by afterloading. J Gynecol 1:13, 1972.

22.   Snelling MD, Lambert HE, Yarnold JR: The treatment of carcinoma of the cervix and endometrium at the Middlesex Hospital. Clin Radiol 30:253,1979.

23.   Stovall M, Shalek RJ: The M.D.Anderson method for the computation of isodose curves around intestitial and intracavitary radiation sources. III. Roentgenograms for input data and the relation of isodose calculations to the Peterson Parker system. Am J Roentgenol 102:667,1968.

24.   Suit HD, Moore EB, Fletcher GH, et al: Modification of the Fletcher ovoid system for afterloading, using standard sized radium tubes. Radiology 81:126-131, 1963.

25.   Wrede D: The relationship between milligram-hours and rads at point A in the treatment of carcinoma of the uterine cervix. Phys Canada 32:298, 1976.

Principles and Practice of Clinical Physics and Dosimetry
Michael L.F. Lim, CMD, ACT
Advanced Medical Publishing, Inc., USA

—— *CHAPTER 48* ——

Emergencies in Radiation Therapy

*The two most common emergencies encountered in radiation therapy are
superior vena cava obstruction (SVC) and spinal cord compression.*

I. SVC OBSTRUCTION

A. Introduction

The common cause of SVC obstruction is from cancer of the lung and lymphoma. The metastatic tumor pushes against the SVC and causes an obstruction. The presentations are shortness of breath, swelling of the truck, upper extremities and face, chest pain, cough, dysphagia and neck vein distention. A single chest X-Ray will reveal the mass. Tissue diagnosis may be attempted after the first treatment to establish diagnosis.

B. Localization

With reference to the patient's chest X-Ray, the mass can be localized under fluoroscopy on the simulator. The field covers the hilar, mediastinal and nearby lesions.

C. Treatment Planning

Treatment must be started immediately giving 400 cGy × 2 followed by 2600 cGy in 13 fractions. The second course total dose depends on the diagnosis. The patient's response is usually obvious in a few days. If the mass is too large to be treated with radiation due to inclusion of large volume of the lungs or if the site has been treated before to the full dose, then chemotherapy may be given instead.

II. SPINAL CORD COMPRESSION

A. Introduction

Spinal cord compression occurs when the tumor extends into the spinal cord. These are usually metastatic tumors from the lung, breast, prostate and lymphoma. If spinal cord compression is not treated, permanent neurological damage is inevitable.

The common presentations are back pain, weakness, autonomic dysfunction, sensory loss, paraplegia and loss of bladder or bowel control.

Diagnosis is by doing a myelogram or CT scan.

B. Localization

With reference to the patient's mylogram and CT films, the mass can be localized under fluoroscopy on the simulator.

C. Treatment Planning

To reduce the pressure from swelling, corticosteroids is given followed immediately by radiation therapy to the spine using a single direct posterior field giving 400 cGy in 2 fractions. A treatment plan is generated to deliver the rest of the radiation giving 3000 cGy in 15 fractions using a pair of wedged fields.

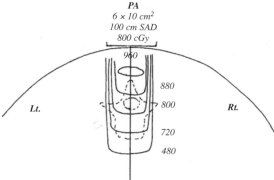

Figure 48.1. Dose distribution for single direct posterior field to treat spinal cord compression. (6 MV photons)

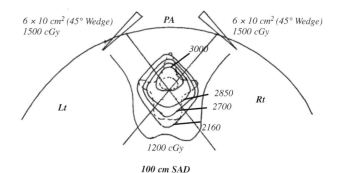

Figure 48.2. Dose distribution for two posterior oblique wedged fields to treat spinal cord compression. (6 MV photons)

III. PUBLICATIONS OF INTERESTS

1. Bach F, Agerlin N, Sorensen JB, et al: Metastatic spinal cord compression secondary to lung cancer. J Clin Oncol 10:1781-1787, 1992.

2. Bruchman JE, Bloomer WE: Management of spinal cord compression. Semin Oncol 5:135,1978.

3. Cairncross JG, Posner JB: Neurologic complications of systemic cancer. In Yarbro JW, Bornstein RS(eds): Oncologic Emergencies, pp 73-96, New Yprk, Grune & Stratton, 1980.

4. Davenport D, Ferree C, Blake D, et al: Radiation therapy in the treatment of superior vena caval obstruction. Cancer 42:2600,1978.

5. Faul CM, Flickinger JC: The use of radiation in the management of spinal metastases. J Neurooncol 23:149-161, 1995.

6. Fisherman WH, Bradfield JS: Superior vena caval syndrome: Response with initially high daily dose irradiation. South Med J 66:667,1973.

7. Helweg-Larsen S, Sorensen PS: Symptoms and signs in metastatic spinal cord compression: A study of

progression from first symptom until diagnosis in 153 patients. Eur J Cancer 30A:396-398, 1994.

8. Herbert SH, Solin LJ, Rate WR, et al: The effect of palliative radiation therapy on epidural compression due to metastatic malignant melanoma. Cancer 67:2472-2476, 1991.

9. Maranzano E, Latini P: Effectiveness of radiation therapy without surgery in metastatic spinal cord compression: Final results from a prospective trial. Int J Radiat Oncol Biol Phys 32:959-967, 1995.

10. Perrin RG: Metastatic tumors of the axial spine. Curr Opin Oncol 4:525-532, 1992.

11. Pigott KH, Baddeley, Maher EJ: Pattern of disease in spinal cord compression on MRI scan and implications for treatment. Clin Oncol 6:7-10, 1994.

12. Schiff D, Shaw EG, Cascino TL: Outcome after spinal reirradiation for malignant epidural spinal cord compression. Ann Neurol 37:583-589, 1995 .

13. Simpson JR, Perez CA, Presant CA, et al: Superior vena cava syndrome. In Yarbro JW, Bornstein RS(eds): Oncologic Emergencies, pp 43-72. New York, Grune & Stratton, 1980.

14. Sorensen PS, Borgesen SE, Rohde K, et al: Metastatic epidural spinal cord compression: Results of treatment and survival. Cancer 65:1502-1508, 1990.

— *CHAPTER 49* —

Quality Assurance in Treatment Planning

I. INTRODUCTION

As explained in chapter 1, the use of radiation in cancer management is to deliver the maximum radiation to the target volume (tumor plus margin) but minimum radiation to the surrounding normal tissues and vital organs that are the limiting factors in radiation therapy.

In order to achieve this, the patient positioning must be accurate and reproducible for target volume localization, simulation for plan verification and daily treatment set-up.

The mechanical and optical qualities of the localization equipment such as the simulator and CT must be within specifications to ensure accuracy and quality images to localize the target volume, normal tissues and vital organs. After the initial acceptance testing and commissioning, regular QA must be performed to ensure their stability and accuracy.

The accuracy of dose distribution of a planning computer depends on the input of measured data such as percentage depth dose, TAR, SAR, TPR, beam profile, CT number verses electron density and the computer algorithms used. In addition, input devices such as the digitizer, joystick, mouse, etc, must be calibrated and checked for accuracy. Output devices such as plotter, monitor display, etc, must also be calibrated and checked for accuracy. A regular QA must be performed to maintain their integrity.

Verification of complex plans using a simulator to mimic the plan field set up is a must. This not only verifies the position of the planned fields but also serves as a record of the plan. Verification may be supplemented with treatment unit port films.

Set up instructions for the plan must be written clearly and accurately and for complex plans, a dosimetrist must be present at first treatment to ensure accurate transfer of the set up instructions.

II. PATIENT POSITIONING

The patient must be in the same position for the fabrication of immobilization shell *(if needed)*, simulation for referencing, CT, plan verification and daily treatment set-up.

The use of well-fitted immobilization shell *(cast)* and polyform cradle help in the reproducibility of patient positioning. The same devices such as hand holder, headrest size, mouth bite, etc, must be used throughout for the individual patient and this must be documented in the patient's set up instructions. These devices must be checked for wear and tear from time to time to ensure accuracy and consistency.

III. TARGET VOLUME LOCALIZATION

The simulator and/or CT are used to localize the target volume. To ensure accuracy of the localization, the parameters of the simulator such as light field coincidence with radiation field, digital display of field size, gantry angle, collimator angle, floor angle, isocenter, wall lazers source film distance and SSD must be checked regularly.

In addition, image quality and film quality must also be checked to ensure sharp images with good contrast. To produce sharp and good contrast simulator films, not only would the kVp and mA of the simulator tube need to be checked but also the film processing unit.

The mechanical and optical qualities of the CT unit must also be checked for deviation from the original specifications. The gantry angle, slice thickness, longitudinal couch movement must be checked for accuracy. Window and level settings must also be checked against known values. Variable inhomogeneity values must be checked using a phantom of known inhomogeneity values.

IV. PLANNING COMPUTER

Input devices such as the digitizer must be checked for scaling accuracy by digitizing a known contour into the computer and checking the contour depth using the depth report function of the computer.

Output devices such as the plotter must be checked for scaling accuracy by plotting the above contour and comparing the plot against the known contour.

Beam data files such as percentage depth dose, TAR, TPR, SAR, beam profile, dose build up region, wedge data, etc, are checked against measured data. Plotted samples of isodose charts and beam dose profiles are compared with the measured charts and printed values of TPR, wedge factors, tray factors, etc may be checked against measured ones.

Dose distribution for multifield plans with and without inhomogeneity correction, equal and unequal weightings, wedged and unwedged fields are checked at regular periods against known and measured stored plans.

V. PLAN AND CALCULATION CHECK

All plans and calculations must be checked by a second dosimetrist and complex plans and calculations must be checked by a physicist before treatment. All plans and verification films must be approved and signed by the radiation oncologist before commencement of treatment.

VI. PLAN VERIFICATION

The plan treatment fields must be verified at simulation by setting the field parameters as planned and obtaining simulator films for the treatment record. The field light and center are drawn on the patient's skin or shell (cast) for treatment set up. The verification may be supplemented with port films on the treatment unit.

VII. SET UP INSTRUCTIONS

The set-up instructions for the plan must be written clearly and accurately and for complex plans, a dosimetrist must be present at first treatment to ensure accurate transfer of the set up instructions. The fields are set up as planned and the field center and field light are checked against the marks drawn on the patient's skin or shell (cast) from simulation.

VIII. III. PUBLICATIONS OF INTERESTS

1. AAPM, TG24-Draft G:Physical aspects of Quality Assurance in Radiation Therapy. June,1982.

2. Essenburg A, Koziarsky A: Allignment of light localized beam and radiographic X-Ray beam. Radiology,104(3):716,1972.

3. Harms WB, Low DA, Purdy JA: Commissioning a three-dimensional dose-calculation algorithm for clinical use. In Purdy JA, Fraass BA, eds: Syllabus: A Categorical Course in Physics. Oak Brook, IL, Radiological Society of North America, 1994

4. Harms WB, Purdy JA, Emami B, et al: Quality assurance for three-dimensional treatment planning. In Purdy JA, Fraass BA, eds: Syllabus: A Categorical Course in Physics. Oak Brook, IL, Radiological Society of North America, 1994

5. Herring DF, Compton DMJ: The degree of precision in the radiation dose delivered in cancer radiotherapy. Computers in Radiotherapy. Br J Radiol. Special report #5,pp51-58,1971.

6. Kelsey CA, Berardo PA, Smith AR, Kligerman MM: CT scanner selection and specification for radiation therapy. Med Phys 7:555-558,1980.

7. Klemp PFB, Perry AM, Hedland-Thomas B, et al: Commissioning of a linear accelerator with independent jaws: Computerized data collection and transfer to a planning computer. Phys Med Biol 33:865, 1988

8. Kutcher GJ, Coia L, Gillin M, et al: Comprehensive QA for radiation oncology: Report of AAPM Radiation Therapy Committee Task Group 40. Med Phys 21:581-618, 1994

9. Leunens G, Verstraete J, Van den Bogaert W, et al: Human errors in data transfer during preparation and delivery of radiation treatment affecting the final result: "Garbage in, garbage out." Radiother Oncol 23:217, 1992

10. Marks JE, Haus AG, Sutton GH, Griem ML: The value of treatment verification films in reducing localization errors in the irradiation of complex fields. Cancer 37:2755,1976.

11. McCullough EC, Krueger AM: Performance evaluation of computerized treatment planning systems for radiotherapy:External photon beams. Int J Radiation Oncology Biol Phys 6:1559-1605,1980.

12. Van Dyk J, Barrett RB, Cygler JE, et al: Commissioning and quality assurance of treatment planning computers. Int J Radiat Oncol Biol Phys 26:261-273, 1993

—— PROBLEMS ——

1. A child is treated for Medulloblastoma on the 6 MV Linear Accelerator at 100 cm SAD employing a 6×30 cm^2 spinal field and 16×16 cm^2 opposed lateral skull fields. What is the collimator angle of the lateral skull fields to match the divergence of the spinal field?

2. Calculate the gap on the skin if two PA fields 32 cm and 34 cm long are used to treat a patient at 100 cm SSD to match at 7 cm depth.

3. For Cobalt-60 unit, the % transmission through a lead block 3.3 cm thick is?

4. A patient was simulated at 80 cm SSD to define a field size to cover a tumor at 6cm depth. The field size was established at 6×14 cm^2. If the patient is treated at 80 cm SAD, what should the collimator setting be?

5. The %DD for 10×10 cm^2 at 80 cm SSD at 10cm depth is 55.45%. D_{max} is 0.5 cm. If the field size is kept the same but the SSD is increased to 120 cm, the new %DD at 10 cm is?

6. Given the following data, calculate the geometric penumbra on the skin.

   Source size = 2 cm

   Source diaphragm distance = 45 cm

   Source skin distance = 110 cm

7. If the source diaphragm distance is 45 cm, the SSD is 80 cm and the source size is 2 cm, the geometry penumbra size is:

8. A 20mCi Cs-137 source sits on a bench in the brachytherapy room. What is the exposure rate at a distance of 30 cm away. *(Exposure Rate Constant for Cs-137 is 3.23 R/h/mCi at 1cm)*

9. The air dose rate for 10×10 cm^2 at 80 cm SSD is 120.5 cGy/min. What is the dose rate if the distance is decreased to 62 cm SSD?

10. If the air dose rate on the Cobalt-60 unit is 180 cGy/min on the 1st July 1991, what is the air dose rate on the 15th Oct 1992?

11. A dose of 2000 cGy in 10 fractions to a depth of 5 cm from a single posterior field is prescribed to treat metastatic disease in the vertebra using an isocentric technique, 80 cm SAD. The patient was incorrectly treated 5 fractions at 80 cm SSD. The approximate dose at 5 cm after 5 fractions is ?

12. The DTD for field # 2 on a plan was 70 cGy using a 10×10 cm^2, 30° wedge on the Cobalt-60 unit at 80 cm SAD. The depth is 7.3 cm and the wedge factor is 0.752. If the wedge is left out, what is the TD given for that day if the same treatment time was used as calculated with the wedge in?

13. The tissue dose rate for 10×12 cm^2 at 10 cm depth is 100 cGy/min. If 1.53 min of treatment time was delivered, what is the dose delivered? *(Timer correction is +0.02 min)*

14. A patient was planned to be treated at 100 cm SSD. The patient was treated at 102 cm SSD by mistake. The error in dose delivered at d_{max} is?

15. Given the following data, calculate the cord dose using the TAR method.

Parallel opposed fields of 10 × 14 cm² field size at 80 cm SAD.

Separation is 22 cm.

Depth to cord from the anterior is 15 cm.

Total tumor dose to mid depth is 4500 cGy.

16. The diagram below shows a treatment field with shielding. The table contains the radaii from the center of the field to the edge of the treated field. From the SAR table and TAR *(zero field)* table for Cobalt-60, calculate the treatment time if 2000 cGy in 10 fractions is prescribed to 5 cm depth at 80 cm SAD. Use the output factor table in the data section. *(Timer correction = +0.02min.)*

Sector	Radii	Sector	Radii	Sector	Radii
0	9	12	7	24	8.5
1	6.5	13	5.5	25	8
2	5.7	14	4.5	26	7.5
3	5.3	15	4	27	7.5
4	5.3	16	3.8	28	7.5
5	5.5	17	3.6	29	8
6	6	18	3.5	30	8.5
7	8	19	3.6	31	9.6
8	7.5	20	3.8	32	11.5
9	7.5	21	10.5	33	10.3
10	7.5	22	11.5	34	9.5
11	8	23	9.8	35	9

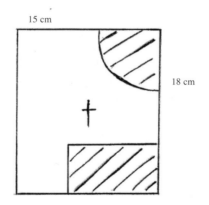

15 cm

18 cm

17. If 5000 cGy in 25 fractions is prescribed to the centre at mid-depth by parallel opposed fields at 80 cm SAD, calculate the treatment time for each field given the TAR *(zero field size) at 10 cm depth is 0.534 and the average SAR after irregular field is 0.195.* The tray factor is 0.939 and the timer correction is +0.02 min. *(Output factor = 136.9 cGy/min)*

18. A patient was set up on the DXR to treat a tumor on the cheek. The applicator is a 6 × 6cm²with a 4 × 4 cm² lead cut-out. The tissue dose rate for 6 × 6 cm² is 180 cGy/min. The BSF for 6 × 6 cm² is 1.178 and for 4 × 4 cm² is 1.126. Calculate the tissue dose rate after shielding. *(The SSD is 50 cm)*

19. A skin lesion is treated on the SXR unit using an applicator 5 cm circle. If the area of the cut out is 15 cm square, calculate the treatment time if the daily given dose is 250 cGy. *(Timer correction is -0.02 min. Output factor for 5 cm circle is 180 cGy/min)*

Diametr	PSF
2cm	1.071
2.5	1.085
3	1.099
3.5	1.112
4	1.124
4.5	1.136
5	1.147

20. With reference to the 16 MeV e- depth dose table, what is the dose to the cord at 7 cm depth from skin surface if 2000 cGy is prescribed to the 90% with 1cm of superflab on the skin?

0 (cm)	93%
1	99
2	100
3	100
4	95
5	93
6	75
7	44
8	13
9	3
10	3

21. Using the items in Column I, match the items in Column II that apply. Items from Column I may be used more than once.

Column I.

        A. Superficial X-Ray beam (HVL 3mm AL.)

        B. Cobalt-60 beam

        C. 4 MV photon beam

        D. 20 MV photon beam

Column II.

        1. Has similar %DD characteristics to Cobalt-60

        2. Has greatest PSF

        3. Has maximum dose at skin

        4. D_{max} is about 4 cm

        5. Has the largest geometric penumbra

        6. Dose rate decreases with time

        7. Has highest exit dose

        8. Commonly used to treat laryngeal tumors

22. With reference to the diagram below, calculate the MU setting to each field if 4000 cGy in 20 fractions is prescribed to the isocenter (100%. correcting for inhomogeneity using Batho's method. The lung density is 0.3 gm/cc. The patient is treated on the 6 MV Linear Accelerator unit at 100 cm SAD.

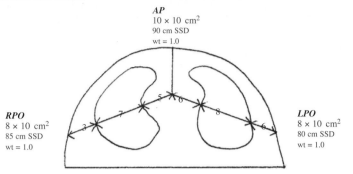

23. The central axis of a 6 MV photon beam traverses 2.5 cm of soft tissue, 11 cm of lung and 3.5 cm of soft tissue. If the density of lung is 0.2 g/cc, what is the effective path length?

24. The distribution for an iridium wire implant shows that the tumor is encompased by the 42cGy/h isodose line. The prescription is 3000 cGy to this level. The treatment started at 08:30h on Sep 22. Calculate the time and date at which the implant should be removed.

25. Calculate the %DD at 12 cm depth for 10×15 cm^2 field at 80 cm SSD *(Cobalt-60. using TAR table)*.

26. Calculate the TAR at 15 cm depth for 12×16 cm^2 field at 80 cm SSD using %DD table.

27. A patient is treated on the 6 MV unit with three fields gantry angles of 0° (AP), 120° (LPO) and 240° (RPO) using 8×10 cm^2 field size at 100 cm SAD. The depths are 13 cm, 15 cm and 16 cm respectively. The weighting at isocenter to all three fields are equal. Total tumor dose of 5000 cGy in 25 treatments is prescribed to the 95% isodose line. Calculate the MU setting to each field.

28. Repeat problem 27 if the weightings at isocenter are 100%, 80%, and 70% respectively.

29. Calculate the treatment and rotation speed if 4000 cGy in 15 treatments is prescribed to the 95% isodose in a 300° arc rotation treatment using 8×8 cm^2 field size at 80 cm SAD on the Cobalt-60 treatment unit. The arc angles and field depths are given below. *(Timer correction = +0.02 min)*

Angle	Depth	Angle	Depth
210	13	10	13
230	14	30	14
250	15	50	14
270	16	70	15
290	16	90	16
310	15	110	16
330	14	130	15
350	14	150	14

30. A patient was planned to receive 5000 cGy in 25 fractions treating 5 fractions a week. After 12 treatments, a rest of 5 days was prescribed. Calculate the daily tumor dose for the remaining 13 treatments to achieve the same TDF.

— ANSWERS —

1. 8.5°

2. 2.31 cm

3. 12.5%

4. 6.5 × 15 cm^2

5. 59.6%

6. 2.9 cm

7. 1.56 cm

8. 0.072 R/h

9. 200.6 cGy/min

10. 151.8 cGy min

11. 886 cGy

12. 93c Gy

13. 151cGy

14. Underdose of 4%

15. 4680 cGy

16. 1.58 min

17. 1.09 min

18. 172.1 cGy/min

19. 1.38 min

20. 289 cGy

21.
   1. C
   2. A
   3. A
   4. D
   5. B
   6. B
   7. D
   8. C

22.
  AP = 86 MU
  RPO = 89 MU
  LPO = 107 MU

23. 8.2 cm

24. 07:54 Sep 25

25. 49.5 %

26. 0.672

27.
  AP = 103 MU
  LPO = 111 MU
  RPO = 116 MU

28.
  AP = 123 MU
  LPO = 107 MU
  RPO = 97 MU

29.
  Treatment time = 3.80 min.
  Arc speed = 0.219 rpm (rev per min)

30. 201 cGy.

Principles and Practice of Clinical Physics and Dosimetry
Michael L.F. Lim, CMD, ACT
Advanced Medical Publishing, Inc., USA

—— APPENDICES ——

—— APPENDIX A ——
COBALT-60

%DD for Co-60

Eq.Sq	5	6	7	8	9	10	11	12	13	14	15	16	17	18	19
Depth															
0.5	100.0	10.0	100.0	100.0	100.0	100.0	100.0	100.0	100.0	100.0	100.0	100.0	100.0	100.0	100.0
1	97.3	97.5	97.6	97.8	97.9	98.0	98.0	98.1	98.1	98.2	98.2	98.2	98.3	98.3	98.3
2	91.6	92.1	92.5	92.9	93.2	93.4	93.6	93.8	93.9	94.0	94.1	94.2	94.3	94.3	94.4
3	85.8	86.5	87.1	87.6	88.1	88.4	88.8	89.0	89.2	89.4	89.6	89.7	89.8	89.9	90.0
4	80.0	80.9	81.7	82.3	82.9	83.3	83.7	84.1	84.4	84.6	84.9	85.0	85.2	85.4	85.5
5	74.5	75.5	76.3	77.0	77.7	78.2	78.7	79.1	79.5	79.8	80.0	80.3	80.5	80.7	80.9
6	69.1	70.2	71.1	71.9	72.6	73.2	73.8	74.3	74.7	75.1	75.4	75.7	75.9	76.2	76.4
7	64.1	65.2	66.2	67.0	67.8	68.4	69.0	69.6	70.0	70.5	70.8	71.2	71.5	71.8	72.0
8	59.4	60.5	61.5	62.4	63.2	63.9	64.5	65.0	65.6	66.0	66.5	66.8	67.2	67.5	67.8
9	54.9	56.0	57.1	58.0	58.8	59.5	60.2	60.8	61.3	61.8	62.3	62.7	63.1	63.4	63.7
10	50.8	51.9	52.9	53.9	54.7	55.5	56.1	56.8	57.4	57.9	58.4	58.8	59.2	59.6	59.9
11	46.9	48.0	49.1	50.0	50.9	51.6	52.3	53.0	53.6	54.1	54.6	55.1	55.5	55.9	56.3
12	43.4	44.5	45.5	46.4	47.3	48.0	48.8	49.4	50.0	50.6	51.1	51.6	52.1	52.5	52.9
13	40.1	41.2	42.2	43.1	43.9	44.7	45.4	46.1	46.7	457.3	47.9	48.4	48.8	49.3	49.7
14	37.0	38.1	39.0	40.0	40.8	41.6	42.3	43.0	43.7	44.2	44.8	45.3	45.8	46.2	46.6
15	34.2	35.2	36.2	37.1	37.9	38.7	39.4	40.1	40.8	41.4	41.9	42.4	42.9	43.4	43.8
16	31.6	32.6	33.5	34.4	35.2	36.0	36.7	37.4	38.1	38.7	39.2	39.8	40.2	40.7	41.1
17	29.2	30.2	31.1	31.9	32.8	33.5	34.2	34.9	35.6	36.2	36.7	37.2	37.7	38.2	38.6
18	27.0	27.9	28.8	29.6	30.4	31.2	31.9	32.6	33.2	33.8	34.4	34.9	35.4	35.9	36.3
19	24.9	25.8	26.7	27.5	28.3	29.0	29.7	30.3	31.0	31.6	32.2	32.7	33.1	33.7	34.1
20	23.0	23.9	24.8	25.5	26.3	27.0	27.7	28.3	29.0	29.6	30.1	30.6	31.1	31.6	32.0

OF FOR Co60 80cm SAD

Eq.Sq	cGy/min	Eq.Sq	cGy/min
5	139.6	17	146.6
6	140.4	18	147.0
7	141.1	19	147.3
8	141.8	20	147.6
9	142.5	21	147.8
10	143.2	22	148.0
11	143.8	23	148.2
12	144.3	24	148.3
13	144.9	25	148.4
14	145.4	26	148.4
15	145.8	27	148.5
16	146.2	28	148.4

OF FOR Co60 80cm SSD

Eq.Sq	cGy/min	Eq.Sq	cGy/min
5	140.4	17	152.7
6	141.7	18	153.4
7	142.9	19	154.1
8	144.1	20	154.7
9	145.2	21	155.3
10	146.3	22	155.8
11	147.4	23	156.3
12	148.4	24	156.7
13	149.3	25	157.1
14	150.2	26	157.4
15	151.1	27	157.7
16	151.9	28	157.9

Wedge Factors for Co-60

30deg		45deg		60deg	
6x15	0.792	6x15	0.678	6x15	0.545
8x15	0.752	8x15	0.628	8x15	0.469
10x15	0.714	10x15	0.583	10x15	0.409

Tray Factor= .959

Eq.Sq	5	6	7	8	9	10	11	12	13	14	15	16	17	18	19
Depth															
0.5	1.108	1.022	1.025	1.029	1.032	1.035	1.038	1.041	1.044	1.047	1.049	1.052	1.054	1.057	1.059
1	1.003	1.008	1.013	1.018	1.022	1.026	1.030	1.034	1.037	1.040	1.043	1.046	1.049	1.050	1.054
2	0.967	0.976	0.983	0.990	0.996	1.000	1.007	1.012	1.016	1.020	1.023	1.027	1.030	1.033	1.036
3	0.927	0.938	0.948	0.956	0.964	0.971	0.977	0.983	0.988	0.993	0.997	1.000	1.005	1.009	1.012
4	0.885	0.897	0.909	0.919	0.928	0.936	0.943	0.950	0.956	0.961	0.960	0.971	0.975	0.979	0.983
5	0.842	0.855	0.868	0.879	0.889	0.898	0.906	0.914	0.920	0.927	0.932	0.938	0.943	0.947	0.951
6	0.799	0.813	0.826	0.838	0.849	0.859	0.868	0.876	0.884	0.890	0.897	0.903	0.908	0.913	0.918
7	0.756	0.771	0.785	0.798	0.809	0.819	0.829	0.838	0.846	0.853	0.860	0.867	0.873	0.878	0.884
8	0.715	0.730	0.745	0.758	0.769	0.780	0.790	0.800	0.808	0.816	0.824	0.831	0.837	0.843	0.849
9	0.675	0.691	0.705	0.718	0.731	0.742	0.753	0.762	0.771	0.780	0.788	0.795	0.802	0.808	0.814
10	0.637	0.653	0.667	0.681	0.693	0.705	0.715	0.726	0.735	0.744	0.752	0.760	0.767	0.774	0.780
11	0.600	0.616	0.631	0.644	0.657	0.669	0.680	0.690	0.700	0.709	0.717	0.725	0.733	0.740	0.747
12	0.566	0.581	0.596	0.609	0.622	0.634	0.645	0.656	0.665	0.675	0.684	0.692	0.700	0.707	0.714
13	0.533	0.548	0.562	0.576	0.588	0.600	0.612	0.622	0.632	0.642	0.651	0.660	0.668	0.676	0.683
14	0.501	0.516	0.530	0.544	0.556	0.568	0.580	0.590	0.601	0.610	0.620	0.628	0.637	0.645	0.652
15	0.472	0.486	0.500	0.513	0.526	0.538	0.549	0.560	0.570	0.580	0.590	0.598	0.607	0.615	0.623
16	0.444	0.458	0.472	0.485	0.497	0.509	0.520	0.531	0.541	0.551	0.560	0.570	0.578	0.586	0.594
17	0.418	0.431	0.445	0.457	0.470	0.481	0.492	0.503	0.513	0.523	0.533	0.542	0.550	0.559	0.567
18	0.392	0.406	0.419	0.431	0.443	0.455	0.466	0.477	0.487	0.497	0.506	0.515	0.524	0.532	0.540
19	0.369	0.382	0.395	0.407	0.419	0.430	0.441	0.451	0.461	0.471	0.481	0.490	0.499	0.507	0.515
20	0.347	0.360	0.372	0.384	0.395	0.406	0.417	0.427	0.437	0.447	0.456	0.465	0.474	0.483	0.491

TAR FOR Co-60

—— *APPENDIX B* ——
6 MV

OF for 6MV

Eq.Sq	cGy/MU	Eq.Sq	cGy/MU	Eq.Sq	cGy/MU
4	0.921	16	1.043	28	1.085
5	0.938	17	1.048	29	1.087
6	0.953	18	1.053	30	1.090
7	0.967	19	1.057	31	1.092
8	0.979	20	1.061	32	1.095
9	0.990	21	1.064	33	1.097
10	1.000	22	1.067	34	1.099
11	1.009	23	1.071	35	1.102
12	1.018	24	1.074	36	1.104
13	1.025	25	1.076	37	1.106
14	1.032	26	1.079	38	1.107
15	1.038	27	1.082	39	1.109

PSF for 6MV

Eq.Sq	PSF	Eq.Sq	PSF	Eq.Sq	PSF
4	1.012	12	1.043	20	1.066
5	1.017	13	1.046	21	1.069
6	1.022	14	1.050	22	1.071
7	1.026	15	1.052	23	1.073
8	1.030	16	1.056	24	1.076
9	1.033	17	1.058	25	1.077
10	1.035	18	1.061	26	1.080
11	1.040	19	1.064	27	1.082

Wedge Factors for 6MV	
30deg	0.682
45deg	0.625
60deg	0.599
TF	0.970

TMR 6 MV, norm at 1.5cm																
Eq.Sq	4	5	6	7	8	9	10	11	12	13	14	15	16	17	18	19	20
Depth																	
1.5	1	1	1	1	1	1	1	1	1	1	1	1	1	1	1	1	1
2	1.010	1.006	1.004	1.002	1.000	0.999	0.998	0.997	0.996	0.996	0.995	0.995	0.995	0.994	0.994	0.994	0.994
3	0.971	0.971	0.971	0.972	0.973	0.973	0.973	0.974	0.974	0.974	0.974	0.974	0.974	0.974	0.974	0.974	0.974
4	0.928	0.932	0.936	0.940	0.942	0.945	0.946	0.948	0.949	0.950	0.951	0.951	0.952	0.953	0.953	0.953	0.953
5	0.889	0.896	0.902	0.908	0.912	0.916	0.919	0.922	0.924	0.925	0.927	0.928	0.929	0.930	0.931	0.931	0.932
6	0.852	0.861	0.869	0.876	0.882	0.887	0.891	0.895	0.897	0.900	0.902	0.904	0.905	0.906	0.908	0.909	0.909
7	0.816	0.827	0.837	0.845	0.852	0.858	0.863	0.867	0.871	0.874	0.877	0.879	0.881	0.882	0.884	0.885	0.886
8	0.782	0.794	0.805	0.814	0.822	0.829	0.835	0.840	0.844	0.848	0.851	0.854	0.856	0.858	0.860	0.862	0.863
9	0.749	0.762	0.773	0.784	0.792	0.800	0.807	0.812	0.817	0.821	0.825	0.828	0.831	0.833	0.836	0.838	0.839
10	0.717	0.730	0.742	0.753	0.763	0.771	0.778	0.785	0.790	0.795	0.799	0.802	0.806	0.808	0.811	0.813	0.815
11	0.686	0.700	0.712	0.724	0.734	0.743	0.750	0.757	0.763	0.768	0.773	0.777	0.780	0.784	0.786	0.789	0.791
12	0.656	0.670	0.683	0.695	0.706	0.715	0.723	0.730	0.736	0.742	0.747	0.751	0.755	0.758	0.762	0.765	0.767
13	0.628	0.642	0.655	0.667	0.678	0.687	0.696	0.703	0.710	0.716	0.721	0.726	0.730	0.734	0.738	0.741	0.744
14	0.600	0.614	0.627	0.639	0.651	0.660	0.669	0.677	0.684	0.690	0.695	0.701	0.705	0.710	0.713	0.717	0.720
15	0.573	0.587	0.601	0.613	0.624	0.634	0.643	0.651	0.658	0.665	0.671	0.676	0.681	0.685	0.690	0.693	0.697
16	0.548	0.562	0.575	0.587	0.598	0.609	0.618	0.626	0.633	0.640	0.646	0.652	0.657	0.662	0.666	0.670	0.674
17	0.524	0.537	0.550	0.562	0.574	0.584	0.593	0.601	0.609	0.616	0.622	0.628	0.633	0.638	0.643	0.647	0.651
18	0.500	0.513	0.526	0.538	0.549	0.560	0.569	0.577	0.585	0.592	0.599	0.605	0.610	0.615	0.620	0.625	0.629
19	0.478	0.491	0.503	0.515	0.526	0.536	0.546	0.554	0.562	0.569	0.576	0.582	0.588	0.593	0.598	0.603	0.607
20	0.456	0.469	0.481	0.493	0.504	0.514	0.523	0.531	0.539	0.547	0.553	0.560	0.560	0.571	0.576	0.581	0.585
21	0.436	0.448	0.460	0.471	0.482	0.492	0.501	0.510	0.518	0.525	0.532	0.538	0.544	0.550	0.555	0.560	0.564
22	0.416	0.428	0.439	0.451	0.461	0.471	0.480	0.489	0.497	0.504	0.511	0.517	0.523	0.529	0.534	0.539	0.544
23	0.397	0.409	0.420	0.431	0.441	0.451	0.460	0.468	0.476	0.484	0.490	0.497	0.503	0.509	0.514	0.519	0.524
24	0.379	0.390	0.401	0.412	0.422	0.431	0.440	0.449	0.456	0.464	0.471	0.477	0.483	0.489	0.495	0.500	0.504
25	0.362	0.373	0.383	0.394	0.403	0.413	0.422	0.430	0.437	0.445	0.452	0.458	0.464	0.470	0.476	0.481	0.486

6 MV %DD						
Eq.Sq	5	10	15	20	25	30
Depth						
1.5	100	100	100	100	100	100
2	98.2	98.5	98.6	98.7	98.6	98.5
3	93.7	94.7	94.9	95.0	95.0	95.1
4	88.8	90.3	91.2	91.4	91.7	92.0
5	83.8	86.1	87.2	87.7	88.2	88.6
6	79.2	82.0	83.3	84.0	84.6	85.1
7	74.5	78.0	79.5	80.3	81.0	81.7
8	70.2	74.1	75.8	76.8	77.7	78.4
9	66.2	70.3	72.3	73.4	74.5	75.2
10	62.3	66.7	68.6	70.1	71.4	72.1
11	58.6	63.1	65.3	67.2	68.4	69.0
12	55.2	60.0	62.3	63.8	65.2	66.0
13	51.8	56.8	59.3	60.7	62.2	63.1
14	48.7	53.7	56.3	57.9	59.4	60.3
15	46.0	50.8	53.3	55.0	56.6	57.6
16	43.4	48.0	50.6	52.2	53.7	54.9
17	40.9	45.5	48.0	49.7	51.2	52.3
18	38.5	43.0	45.6	47.3	48.9	50.0
19	36.3	40.6	43.2	45.1	46.9	47.7
20	34.4	38.4	41.0	42.9	44.5	45.7

— APPENDIX C —
15 MV

15 MV %DD				
Eq.Sq	5	10	20	30
Depth				
3	100.0	100.0	100.0	100.0
10	76.0	77.4	78.5	78.9
15	60.6	62.6	64.6	65.5
20	48.3	50.5	53.1	54.2
25	38.7	40.9	43.6	44.7

OF for 15MV					
Eq.Sq	cGy/MU	Eq.Sq	cGy/MU	Eq.Sq	cGy/MU
4	0.892	16	1.039	28	1.057
5	0.917	17	1.041	29	1.058
6	0.939	18	1.044	30	1.060
7	0.958	19	1.045	31	1.061
8	0.974	20	1.047	32	1.063
9	0.988	21	1.048	33	1.065
10	1.000	22	1.049	34	1.066
11	1.010	23	1.050	35	1.068
12	1.018	24	1.051	36	1.069
13	1.025	25	1.053	37	1.069
14	1.031	26	1.054	38	1.069
15	1.035	27	1.055	39	1.068

Wedge Factors for 15MV	
15deg	0.796
30deg	0.774
45deg	0.644
60deg	0.604
TF	0.980

PSF for 15MV					
Eq.Sq	PSF	Eq.Sq	PSF	Eq.Sq	PSF
4	1.013	12	1.033	20	1.049
5	1.015	13	1.035	21	1.050
6	1.018	14	1.037	22	1.051
7	1.021	15	1.039	23	1.053
8	1.023	16	1.041	24	1.054
9	1.026	17	1.043	25	1.055
10	1.028	18	1.045	26	1.056
11	1.031	19	1.047	27	1.056

TPR 15 MV, norm at 4cm																
Eq.Sq	5	6	7	8	9	10	11	12	13	14	15	16	17	18	19	20
Depth																
4	1.000	1.000	1.000	1.000	1.000	1.000	1.000	1.000	1.000	1.000	1.000	1.000	1.000	1.000	1.000	1.000
5	0.977	0.978	0.979	0.979	0.980	0.980	0.985	0.985	0.986	0.986	0.987	0.982	0.982	0.983	0.983	0.984
6	0.958	0.960	0.961	0.962	0.963	0.963	0.964	0.964	0.965	0.965	0.966	0.966	0.967	0.967	0.968	0.968
7	0.930	0.933	0.935	0.937	0.939	0.940	0.942	0.943	0.945	0.947	0.948	0.949	0.949	0.950	0.950	0.951
8	0.906	0.910	0.913	0.915	0.917	0.918	0.920	0.922	0.923	0.924	0.925	0.926	0.927	0.928	0.929	0.930
9	0.884	0.885	0.889	0.893	0.896	0.899	0.901	0.903	0.905	0.907	0.908	0.909	0.910	0.911	0.912	0.913
10	0.861	0.866	0.870	0.873	0.876	0.879	0.881	0.883	0.885	0.887	0.888	0.889	0.889	0.890	0.892	0.894
11	0.832	0.838	0.843	0.848	0.853	0.857	0.859	0.860	0.863	0.863	0.868	0.870	0.871	0.873	0.874	0.875
12	0.813	0.819	0.824	0.828	0.831	0.834	0.838	0.841	0.844	0.846	0.848	0.850	0.852	0.854	0.856	0.858
13	0.787	0.793	0.798	0.803	0.808	0.813	0.816	0.818	0.822	0.825	0.828	0.830	0.832	0.834	0.836	0.838
14	0.769	0.775	0.780	0.785	0.789	0.793	0.797	0.801	0.804	0.807	0.810	0.812	0.814	0.816	0.818	0.820
15	0.743	0.750	0.756	0.761	0.766	0.770	0.774	0.778	0.782	0.786	0.789	0.792	0.794	0.796	0.798	0.800
16	0.722	0.730	0.736	0.741	0.746	0.751	0.756	0.760	0.764	0.767	0.770	0.774	0.776	0.778	0.780	0.782
17	0.701	0.709	0.715	0.720	0.725	0.730	0.734	0.738	0.742	0.746	0.750	0.752	0.755	0.758	0.760	0.762
18	0.681	0.689	0.695	0.701	0.706	0.711	0.716	0.720	0.724	0.726	0.731	0.734	0.737	0.740	0.742	0.746
19	0.661	0.668	0.675	0.682	0.688	0.693	0.697	0.701	0.705	0.709	0.713	0.716	0.719	0.722	0.724	0.727
20	0.641	0.650	0.659	0.668	0.671	0.674	0.680	0.685	0.690	0.694	0.697	0.700	0.703	0.706	0.708	0.711
21	0.622	0.630	0.637	0.644	0.650	0.656	0.661	0.665	0.670	0.674	0.678	0.681	0.684	0.687	0.690	0.692
22	0.603	0.612	0.620	0.627	0.633	0.638	0.643	0.648	0.653	0.657	0.660	0.664	0.667	0.671	0.674	0.678
23	0.586	0.594	0.601	0.607	0.614	0.620	0.624	0.629	0.633	0.638	0.642	0.645	0.649	0.652	0.655	0.658
24	0.568	0.576	0.583	0.590	0.596	0.602	0.607	0.611	0.616	0.621	0.625	0.628	0.632	0.635	0.638	0.642
25	0.552	0.560	0.567	0.574	0.581	0.587	0.592	0.596	0.600	0.605	0.610	0.613	0.616	0.619	0.622	0.626

— APPENDIX D —
TDF

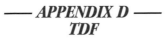

TDF FACTORS FOR ONE FRACTION PER WEEK																
Dose/	Number of fractions															
fraction	4	5	6	7	8	9	10	11	12	13	14	15	16	17	18	19	20
20	0	0	0	1	1	1	1	1	1	1	1	1	1	1	1	1	1
40	1	1	1	2	2	2	2	2	3	3	3	3	3	4	4	4	4
60	2	2	2	3	3	4	4	4	5	5	6	6	6	7	7	8	8
80	3	3	4	4	5	6	6	7	8	8	9	9	10	11	11	12	13
100	4	4	5	6	7	8	9	10	11	12	12	13	14	15	16	17	18
110	4	5	6	7	8	9	10	11	12	13	14	15	16	18	19	20	21
120	5	6	7	8	9	11	12	13	14	15	16	18	19	20	21	22	24
130	5	7	8	9	11	12	13	15	16	17	19	20	21	23	24	25	27
140	6	7	9	10	12	13	15	16	18	19	21	22	24	25	27	28	30
150	7	8	10	12	13	15	17	18	20	22	23	25	27	28	30	32	33
160	7	9	11	13	15	17	18	20	22	24	26	28	29	31	33	35	37
170	8	10	12	14	16	18	20	22	24	26	28	30	32	34	36	38	40
180	9	11	13	15	18	20	22	24	26	29	31	33	35	37	40	42	44
190	10	12	14	17	19	22	24	26	29	31	33	36	38	41	43	45	48
200	10	13	16	18	21	23	26	28	31	34	36	39	41	44	47	49	52
210	11	14	17	20	22	25	28	31	33	36	39	42	45	47	50	53	56
220	12	15	18	21	24	27	30	33	36	39	42	45	48	51	54	57	60
230	15	16	19	22	26	29	32	35	38	42	45	48	51	54	58	61	64
240	14	17	21	24	27	31	34	38	41	44	48	51	55	58	62	65	68
250	15	18	22	26	29	33	36	40	44	47	51	55	58	62	66	69	73
260	16	19	23	27	31	35	39	43	46	50	54	58	62	66	70	74	77
270	16	21	25	29	33	37	41	45	49	53	57	62	66	70	74	78	82
280	17	22	26	30	35	39	43	48	52	56	61	65	69	74	78	82	87
290	18	23	27	32	37	41	46	50	55	60	64	69	73	78	82	87	92
300	19	24	29	34	39	43	48	53	58	63	68	72	77	82	87	92	96

TDF FACTORS FOR TWO FRACTIONS PER WEEK																
Dose/	Number of fractions															
faction	4	5	6	7	8	9	10	11	12	13	14	15	16	17	18	19	20
20	0	0	0	1	1	1	1	1	1	1	1	1	1	1	1	2	2
40	1	1	1	2	2	2	3	3	3	3	4	4	4	4	5	5	5
60	2	2	3	3	4	4	4	5	5	6	6	7	7	8	8	9	9
80	3	4	4	5	6	6	7	8	8	9	10	10	11	12	13	13	14
100	4	5	6	7	8	9	10	11	12	13	14	15	16	17	18	19	20
110	5	6	7	8	9	10	11	13	14	15	16	17	18	19	21	22	23
120	5	7	8	9	10	12	13	14	16	17	18	20	21	22	23	25	26
130	6	7	9	10	12	13	15	16	19	21	22	24	25	27	28	30	31
140	7	8	10	12	13	15	17	18	20	21	23	25	26	28	30	31	33
150	7	9	11	13	15	17	18	20	22	24	26	28	29	31	33	35	37
160	8	10	12	14	16	18	20	22	24	26	28	30	32	35	37	39	41
170	9	11	13	16	18	20	22	25	27	29	31	33	36	38	40	42	45
180	10	12	15	17	19	22	24	27	29	32	34	37	39	41	44	46	49
190	11	13	16	19	21	24	26	29	32	34	37	40	42	45	47	50	53
200	11	14	17	20	23	26	29	31	34	37	40	43	46	49	52	54	57
210	12	15	19	22	25	28	31	34	37	40	43	46	49	52	56	59	62
220	13	17	20	23	27	30	33	36	40	43	46	50	53	56	60	63	66
230	14	18	21	25	28	32	35	39	43	46	50	53	57	60	64	67	71
240	15	19	23	27	30	34	38	42	45	49	53	57	61	64	68	72	76
250	16	20	24	28	32	36	40	44	48	52	56	61	65	69	73	77	81
260	17	21	26	30	34	39	43	47	51	56	60	64	69	73	77	81	86
270	18	23	27	32	36	41	45	50	54	59	64	68	73	77	82	86	91
280	19	24	29	34	38	43	48	53	58	62	67	72	77	82	86	91	96
290	20	25	30	35	41	46	51	56	61	66	71	76	81	86	91	96	101
300	21	27	32	37	43	48	53	59	64	69	75	80	85	91	96	101	107

TDF FACTORS FOR THREE FRACTIONS PER WEEK

Dose/ fraction	Number of fractions																
	4	5	6	8	10	12	14	15	16	18	20	22	24	25	26	28	30
20	0	0	1	1	1	1	1	1	1	2	2	2	2	2	2	2	3
40	1	1	2	2	3	3	4	4	4	5	5	6	6	6	7	7	8
60	2	2	3	4	5	6	7	7	8	9	10	10	11	12	12	13	14
80	3	4	4	6	7	9	10	11	12	13	15	16	18	19	19	21	22
100	4	5	6	8	10	13	15	16	17	19	21	23	25	26	27	29	31
110	5	6	7	10	12	15	17	18	19	22	24	27	29	30	32	34	36
120	6	7	8	11	14	17	19	21	22	25	28	30	33	35	36	39	42
130	6	8	9	13	16	19	22	24	25	28	31	34	38	39	41	44	47
140	7	9	11	14	18	21	25	26	28	32	35	39	42	44	46	49	53
150	8	10	12	16	20	23	27	29	31	35	39	43	47	49	51	55	59
160	9	11	13	17	22	26	30	32	35	39	43	47	52	54	56	60	65
170	9	12	14	19	24	28	33	36	38	43	47	52	57	59	62	66	71
180	10	13	16	21	26	31	36	39	41	47	52	57	62	65	67	72	78
190	11	14	17	22	28	34	39	42	45	51	56	62	67	70	73	79	84
200	12	15	18	24	30	36	43	46	49	55	61	67	73	76	79	85	91
210	13	16	20	26	33	39	46	49	52	59	66	72	79	82	85	92	98
220	14	18	21	28	35	42	49	53	56	63	70	77	84	88	92	99	106
230	15	19	23	30	38	45	53	57	60	68	75	83	90	94	98	106	113
240	16	20	24	32	40	48	56	60	64	72	80	89	97	101	105	113	121
250	17	21	26	34	43	51	60	64	69	77	86	94	103	107	111	120	129
260	18	23	27	36	46	55	64	68	73	82	91	100	109	114	118	127	137
270	19	24	29	39	48	58	68	72	77	87	96	106	116	121	125	135	145
280	20	25	31	41	51	61	71	76	82	92	102	112	127	133	143	153	
290	22	27	32	43	54	65	75	81	86	97	108	118	129	135	140	151	
300	23	28	34	45	57	68	79	85	91	102	113	125	136	142	147	159	

TDF FACTORS FOR FOUR FRACTIONS PER WEEK

Dose/ fraction	Number of fractions																
	4	5	6	8	10	12	14	15	16	18	20	22	24	25	26	28	30
20	0	0	1	1	1	1	1	1	1	2	2	2	2	2	2	3	3
40	1	1	2	2	3	3	4	4	4	5	5	6	6	7	7	8	8
60	2	3	3	4	5	6	7	8	8	9	10	11	12	13	13	14	15
80	3	4	5	6	8	9	11	12	13	14	16	17	19	20	20	22	23
100	4	6	7	9	11	13	15	17	18	20	22	24	26	28	29	31	33
110	5	6	8	10	13	15	18	19	20	23	26	28	31	32	33	36	38
120	6	7	9	12	15	18	20	22	23	26	29	32	35	36	38	41	44
130	7	8	10	13	16	20	23	25	26	30	33	36	40	41	43	46	49
140	7	9	11	15	18	22	26	28	30	33	37	41	44	46	48	52	55
150	8	10	12	16	21	25	29	31	33	37	41	45	49	51	53	58	62
160	9	11	14	18	23	27	32	34	36	41	45	50	54	57	59	64	68
170	10	12	15	20	25	30	35	37	40	45	50	55	60	62	65	70	75
180	11	14	16	22	27	33	38	41	44	49	54	60	65	68	71	76	82
190	12	15	18	24	30	35	41	44	47	53	59	65	71	74	77	83	89
200	13	16	19	26	32	38	45	48	51	58	64	70	77	80	83	90	96
210	14	17	21	28	34	41	48	52	55	62	69	76	83	86	90	97	103
220	15	19	22	30	37	44	52	56	59	67	74	82	89	93	96	104	111
230	16	20	24	32	40	48	56	60	63	71	79	87	95	90	103	111	119
240	17	21	25	34	42	51	59	64	68	76	85	93	102	106	110	119	127
250	18	23	27	36	45	54	63	68	72	81	90	99	108	113	117	126	135
260	19	24	29	38	48	57	67	72	77	86	96	105	115	120	125	134	144
270	20	25	30	41	51	61	71	76	81	91	102	112	122	127	132	142	152
280	21	27	32	43	54	65	75	81	86	97	107	118	129	134	140	150	161
290	23	28	34	45	57	68	79	85	91	102	113	125	136	142	147	159	
300	24	30	36	48	60	72	84	90	96	107	119	131	143	149	155		

TDF FACTORS FOR FIVE FRACTIONS PER WEEK																	
Dose/	Number of fractions																
fraction	4	5	6	8	10	12	14	15	16	18	20	22	24	25	26	28	30
20	0	1	1	1	1	1	1	2	2	2	2	2	2	2	3	3	3
40	1	1	2	2	3	3	4	4	4	5	6	6	7	7	7	8	8
60	2	3	3	4	5	6	7	8	8	9	10	11	12	13	13	15	16
80	3	4	5	6	8	10	11	12	13	15	16	18	19	20	21	23	24
100	5	6	7	9	11	14	16	17	18	20	23	25	27	28	30	32	34
110	5	7	8	11	13	16	18	20	21	24	26	29	32	33	34	37	39
120	6	8	9	12	15	18	21	23	24	27	30	33	36	38	39	42	45
130	7	9	10	14	17	20	24	26	27	31	34	37	41	43	44	48	51
140	8	10	11	15	19	23	27	29	31	34	38	42	46	48	50	53	57
150	9	11	13	17	21	25	30	32	34	38	42	47	51	53	55	59	64
160	9	12	14	19	23	28	33	35	37	42	47	51	56	58	61	66	70
170	10	13	15	21	26	31	36	39	41	46	51	57	62	64	67	72	77
180	11	14	17	22	28	34	39	42	45	50	56	62	67	70	73	79	84
190	12	15	18	24	31	37	43	46	49	55	61	67	73	76	79	85	97
200	13	17	20	26	33	40	46	49	53	59	66	73	79	82	86	92	99
210	14	18	21	28	36	43	50	53	57	64	71	78	85	89	92	99	107
220	15	19	23	31	38	46	53	57	61	69	76	84	92	95	99	107	115
230	16	20	25	33	41	49	57	61	65	74	82	90	98	102	106	114	123
240	17	22	26	35	44	52	61	65	70	79	87	96	105	109	113	122	131
250	19	23	28	37	46	56	65	70	74	84	93	102	112	116	121	130	139
260	20	25	30	40	49	59	69	74	79	89	99	109	118	123	128	138	148
270	21	26	31	42	52	63	73	78	84	94	105	115	126	131	136	146	157
280	22	28	33	44	55	66	77	83	89	100	111	122	133	138	144	155	
290	23	29	35	47	58	70	82	88	93	105	117	128	140	146	152		
300	25	31	37	49	62	74	86	92	98	111	123	135	148	154			

Decay factors" for use with TDF with rest breaks											
T (days)	Rest Period (R days)										
	10	15	20	25	30	35	40	50	60	80	100	
5	0.93	0.89	0.86	0.84	0.82	0.81	0.80	0.79	0.77	0.75	0.73	0.72
10	0.96	0.93	0.90	0.89	0.87	0.86	0.85	0.84	0.82	0.81	0.79	0.77
15	0.97	0.95	0.93	0.91	0.90	0.89	0.88	0.87	0.85	0.84	0.82	0.80
20	0.98	0.96	0.94	0.93	0.91	0.90	0.89	0.89	0.87	0.86	0.84	0.82
25	0.98	0.96	0.95	0.94	0.93	0.92	0.92	0.90	0.89	0.87	0.85	0.84
30	0.98	0.97	0.96	0.95	0.94	0.93	0.92	0.91	0.90	0.89	0.87	0.85
35	0.99	0.97	0.96	0.95	0.94	0.93	0.93	0.92	0.91	0.90	0.88	0.86
40	0.99	0.98	0.97	0.96	0.95	0.94	0.93	0.93	0.91	0.90	0.89	0.87
45	0.99	0.98	0.97	0.96	0.95	0.95	0.94	0.93	0.92	0.91	0.89	0.88
50	0.99	0.98	0.97	0.96	0.96	0.95	0.94	0.94	0.93	0.92	0.90	0.89

—— *APPENDIX E* ——
TAR ZERO

TAR for CO-60 unit					
DEPTH	TAR	DEPTH	TAR	DEPTH	TAR
0	0.377	10	0.534	20	0.277
0.5	1	10.5	0.518	20.5	0.27
1	0.965	11	0.501	21	0.262
1.5	0.935	11.5	0.484	21.5	0.254
2	0.904	12	0.469	22	0.246
2.5	0.875	12.5	0.454	22.5	0.239
3	0.845	13	0.439	23	0.23
3.5	0.819	13.5	0.426	23.5	0.222
4	0.792	14	0.412	24	0.214
4.5	0.767	14.5	0.398	24.5	0.207
5	0.742	15	0.386	25	0.2
5.5	0.718	15.5	0.373	25.5	0.193
6	0.693	16	0.36	26	0.187
6.5	0.672	16.5	0.349	26.5	0.182
7	0.649	17	0.338	27	0.176
7.5	0.629	17.5	0.327	27.5	0.17
8	0.607	18	0.316	28	0.164
8.5	0.589	18.5	0.307	28.5	0.158
9	0.569	19	0.297	29	0.153
9.5	0.552	19.5	0.286	29.5	0.148
				30	0.144

—— *APPENDIX F* ——
SAR FOR COBALT-60

SAR for Co-60 unit										
RAD II Depth	2	4	8	12	16	24	28	32	36	40
0	0.004	0.004	0.018	0.035	0.047	0.053	0.059	0.056	0.056	0.055
1	0.026	0.048	0.078	0.098	0.109	0.122	0.123	0.123	0.123	0.125
2	0.050	0.080	0.116	0.139	0.152	0.166	0.168	0.168	0.166	0.167
3	0.070	0.103	0.147	0.172	0.187	0.204	0.179	0.203	0.205	0.203
4	0.081	0.121	0.170	0.197	0.215	0.237	0.239	0.239	0.241	0.240
5	0.085	0.134	0.189	0.218	0.240	0.264	0.266	0.268	0.269	0.270
6	0.089	0.141	0.201	0.234	0.257	0.282	0.185	0.286	0.288	0.288
7	0.090	0.143	0.209	0.246	0.273	0.302	0.306	0.308	0.309	0.313
8	0.089	0.142	0.214	0.254	0.285	0.313	0.317	0.322	0.326	0.328
9	0.086	0.140	0.216	0.260	0.292	0.324	0.329	0.334	0.337	0.339
10	0.082	0.136	0.215	0.262	0.295	0.333	0.338	0.343	0.345	0.353
11	0.076	0.132	0.213	0.262	0.296	0.337	0.343	0.346	0.349	0.355
12	0.074	0.128	0.210	0.261	0.297	0.340	0.344	0.348	0.353	0.356
13	0.070	0.124	0.207	0.260	0.298	0.341	0.345	0.352	0.355	0.356
14	0.066	0.120	0.204	0.258	0.297	0.344	0.352	0.355	0.361	0.369
15	0.062	0.116	0.200	0.255	0.295	0.344	0.352	0.355	0.361	0.369
16	0.060	0.112	0.196	0.252	0.292	0.341	0.349	0.355	0.360	0.369
17	0.058	0.108	0.191	0.248	0.288	0.338	0.343	0.352	0.359	0.364
18	0.056	0.104	0.186	0.244	0.284	0.334	0.342	0.352	0.359	0.369
19	0.053	0.101	0.181	0.239	0.280	0.330	0.341	0.350	0.356	0.366
20	0.049	0.097	0.176	0.234	0.275	0.325	0.334	0.344	0.348	0.356

— APPENDIX G —
OUTPUT FACTORS FOR SXR

Output Factors for SXR		
Cone diameter(cm)	Output factor in air cGy/min	Output factor on tissue surface cGy/min
1	270	281
1.2	270	282
1.4	271	285
1.6	272	288
1.8	273	291
2	282	302
2.5	283	307
3	283	311
3.5	284	316
4	284	319
4.5	286	325
5	287	329
5.5	288	334
6	292	341
6.5	292	344
7	292	347
7.5	292	349
8	292	350

— APPENDIX II —
BSF FOR SXR

BSF for SXR			
Circular cut out	HVL(mmAL)		
	0.620	1.650	6.800
1	1.022	1.039	1.048
1.2	1.028	1.045	1.058
1.4	1.032	1.051	1.067
1.6	1.036	1.058	1.076
1.8	1.041	1.065	1.085
2	1.045	1.071	1.095
2.5	1.057	1.096	1.116
3	1.067	1.099	1.138
3.5	1.076	1.112	1.159
4	1.086	1.124	1.178
4.5	1.096	1.135	1.196
5	1.106	1.147	1.212
5.5	1.114	1.158	1.228
6	1.120	1.168	1.243
6.5	1.124	1.179	1.257
7	1.130	1.187	1.269
7.5	1.135	1.194	1.281
8	1.140	1.200	1.292

—— *APPENDIX I* ——
OUTPUT FACTORS FOR ELECTRONS

Output Factors for Electrons						
Cone Size(cm)						
MeV	4X4	6X6	10X10	15X15	20X20	25X25
4	0.969	0.976	1.000	1.021	1.056	1.115
6	0.978	0.998	1.000	1.004	1.026	1.069
9	0.966	1.030	1.000	0.921	0.904	0.908
12	0.954	1.012	1.000	0.958	0.937	0.913
16	1.021	1.057	1.000	0.919	0.871	0.836